Facing
Cancer

NOTICE

Medicine is an ever-changing science. As new research and clinical experience broaden our knowledge, changes in treatment and drug therapy are required. The editors and the publisher of this work have checked with sources believed to be reliable in their efforts to provide information that is complete and generally in accord with the standards accepted at the time of publication. However, in view of the possibility of human error or changes in medical sciences, neither the editors nor the publisher nor any other party who has been involved in the preparation or publication of this work warrants that the information contained herein is in every respect accurate or complete, and they disclaim all responsibility for any errors or omissions or for the results obtained from use of the information contained in this work. Readers are encouraged to confirm the information contained herein with other sources. For example and in particular, readers are advised to check the product information sheet included in the package of each drug they plan to administer to be certain that the information contained in this work is accurate and that changes have not been made in the recommended dose or in the contraindications for administration. This recommendation is of particular importance in connection with new or infrequently used drugs.

Facing Cancer

A Complete Guide for People

with Cancer, Their Families,

and Caregivers

Editors

THEODORE A. STERN, M.D.

PSYCHIATRIST AND CHIEF
PSYCHIATRIC CONSULTATION SERVICE
MASSACHUSETTS GENERAL HOSPITAL
PROFESSOR OF PSYCHIATRY
HARVARD MEDICAL SCHOOL
BOSTON, MASSACHUSETTS

MIKKAEL A. SEKERES, M.D., M.S.

LEUKEMIA PROGRAM
DEPARTMENT OF HEMATOLOGY AND MEDICAL ONCOLOGY
THE CLEVELAND CLINIC FOUNDATION
ASSISTANT PROFESSOR OF MEDICINE
CLEVELAND CLINIC LERNER COLLEGE OF MEDICINE
CLEVELAND, OHIO

McGRAW-HILL

MEDICAL PUBLISHING DIVISION

New York   Chicago   San Francisco   Lisbon   London   Madrid   Mexico City
Milan   New Delhi   San Juan   Seoul   Singapore   Sydney   Toronto

The *McGraw·Hill* Companies

Facing Cancer: A Complete Guide for People with Cancer,
Their Families, and Caregivers

1234567890   DOC DOC   09876543

ISBN: 0-07-141491-6

This book was set in Minion by Binghamton Valley Composition.
The editors were Marc Strauss, Lisa Silverman, and Lester A. Sheinis.
The production supervisor was Richard C. Ruzycka.
The cover designer was John Vario.
The indexer was Alexandra Nickerson.
RR Donnelley was printer and binder.
This book is printed on acid-free paper.

Cataloging-in-publication data is on file for this title at the Library of Congress.

To the most important people in the world to us,
our wives (Kathy and Lynda) and
our sons (Tommy and Gabriel),
for their unflagging love and support;
to our patients, who provide us with inspiration;
and to our teachers.

Contents

Contributors

ANNAH N. ABRAMS, M.D.
Clinical Assistant in Psychiatry
Massachusetts General Hospital
Instructor in Psychiatry
Harvard Medical School
Boston, Massachusetts
Chapter 9

MENEKSE ALPAY, M.D.
Clinical Assistant in Psychiatry
Massachusetts General Hospital
Instructor in Psychiatry
Harvard Medical School
Boston, Massachusetts
Chapter 22

EYAL ATTAR, M.D.
Dana-Farber CancerCare
Massachusetts General Hospital Cancer Center
Laboratory of Experimental Hematology
Clinical and Research Fellow in Medicine
Harvard Medical School
Boston, Massachusetts
Chapter 18

EUGENE V. BERESIN, M.D.
Director of Child and Adolescent Psychiatry Residency Training
Massachusetts General and McLean Hospitals
Co-Director, Harvard Medical School Center for Mental Health and Media
Associate Professor of Psychiatry, Harvard Medical School
Boston, Massachusetts
Chapter 28

HAROLD J. BURSTEIN, M.D., PH.D.

Breast Oncology Center
Dana-Farber Cancer Institute
Assistant Professor of Medicine
Harvard Medical School
Boston, Massachusetts
Chapter 21

NED H. CASSEM, M.D., S.J.

Psychiatrist
Massachusetts General Hospital
Professor of Psychiatry
Harvard Medical School
Boston, Massachusetts
Chapter 33

BRIAN CHON, M.D.

Massachusetts General Hospital
Department of Radiation Oncology
Boston, Massachusetts
Chapter 16

COREY CUTLER, M.D., M.P.H., F.R.C.P.C.

Associate Staff
Dana-Farber Cancer Institute
Instructor in Medicine
Harvard Medical School
Boston, Massachusetts
Chapter 20

ROBERT DEAN, M.D.

Clinical Associate
Warren G. Magnuson Clinical Center
National Institutes of Health
Clinical Fellow, Medical Oncology Clinical Research Unit
Center for Cancer Research, National Cancer Institute
Bethesda, Maryland
Chapter 12

STEPHEN DURANT, ED.D.

Assistant Psychologist
Massachusetts General Hospital
Instructor in Psychiatry
Harvard Medical School
Boston, Massachusetts
Chapter 10

AMY E. GAGLIARDI, M.D.

Clinical Instructor in Psychiatry
Harvard Medical School
McLean Hospital
Boston, Massachusetts
Chapter 31

TIMOTHY GILLIGAN, M.D.

Genitourinary Oncologist
Department of Medical Oncology
Dana-Farber Cancer Institute
Instructor in Medicine
Harvard Medical School
Boston, Massachusetts
Chapter 5

WOLFRAM GOESSLING, M.D., PH.D.

Chief Medical Resident
Department of Medicine, Brigham and Women's Hospital
Fellow in Hematology/Oncology
Dana-Farber Cancer Institute
Instructor in Medicine
Harvard Medical School
Boston, Massachusetts
Chapter 24

SARAH HALL, B.A.

Research Assistant
Department of Psychiatry
Massachusetts General Hospital
Boston, Massachusetts
Chapter 28

PAUL HAMMERNESS, M.D.

Clinical Fellow in Child and Adolescent Psychiatry
Massachusetts General Hospital/McLean Hospital
Harvard Medical School
Boston, Massachusetts
Chapter 33

JASON HERSHBERGER, M.D.

New York University Forensic Psychiatry Fellow
Clinical Fellow in Psychiatry and the Law
New York University School of Medicine
New York, New York
Chapter 15

VINCENT T. HO, M.D.
Associate Staff
Center for Hematologic Oncology
Dana-Farber Cancer Institute
Instructor in Medicine
Harvard Medical School
Boston, Massachusetts
Chapter 14

EPHRAIM HOCHBERG, M.D.
Associate Staff
Dana-Farber Cancer Institute
Instructor in Medicine
Harvard Medical School
Boston, Massachusetts
Chapter 3

WILLIAM KIM, M.D.
Associate Staff
Dana-Farber Cancer Institute
Instructor in Medicine
Harvard Medical School
Boston, Massachusetts
Chapter 11

GEOFFREY LIU, M.D.
Assistant in Medicine
Massachusetts General Hospital Cancer Center
Instructor in Medicine
Harvard Medical School
Boston, Massachusetts
Chapter 6

FRED H. MILLHAM, M.D., M.B.A.
Associate Director, Surgical ICU
Boston Medical Center
Associate Professor of Surgery
Boston University School of Medicine
Boston, Massachusetts
Chapters 26, 29

DAVID MISCHOULON, M.D., PH.D.
Assistant in Psychiatry
Massachusetts General Hospital
Assistant Professor of Psychiatry
Harvard Medical School
Boston, Massachusetts
Chapters 17, 21

ANNA C. MURIEL, M.D., M.P.H.
Clinical Assistant in Psychiatry
Massachusetts General Hospital
Instructor in Psychiatry
Harvard Medical School
Boston, Massachusetts
Chapter 4

KRISTIN BAKER NIENDORF, M.S., C.G.C.
Senior Genetic Counselor
Massachusetts General Hospital
Center for Cancer Risk Analysis
Boston, Massachusetts
Chapter 8

OLIVIA OKEREKE, M.D.
Geriatric Fellow, McLean Hospital
Geriatric Psychiatry Fellow, Clinical Fellow in Psychiatry
Harvard Medical School
Boston, Massachusetts
Chapters 23, 27

RICHARD T. PENSON, M.D.
Clinical Director
Medical Gynecologic Oncology
Massachusetts General Hospital
Instructor in Medicine
Harvard Medical School
Boston, Massachusetts
Chapter 8

LAURA M. PRAGER, M.D.
Clinical Instructor in Psychiatry
Massachusetts General Hospital
Instructor in Psychiatry
Harvard Medical School
Boston, Massachusetts
Chapters 26, 29

LISA F. PRICE, M.D.
Fellow, Department of Child and Adolescent Psychiatry
Massachusetts General Hospital/McLean Hospital
Harvard Medical School
Boston, Massachusetts
Chapters 19, 25

JOHN QUERQUES, M.D.

Assistant Medical Director and Attending Psychiatrist
Erich Lindemann Mental Health Center
Clinical Assistant in Psychiatry
Massachusetts General Hospital
Instructor in Psychiatry
Harvard Medical School
Boston, Massachusetts
Chapter 2

TERRY RABINOWITZ, M.D., D.D.S.

Director, Psychiatric Consultation Service
Fletcher Allen Health Care
Associate Professor of Psychiatry and of Family Practice
University of Vermont College of Medicine
Burlington, Vermont
Chapters 30, 32

PAULA K. RAUCH, M.D.

Chief, Child Psychiatry Consultation Service
Director, MGH Cancer Center Parenting Program
Massachusetts General Hospital
Assistant Professor of Psychiatry
Harvard Medical School
Boston, Massachusetts
Chapters 4, 10

PAULA D. RYAN, M.D. PH.D.

Medical Director
Breast and Ovarian Cancer Genetics and Risk Assessment Program
Massachusetts General Hospital
Instructor in Medicine
Harvard Medical School
Boston, Massachusetts
Chapter 8

ERIKA RYST, M.D.

Clinical Fellow in Psychiatry
Massachusetts General Hospital
Harvard Medical School
Boston, Massachusetts
Chapter 7

MIKKAEL A. SEKERES, M.D., M.S.

Leukemia Program
Department of Hematology and Medical Oncology
The Cleveland Clinic Foundation
Assistant Professor of Medicine
Cleveland Clinic Lerner College of Medicine
Cleveland, Ohio
Chapter 1

KRISTEN MAHONEY SHANNON, M.S., C.G.C.

Senior Genetic Counselor
Massachusetts General Hospital
Center for Cancer Risk Analysis
Boston, Massachusetts
Chapter 8

SCOTT SHAPIRO, M.D.

Attending in Psychiatry and Medicine
Assistant Clinical Instructor, St. Vincent's Hospital
New York, New York
Chapter 22

DAVID R. SPIGEL, M.D.

Fellow Staff
Dana-Farber Cancer Institute
Clinical Fellow in Medicine
Harvard Medical School
Boston, Massachusetts
Chapter 13

THEODORE A. STERN, M.D.

Psychiatrist and Chief
Psychiatric Consultation Service
Massachusetts General Hospital
Professor of Psychiatry
Harvard Medical School
Boston, Massachusetts
Chapters 2, 15

Preface

M any patients don't want to utter the word (cancer). For that matter, many doctors don't want to say it either. They struggle for euphemisms, such as, "You have a growth," or "We see an abnormality on your x-rays."

Eventually, most people who have been given the diagnosis, their friends and family members, and the medical staff who take care of them come to terms with the diagnosis. However, it is often difficult to weather the emotional storm created by being told you have cancer. This is especially true when you are first trying to understand the nuances of evaluating the extent of the cancer, the treatment options, the potential side effects of those treatments, and the ways in which cancer and cancer therapy will be integrated into the other aspects of your life. Simply absorbing the information that you acquire from the Internet or from your doctor when the diagnosis of cancer is broached can be daunting. Early on in this process many individuals are in a state of shock about their diagnosis; they cannot believe it has happened to them.

The people we have cared for over the years have taught us about this trying process. For them and for others like them, we have compiled a series of chapters written by experts in the fields of medical oncology, radiation oncology, surgical oncology, and psychiatry. Our authors have tried to write in plain English, as if they were sitting across a kitchen table from members of their own family, engaged in a discussion about some aspect of cancer. We have tried to avoid being overly simplistic or patronizing.

The first section of the book, "Facing a Cancer Diagnosis" (Chapters 1–13), takes you through the medical and psychological aspects of hearing the news, and learning how you can deal with that news. This section also describes how a cancer diagnosis will affect other members of your family. The next section, "Facing Cancer Therapy" (Chapters 14–25) discusses common treatments for cancer, potential side effects of those treatments (and how to manage the side effects from those treatments), and complementary interventions (such as support groups, faith, and alternative therapies). The final section of the book, "Facing the Impact of Cancer" (Chapters 26–33), addresses everything from how cancer is portrayed in the media, to living wills, and to issues that are raised at the end of life.

We have also included a glossary of terms to help define many of the terms and medical jargon you will inevitably encounter and have added a few blank pages at the book's end for note taking. Our intent was to create a useful reference book that could be taken to your appointments. It is a book that you could refer to while in the waiting room, a book that you can write notes in while in your doctor's office, and a book that provides you with information and resources (such as other books, movies, and Internet sites) about your particular cancer and its treatment. In addition, we hope that it will stimulate you to ask more questions about your condition.

We welcome your feedback about the content of this book, so that we can make future editions even better. Please e-mail your comments to our editor, Marc Strauss: Marc_Strauss@McGraw-Hill.com.

Everyone, either directly or through a friend or family member, is touched by cancer. We hope that our collective experiences can make the journey less frightening, less painful, and less lonely.

T.A.S.

M.A.S.

Acknowledgments

OUR THANKS

This book would not have come into being if not for our patients. They expressed to us their need for a guide to the experience of having cancer and were so generous in including us in their day-to-day triumphs and struggles. We hope we were able to return the favor.

Without the participation of so many physicians, this book would never have been completed. We thank our contributors for their thoughtfulness and gifted writing, as well as their tolerance of our deadlines and edits. We also thank our teachers and mentors for imbuing in us a sense of responsibility to educate, to write with rigor, and most importantly to provide exceptional care to our patients: Tom Hackett and Ned Cassem at the Massachusetts General Hospital; Brian Strom at the University of Pennsylvania; Rich Stone and Bob Mayer at the Dana–Farber Cancer Institute; and Matt Kalaycio and Brian Bolwell at The Cleveland Clinic Foundation

Many individuals outside of medicine reviewed parts of this manuscript and/or provided input about its content and helped to make it more readable and vibrant. Our deep thanks go to Lynda Montgomery, Joanna Spencer, Caleb Sekeres, Douglas Neu, Fran Palasak, and of course our parents. We are sure they will find the results of their comments and edits sprinkled throughout the text. We gratefully thank Melissa Mason and Eric Shetler for their enormous efforts and generous help with the photographs in the book. They helped to give the book its depth. We also thank our medical colleagues, who contributed mightily by virtue of their experiences and example.

We are also grateful to Judy Byford for her unflagging assistance with administrative matters and transmittal of our manuscripts to McGraw-Hill.

At McGraw-Hill, we thank Lester A. Sheinis for his attention to detail and Marc Strauss, who nurtured our project and added—with a gentle but firm hand—perspective. His humor and vibrant laughter were a godsend. To him, we owe our special thanks.

T.A.S.
M.A.S.

Facing Cancer

CHAPTER 1

What Is Cancer?

MIKKAEL A. SEKERES, M.D., M.S.

OUTLINE

WHAT IS CANCER?

Put simply, cancer is the abnormal growth of cells. Cancers arise from an organ or body structure and are composed of tiny cells that have lost the ability to stop growing. This growing mass of cells then projects from that organ or body structure until it becomes large enough to be noticed by a patient or physician. Occasionally, cancer may be detected "incidentally" by a laboratory test or x-ray—that is, the test or x-ray may have been ordered for purposes of routine screening or for an entirely different reason; in such a case, the cancer gets noticed almost by accident. At this point, it may be referred to as a "mass," "growth," "tumor," "nodule," "spot," "lump," "lesion," or "malignancy."

In general, the cancer must reach a size of 1 centimeter (that is, between ⅓ and ½ inch), or be made up of 1 million cells, before it is detected. Exceptions to this general rule include cancers of the blood and bone marrow—called lymphomas, leukemias, and multiple myeloma—which frequently do not produce a mass but will be evident on laboratory tests; these cancers still require more than a million cells to be present before they are detected. Lymphomas and leukemias are examples of "liquid tumors," or cancers present in body fluids (the blood and bone marrow), and are detectable by laboratory tests of the blood. "Solid tumors"—including cancers of the lung, breast, prostate, colon, rectum, and bladder—are not present in large enough numbers in body fluids to be detected with a blood test. However, they may release chemicals that are detectable in body fluids. A person with prostate cancer, for example, may have an elevated level of prostate-specific antigen, or PSA, in the blood-stream (Table 1-1).

WHERE IN THE BODY CAN CANCER DEVELOP?

Cancer can occur anywhere in the body. Any area of the body that you can name can be the target for a cancer. Some cancers even arise in parts of the body that contained structures only when the person was just an embryo—just weeks after conception! Cancer cells—those abnormal cells that have lost the ability to stop

TABLE 1-1 Examples of Tumor Types and How They Are Categorized

Liquid Tumors	Solid Tumors
Lymphoma	Lung cancer
Leukemia	Breast cancer
Multiple myeloma	Prostate cancer
	Colon cancer
	Rectal cancer
	Bladder cancer
	Brain cancer

growing—arise from cells that used to be normal components of organs and tissues. What causes cells to become cancerous? Cells grow abnormally because of environmental factors (such as cigarette smoking or radiation exposure), a genetic predisposition, "dumb luck," and as yet unexplained causes. Just "dumb luck" accounts for the majority of cancers.

WHAT MAKES CANCEROUS CELLS STOP GROWING?

Cancers continue to grow unless one of four things occurs: (1) The cancerous mass is removed by a surgeon; (2) chemotherapy or another type of cancer-specific medication, such as hormonal therapy, is given to the person with cancer; (3) a person with cancer receives radiation therapy; or (4) the cancer cells shrink and disappear on their own. This last event, while extremely rare, can occur with some melanomas (a type of skin cancer) or some kidney cancers (Table 1-2).

WHY NOT JUST LET THE CANCER GROW?

In some cases, this may be the right thing to do. As some people have cancers that grow slowly, exposing them to either surgery or chemotherapy may make them sick without doing much to improve their survival. Older adults, in particular, are more prone to experience the side effects of therapy; if those side effects outweigh the potential benefit of therapy or the potential harm of living with cancer, the proposed therapy may not be of benefit. This is where the notion of "quality of life" becomes important. Alternatively, a person may be ideologically opposed to therapy; for such an individual, letting the cancer grow might be the right thing to do.

In other cases, letting the cancer grow may not be the right thing to do. Unfortunately, many cancer cells do not respect the boundaries of other organs or body structures. A growing cancer might press on another organ and prevent that organ from functioning normally, or it might actually invade an organ and impair that organ's function. Then, a situation may arise in which bleeding or an infection occurs. A lung cancer, for example, might press on the esophagus (the tube that carries food from the mouth to the stomach) and block the transit of food. A person with such a cancer might describe a sensation of "food getting caught in my throat—I just can't get it down." Alternatively, if the cancer invaded a blood

TABLE 1-2 **What Makes Cancerous Cells Stop Growing?**

1. Removal of the cancerous mass by a surgeon
2. Administration of chemotherapy or another type of cancer-specific medication
3. Radiation therapy
4. Spontaneous shrinkage and disappearance due to an unknown mechanism

vessel in the lungs, bleeding would occur, and the person might describe episodes of "coughing up blood."

WHY DOES HAVING CANCER MAKE A PERSON FEEL SICK?

Some types of cancer release chemicals that make a person feel ill. These chemicals, called *cytokines*, may cause fevers, chills, sweats, fatigue, anorexia (loss of appetite), or even nausea and vomiting. These are the same chemicals that are released into the bloodstream when a person has the flu, which explains why the symptoms of flu and of cancer often are similar. One of these cytokines, called *tumor necrosis factor*, or TNF, used to be called *cachexin*, because its release from cancer cells was associated with cachexia, or wasting. These symptoms are, in fact, the ones that often bring a person with cancer to a doctor's attention in the first place. As a cancer continues to grow, these chemicals continue to be released. Treating the cancer should alleviate these symptoms.

IS CANCER CURABLE?

The short answer to this question is yes. In fact, all cancers are curable *if they are caught early enough*. That is the justification for screening tests (such as mammograms, colonoscopies, and prostate exams). These tests are explained in more detail in Chap. 5. When cancers are caught early, they tend to be smaller; they are thus either easier to remove surgically or more likely to shrink in response to chemotherapy or radiation therapy.

Cancers not caught early enough (when they are no longer small in size or few in number) still may be curable and almost certainly are treatable. Even advanced cancers—malignancies that have spread to different parts of the body, or have *metastasized*—usually are treatable. Often, they are thought of as "chronic diseases," or diseases that a person will live with over a long period. While a given therapy may not cure a disease, it may extend a person's life until a more promising and potentially curative therapy becomes available.

WHAT IS THE NORMAL STRUCTURE AND FUNCTION OF AN ORGAN IN THE BODY?

Every organ in the body performs specific duties. Each organ functions as a member of a community of organs, all contributing to the good of the body as a whole. The brain, the "high commander," dictates the functions of most organs. The heart pumps blood (at varying rates and pressures, depending on the brain's signals) to other tissues and organs, the lungs breathe air (providing necessary oxygen to tissues and organs via the bloodstream), and the stomach digests food (providing nutrients to itself and other organs and tissues in the body). The pancreas and gall-bladder assist with that digestion, while the liver and kidneys help to process and excrete toxins from the body. The reproductive organs (ovaries in a woman and testes in a man) ensure that the elements that define the individuality of a person (the genes) get passed on to the next generation. Every organ is composed of tissues; tissues are, in turn, composed of cells.

The human body has evolved with a complicated set of organs, each of which performs specific functions and each of which relies on and communicates with other organs for the good of the whole individual. The brain, for example, controls higher-order functioning (memory, thought, sensory input and output) and basic bodily functions (breathing, the beating of the heart, the drive to eat and sleep). It transmits electrical signals to the heart to beat faster or slower, to the lungs to vary the rate of respiration, and to the muscles to facilitate or prevent movement. It also sends out hormonal signals through the release of chemicals from the pituitary gland. These signals affect other organs, including the heart, lungs, kidneys, reproductive organs, and thyroid gland. The organs affected by the brain then vary their function, in turn sending out signals (either electrical, chemical, or both) to still other organs, then back to the brain to provide "feedback" about how the organ is responding to the brain's initial stimulus.

A scenario may clarify these interactions. You are walking in the forest one day when a tiger jumps out from the bushes. Your brain thinks, "Oh my god, it's a tiger! I'm in trouble!"—a process known as "higher-order functioning." It then transmits electrical signals to the heart to beat faster, to the lungs to breathe harder (basic bodily functions), and to the muscles to tense up, preparing you to flee from or to fight the tiger (your choice!). At the same time, the brain triggers the pituitary gland (also located in the skull) to release hormones, including one that stimulates the adrenal glands to produce adrenaline (epinephrine). Adrenaline also stimulates the heart to beat faster and the lungs to breathe harder. These organs, in turn, send signals back to the brain to tell it "Okay—we're really moving now! You can stop signaling us to work harder. We're already doing it!" (feedback). These organs work together to ensure survival.

Organs, then, perform specific functions, but they also respond to both electrical and chemical stimuli from other organs, all for the good of the individual.

HOW DO CELLS FUNCTION?

Cells are the basic building blocks of the bodily structures. Cells attach to and interact with each other to form, say, the liver, the lungs, or the bones. Each cell, in turn, functions as its own minifactory, contributing to the general function of the organ it is a part of (for example, enabling the stomach to digest food) and ensuring its own self-preservation. A single organ contains billions of cells. The cells comprised by an organ, however, differ from each other and may contribute to different types of tissues within that organ. For example, certain cells within the lungs form the major lung tissue, called lung *parenchyma*, that gives lungs their substance. Other cells within the lungs form the tough, fibrous structures that surround the lungs and give them their shape. Still other cells contribute to the blood vessels that supply the lung tissue with blood, while entirely different cells make up the nerves associated with the lungs. Any one of these cells could potentially develop into a cancerous cell; this explains why so many different types of cancers might arise in the same organ.

The blueprints for a cell's function, development, reproduction, and eventual death are contained in structures called DNA (short for *deoxyribonucleic acid*). The DNA, in turn, is combined to form *chromosomes*, and chromosomes are housed in a central cell structure called the *nucleus*. The machinery that carries out the cell's functions is found in the area surrounding the nucleus, called the *cytoplasm*.

Cells reproduce by dividing into identical halves. These halves then mature, carry out the same functions as their parent, and in turn divide to form four identical cells, and so on. As an individual grows from an embryo into a fetus and then into infancy, childhood, and finally adulthood, the number of these dividing cells exceeds the cells that are being replaced (older, dying cells), and organs and tissues grow. Once an individual reaches adulthood, though, cell division slows to keep pace with cell loss, and organs and tissues maintain their size.

Most cells live for a given amount of time (this can vary from minutes to years) and then undergo programmed cell death, a process called *apoptosis*. It is as if each cell came with its own, predetermined expiration date, brought about by its own DNA. As cells age, they lose some or all of their ability to function. They then can no longer contribute as much to the organ or body part to which they belong, and that organ or body part will therefore not function as well. For example, an aging platelet (a cell in the bloodstream whose job is to facilitate blood clotting) will not stem bleeding as well as a young platelet that has freshly entered the bloodstream from the bone marrow. Apoptosis is the body's built-in mechanism for removing these dysfunctional cells so as to keep its organs operating as efficiently as possible.

WHAT OCCURS WHEN THE STRUCTURE AND FUNCTION OF ORGANS BECOME ABNORMAL?

As already described, cells eventually undergo apoptosis, or programmed cell death. Occasionally, a cell ignores its expiration date; it not only continues to live but continues to divide, creating offspring identical to itself. When a cell fails to undergo apoptosis (because of an error in the DNA "blueprints" for apoptosis) its progeny inherit this tendency as well, so that they, too, continue to divide and fail to undergo apoptosis. Soon, the growth of these cells outstrips the normal apoptosis of other cells in the same area of the body or in the same organ, and a mass develops. This mass is a cancer.

HOW DOES A CANCER CELL IN, SAY, THE BONE MARROW DIFFER FROM OTHER, NORMAL CELLS IN THE BONE MARROW?

Can't cancer cells, because they constantly grow and divide, turn regular organs into "superorgans?" Well, yes and no. A person with leukemia has a cancer of the cells in the bone marrow. In particular, leukemia is predominantly a cancer of the white blood cells, which fight infections. A normal white blood cell count might be 6000 white blood cells per cubic millimeter. A person with leukemia might have a white blood cell count of 20,000 or even 200,000 cells per cubic millimeter! In a way, then, the bone marrow in a person with leukemia *is* functioning as a super-organ. With that number of white blood cells, the body should be able to fight even the plague!

But that large number of cells comes at a price. With leukemia, as with many cancers, the abnormal cells do not function well and may not function at all. Leukemia cells, for example, contain a defect that stops their maturation but promotes their ability to divide and reproduce. These thousands or even hundreds of thousands of immature cells are incapable of fighting even simple infections and leave a person with leukemia *functionally* immunosuppressed and thus susceptible to infections.

At the same time, the immature, nonfunctioning leukemia cells that develop in the bone marrow take up valuable space and crowd out normal cells. As a result, red blood cells (which deliver much-needed oxygen to tissues via the bloodstream) and platelets (which help to stop bleeding), both of which are normally produced from cells in the bone marrow, decrease in number. This can be likened to crab-grass taking over a normal, plush lawn. A person with leukemia, then, has too many nonfunctioning white blood cells, and possibly too few functioning red blood cells (leaving him or her anemic) and too few platelets (leaving him or her at risk for bleeding). In other types of cancer, the immature cancer cells may crowd out normally functioning cells in the same organ, preventing that organ from performing its usual role.

On the flip side, certain cancers function too well or produce chemicals entirely unrelated to their organ's normal functions. Ordinarily, the adrenal glands produce a steroid, called cortisol, in small amounts. One type of cancer of the adrenal glands, called an adrenal cortical neoplasm, produces excess amounts of cortisol; it, in turn, causes a person to appear as if he or she were taking steroids. Signs of this disorder include weight gain, thinning hair, and muscle atrophy. Similarly a rare cancer of the pancreas, called an insulinoma, produces too much insulin, with a consequent drop in that person's sugar levels, as if he or she had been given an insulin overdose.

Most cancers that produce chemicals unrelated to their organ's function arise in the lungs. "Small cell" cancers of the lung are notorious for this phenomenon; when this cell behavior occurs in an individual, he or she is said to have a "paraneoplastic syndrome." One type of paraneoplastic syndrome involves production of a chemical that stimulates the adrenal glands to produce too much cortisol, just as if that person had an adrenal cortical neoplasm. Another type, called the Eaton-Lambert syndrome, produces a chemical that causes muscle weakness, as if that person had a disease called myasthenia gravis. Often, these symptoms prompt a diagnosis of lung cancer to be made. The diagnosis may even be made earlier in this case than in the case of a person who did not have these symptoms.

Finally, cancers can interfere with an organ's normal function through mechanical obstruction, simply, by getting in the way. Cholangiocarcinoma, or cancer of the gallbladder, often is diagnosed either when a person complains of a mass or a pain in a particular area of the abdomen (the right upper quadrant of the belly) or when the cancer grows big enough to obstruct the normal flow of bile into the intestines. Bile then backs up through the liver and into the bloodstream. Bile in the blood causes a person's skin to turn yellow, a condition called *jaundice*. Cancer of the pancreas, an organ located on the other side of the bile ducts, can also cause a mechanical obstruction when it grows to a certain size, forcing bile into the bloodstream and again causing jaundice.

Cancer cells do not function the same way as other, normal cells in the same organ. Their presence may inhibit proper organ function through simple mechanical interference; this, in turn, often leads to the diagnosis of cancer.

WHAT ARE GENETIC FACTORS THAT INFLUENCE THE DEVELOPMENT OF CANCER?

Why is it that a cancer cell fails to undergo apoptosis (programmed cell death) or it acquires some selective advantage to growing and dividing? As mentioned previously, the blueprints for a cell's function, development, reproduction, and eventual death are contained in the DNA. On an elemental level, something goes wrong in the DNA to prevent apoptosis or to promote cell growth and division.

DNA is grouped into packets called *genes*, which, in turn, are contained in chromosomes. When a cell divides, thus reproducing, the chromosomes and the DNA they contain must be copied exactly in order to create two new cells (with the same structure and function as the parent cell). Rarely, the copying process is imperfect, and errors in DNA result. This makes sense statistically: if a cell is able to copy its own genetic information with an accuracy of 99.9 percent, then one time in 1000 it will copy its information incorrectly. And one cell contains thousands of genes.

Luckily, cells contain quality-control mechanisms that scan genetic information for errors. Cells also contain repair mechanisms to fix those errors, allowing a cell to copy its DNA with amazing accuracy. Playing the statistics game again, though, we can see how errors still might occur: if both the quality control mechanism and the repair mechanism have a combined accuracy of 99.9 percent, combining the two will yield an error rate of one time in 1000. These are still excellent odds, but the transmission of crucial information is not perfect. If a cell contains 1000 genes and divides 1000 times, statistics predict that an error will be passed on to one of its progeny.

Sometimes that "error" provides an advantage to the survival of the species; this is the basis for the theories of Charles Darwin. The new cell might allow the species to have improved vision (which might help the species to avoid predators or to find food better than its peers might)—a characteristic that will be passed on to its offspring. Most of the time, these errors have no consequence: the erroneously copied genetic information does not play a major role in the cell's survival. Rarely, however, the genetic error creates a cancer cell that continues to pass the error on to its offspring, and a mass of cancer cells develops.

One classic example that illustrates this chain of events is chronic myelogenous leukemia, or CML. The cancer cells in this disorder come from a "grandfather" cell, called a stem cell, located in the bone marrow. When a cell such as this divides, its chromosomes come very close to each other in the middle of the cell, duplicate (by a process called *transcription*), and then separate toward opposite ends of the cell as the cell pinches itself off in the middle. This process creates two new cells. When the stem cell in CML divides, two of its chromosomes, numbers 9 and 22, come close to each other in the middle of the cell and actually trade DNA by accident! It's as if the two were dancing in the middle of a ballroom and then suddenly exchanged legs or arms. When the chromosomes separate toward opposite ends of the cell and two new cells are created, each new cell then contains chromosome 9 with a piece of chromosome 22 and chromosome 22 with a piece of 9. The presence of this genetic "swapping" was first described by Drs. Nowell and Hungerford in 1960.

For some reason, the stem cell's quality-control mechanism does not correct the new approximation of pieces of chromosome 9 and 22, and the repair mechanism is not even called into action. This approximation results in the production of a protein, tyrosine kinase, that gives the CML cell a survival advantage over its normal brethren. The CML cell is a white blood cell that may fail to fight infections properly and that crowds out normal cells from the bone marrow, resulting in fewer normal white blood cells, red blood cells, and platelets.

Understanding the genetic basis for cancer cell growth and reproduction, scientists have designed chemotherapy regimens that target cancer masses at the cellular level, trying to stop the cell's machinery from continuing its out-of-control division. Alkylating agents, such as cyclophosphamide, and platinum compounds, such as cisplatin, either cause the DNA to become too sticky, so it cannot be copied, or cause breaks in the DNA, which prevent it from being copied. Another drug, 5-fluorouracil (5-FU), trips up cancer cells by acting as a "Trojan horse." It resembles one of the most basic units of DNA, called a *base*, and is incorporated into

DNA as if it were a normal base. Once inside the DNA, however, it renders the DNA uncopyable. As a result, division and replication of the cell cannot be accomplished. The different types of chemotherapy are explained in more detail in Chap. 14.

Newer chemotherapy drugs actually "target" the specific genetic error known to cause a cell to become cancerous. In CML, the new drug Gleevec, formerly called STI-571 prior to its approval by the U.S. Food and Drug Administration, specifically blocks the actions of tyrosine kinase, the protein produced by the approximation of pieces of chromosomes 9 and 22. These types of drugs are being studied in all cancers and represent the future of cancer chemotherapy.

HOW DO ENVIRONMENTAL FACTORS INFLUENCE CANCER DEVELOPMENT?

It has long been recognized that cancers do not arise in a vacuum. While genetics certainly play the primary role in cancer development, the environment—including the colds we've suffered through, the foods we eat, the toxic substances we knowingly or unknowingly have been exposed to—contributes in a major way to our chance of getting cancer (Table 1-3).

Consider this. If genetics were the only cause of cancer, then all identical twins (who have identical DNA and chromosomes) would get the same cancers. They don't.

Similarly, if only specific combinations of DNA gave rise to cancer and we are born with our entire library of DNA, then babies under the age of 1 or 2 years would be dying of lung cancer. They aren't.

TABLE 1-3 **Environmental Factors That Influence Cancer Development**

Lifestyle factors
  Cigarette smoking
  Diets high in fat and/or in smoked or salted meats and fish
  Alcohol use
  Obesity
  Lack of physical activity
Exposures
  Radiation
  Radon
  Certain drugs, including chemotherapy agents (e.g., alkylating agents or topoisomerase inhibitors); hormones (e.g., estrogen); or immunosuppressants (e.g., cyclosporine)
  Certain chemicals (e.g., arsenic, asbestos, benzene, vinyl chloride)
  Certain infections (e.g., HIV, human papillomavirus, Epstein-Barr virus, *Helicobacter pylori,* hepatitis B and C)
Congenital conditions
  Down's syndrome
  Fanconi's anemia

On the flip side, if the environment were the only cause of cancer, then entire families who have lived under the same roof for more than 50 years should all develop the same cancers. Or everyone who smoked the same number of cigarettes over a lifetime would develop lung cancer or bladder cancer at the same rate. Neither of these situations occurs.

In truth, a combination of genetic and environmental factors causes cancer. The situation is a little more complicated because we are born with some genetic factors and others develop as a result of the environment. The relative contribution of genetic and environmental influences differs for each person. In addition, whereas the contribution of genetics to cancer arises from a one-time error of DNA copying, most environmental contributions to cancer development depend on either a prolonged exposure or a large one-time dose.

An example is radiation exposure. Radiation causes errors in a cell's ability to copy DNA accurately and subsequently to divide. Exposure to radiation that occurs over a long time similarly increases the chance that errors in DNA copying will not be caught by the cell's quality control mechanisms or will not be corrected by the cell's repair mechanism. Exposure to a large dose of radiation all at once may overwhelm the body's surveillance and corrective mechanisms, allowing an error to slip though. Children given radiation therapy to the thymus gland or teenagers given radiation therapy for acne (both "therapies" are no longer practiced) are placed at risk for developing cancer of the thyroid gland as adults. Similarly, the Nobel Prize winner Marie Curie, one of the first people to experiment extensively with substances that emit radiation, died of leukemia. These are examples of radiation exposure that took place over a prolonged period. Brief exposure to high doses of radiation is also problematic. Survivors of the nuclear bomb explosions in Hiroshima and Nagasaki in 1945 had a higher incidence of a number of cancers in the following years.

Probably the most notorious environmental influence on cancer is cigarette smoking. Doctors have developed a terminology to incorporate the duration of exposure and the dose of smoking, called the *pack-year*. Thus, a person who smokes two packs of cigarettes per day for 20 years has a smoking history of 40 pack-years (2 times 20). The higher the number of pack-years, the more likely a person is to develop cancer. This is known as a "dose-response" effect, lending further credence to the causal relationship between smoking and cancer. In fact, smoking plays a role in a number of cancers, including cancers of the lung, head and neck, esophagus, pancreas, cervix, kidney, and bladder.

Both radiation and tobacco smoke are examples of toxic exposures that contribute to cancer. Diet also plays a role in much the same way: the degree to which the foods we eat cause cancer depends on the duration of the exposure as well as the dose. This is a much more difficult area to study, however, because it is difficult to quantify exactly how much of a certain food a person has eaten over a lifetime and what component of that food contributes to the development of cancer. For that reason, many studies indicate an association between a type of food and cancer, but they will not come out and say, for example, "Ban hot dogs—they cause cancer!"

Examples of associations between food and cancer abound. Diets high in fat have been linked to an increased risk of cancers of the breast, colon, and prostate and possibly to cancers of the pancreas, ovary, and endometrium. Salted, pickled, or smoked foods may contribute to cancer of the stomach. On the other hand, diets high in fiber may decrease the risk of cancer.

Finally, certain infections may contribute to the development of cancer. People infected with human immunodeficiency virus (HIV), for example, are much more likely to develop lymphoma and other cancers as a result of being immunosuppressed. The immune system is part of the body's surveillance system for detecting and eliminating cancerous cells. If the immune system is not functioning well, cancer cells may have free reign. Other infections lead more directly to cancer. The human papillomavirus (HPV), the cause of genital warts, plays a major role in the etiology of cervical cancer. Epstein-Barr virus (EBV), the virus responsible for infectious mononucleosis (commonly called "mono"), also plays a role in the etiology of lymphoma. With infections, as with other environmental factors, genetic factors must also contribute to cancer development. Certainly, not everyone with the "kissing disease" gets lymphoma!

SUMMARY

Cancer is the abnormal growth of cells. Cells are the basic building blocks of organs, and any normal cell in the body has the potential of becoming a cancerous cell. Cancer arises through errors in copying genetic information in a cell, through environmental influences, and through a combination of the two. Cancer cells grow and divide faster than normal cells, and they fail to undergo programmed cell death (apoptosis). Chemotherapy targets these characteristics of cancer cells.

CHAPTER 2

Hearing the News: Reactions to Receiving the Diagnosis of Cancer

JOHN QUERQUES, M.D.
THEODORE A. STERN, M.D.

OUTLINE

WHAT IS THE "NORMAL" WAY TO REACT TO NEWS OF A CANCER DIAGNOSIS?

There is no "right" or "normal" way to react to the diagnosis of cancer. However, it is possible to make some general statements about likely or usual reactions. Most if not all people will be shocked by the news; disbelief and devastation may develop. Common expressions that convey the visceral impact of this news include "It took my breath away," "It feels like a blow," "I feel like I've been kicked in the stomach." For some, the entire experience feels surreal; it is as if someone else had just been diagnosed with cancer (see Fig. 2-1).

Thus, the initial response to a cancer diagnosis is typically an emotional one, associated with feelings of disbelief, sadness, and even anger. Over time, however, you can expect this emotional response to subside and to change. You then may realize you have many questions about your diagnosis and the next steps that you and your doctor need to take.

Information and knowledge become powerful weapons as the person newly diagnosed with cancer assumes a fighting stance against the enemy—cancer. You may find yourself turning to the Internet (see Chap. 12), to friends and family

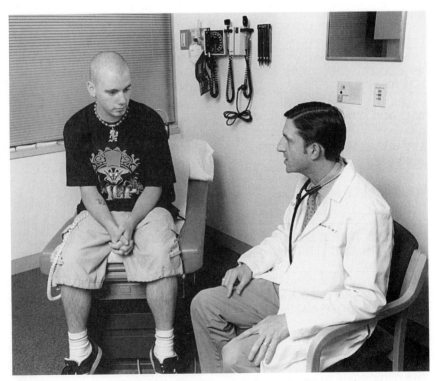

FIGURE 2-1 There is no "right" or "normal" way to react to the diagnosis of cancer.

members with cancer, and perhaps even to the medical library at a local hospital for answers to your many questions. In this phase, you may attempt to learn as much as you can about your diagnosis and to learn more about what the future may hold for you and for your family.

WHY DON'T I BELIEVE WHAT MY DOCTOR SAYS?

Shock, devastation, and disbelief in reaction to the news of cancer may be accompanied by a sense of loss; it may feel as if someone close to you has died. Sometimes, however, the initial reaction to a loss (e.g., the death of a loved one) is denial. Elisabeth Kübler-Ross popularized this idea in her 1969 book *On Death and Dying*. Dr. Kübler-Ross described five stages associated with the grieving process: denial, anger, bargaining, depression, and acceptance (see Table 2-1). At first, news of a loved one's death or one's own diagnosis of a potentially terminal medical condition can be so psychologically painful and jarring that an individual actually denies that the news is true. Denial is one of our most potent defenses against bad news, as it actually casts the news out of one's mind. Unfortunately, it is impossible to deny the reality of a cancer diagnosis and simultaneously believe what your doctor is telling you; thus, if you are in the denial stage, it may be difficult or impossible for you to believe what he or she is telling you.

WHY DO I FEEL SO ANGRY?

As Kübler-Ross pointed out, the second stage of grieving is anger. An individual may feel cheated out of a full and productive life. A person's view of his or her future usually does not provide room for a life-threatening illness. You may even blame God and focus the anger on a higher power. "Why me?" is a frequently asked question. Your anger may become *displaced*, that is, taken out on others or on circumstances completely unrelated to the real source of your anger. You may get mad at your spouse, at one of your children, or at your boss over a trivial matter that you would ordinarily shrug off as a mere annoyance. However, if you are upset at the diagnosis or even mad at yourself (as if somehow you were at fault for

TABLE 2-1 **Stages Commonly Encountered after Learning about a Diagnosis of Cancer (per Kübler-Ross)**

Denial
Anger
Bargaining
Depression
Acceptance

having cancer), you may find yourself "taking it out" on one of these people, including your physician (for giving you terrible news).

ARE MY FEELINGS OF DEPRESSION NORMAL?

Feeling sad, blue, or depressed can be an understandable reaction to learning that you have cancer. However, the syndrome of clinical or major depression is never a normal reaction to receiving bad news. Sadness is integrally related to the idea of loss; a diagnosis of cancer connotes a loss of health, a loss of plans and hopes, and perhaps a loss of life. You may find yourself grieving the life you enjoyed "before your diagnosis" as well as mourning the life you had planned—a life that now feels radically transformed by the diagnosis.

WHAT SHOULD I DO IF I FEEL HOPELESS?

Hopelessness is not a comfortable state of being. Moreover, it can be associated with a perceived loss of control and with notions of suicide. At times, hopelessness reflects a serious medical condition called *major depressive disorder;* fortunately, this condition can be treated effectively with medication, psychotherapy, or a combination of the two. Other symptoms of depression include a disturbance of sleep and appetite, an inability to experience pleasure or to think clearly, a feeling of worthlessness or guilt (e.g., the thought that you are somehow responsible for being stricken with cancer), and low energy. Feelings of hopelessness, helplessness, and worthlessness, as well as thoughts of harming yourself, are particularly ominous features of depression. If you notice that you are experiencing a number of these symptoms every day for more than a week, you should tell your doctor (see Table 2-2).

TABLE 2-2 **Symptoms of Major Depressive Disorder, Recalled by the Mnemonic SIG: E CAPS***

Sleep disturbed (increased or decreased)
Interests reduced, with a loss of pleasure
Guilt, or a preoccupation of thoughts
Energy reduced
Concentration ability reduced
Appetite disturbed (increased or decreased)
Psychomotor changes (i.e., feeling agitated or "like a bump on a log")
Suicidal thoughts, or thoughts of death

Note: Four or more of the above symptoms in the presence of depressed mood for 2 weeks or longer qualifies for a diagnosis of major depressive disorder.
*These criteria form the basis for a mnemonic, **SIG: E CAPS** (e.g., as in the label on a prescription [**SIG:**] for energy [**E**] capsules [**CAPS**]). Each letter of the mnemonic acts as a reminder of the diagnostic criteria.

WHAT WILL IT TAKE FOR ME TO ACCEPT THE FACT THAT I HAVE CANCER?

The passage of time is probably all that it will take for you to accept your diagnosis—not that acceptance is this easy. Over time, you will pass through various stages of reaction, whether it be Kübler-Ross's five stages or some other series of responses. Your rate of progression through various stages will depend on your personality, on your experience with similar trying circumstances, and the extent of your support system (e.g., family and friends).

Although your personality during your adult years is relatively fixed and your experience in the world has already taken place, you can modify your support system. Probably your most important source of support will be your family and friends; you can rely on them for help, for advice, and for love. Simply knowing that someone else is there for you can result in tremendous rewards. You may even supplement this "support team" with the assistance of various professionals: clergy, therapists, and counselors (see below). You may also find support groups (composed of people who currently have or have had cancer) helpful. By surrounding yourself with others, your spirits and determination can be buoyed. Over time you will feel more hopeful and optimistic.

HOW LONG WILL IT TAKE ME TO REGAIN MY EMOTIONAL EQUILIBRIUM?

This is a difficult question; the answer depends on your personality, your experience with trying and stressful situations, and the extent and strength of your support system. People who tend to be resilient, flexible, and optimistic in the face of trying circumstances and who are tolerant of change predictably will fare better than those with a rigid, controlling, or pessimistic (the proverbial "glass half empty") approach to life. If your adaptive personality traits have weathered storms in the past, all the better; your ability to approach your diagnosis of cancer will be supported by your confidence and by tested psychological mettle.

THE FIRST STEP IS TO TAKE A DEEP BREATH—WHY IS CANCER NOT THE END OF THE WORLD?

Cancer is not the end of the world, because some cancers can be cured, and those that cannot be eradicated completely can often be held in check for various lengths of time (depending on the type, aggressiveness, and extent of spread of the cancer)—even years or decades in some cases! In addition, the diagnosis of cancer does not necessarily portend months of discomfort, suffering, and pain. Some cancers (as is the case with some prostate cancers) grow extremely slowly, causing no symptoms in a person even without therapy. Even with cancers that cause symptoms or with the therapies (chemotherapy, radiation treatments, or surgery) for cancers, doctors and nurses have become quite skilled at making patients comfortable and treating seemingly intolerable side effects. For example, new antinausea medications are a tremendous boon to people with cancer who are receiving chemotherapy, while patient-controlled analgesia puts control of pain and its relief literally in the cancer patient's hand.

SHOULD I RESIGN MYSELF TO MY FATE?

The answer to this question is a resounding no! Your future is probably brighter than you may think it is. Resignation to a presumed negative outcome in the face of a host of reasons to be hopeful and optimistic is an example of a defeatist personality style. The popular expression "The glass looks half empty" (when it could just as easily be seen as half full) can aptly be applied to this psychological stance.

SHOULD I GATHER MORE INFORMATION ABOUT THE DIAGNOSIS AND TREATMENT?

This depends on what kind of person you are. You might thrive on information and seek it wherever you can. If so, the more information at your disposal, the better, because you can then feel armed for impending battles and in control of them. (If you are this type of person, see Chap. 12.) In contrast, you might do considerably worse with each bit of information that comes your way, either because it provides you with more sources of worry or apprehension or because you would become emotionally overwhelmed by the information. You know what type of person you are and how you best cope with adversities. Use whatever techniques you have found helpful in previous trying circumstances.

SHOULD I GET A SECOND OPINION?

Again, this depends on what kind of person you are. If you're the type who would just as soon leave major decisions to someone else and put ultimate faith and trust in your own physician, you may feel more comfortable opting for whatever he or she deems best. If, however, you would feel more secure by availing yourself of any and all potentially varying opinions and, ultimately, options for treatment, a second, third, or even fourth opinion may be the way for you to go. Most importantly, you should not feel guilty about seeking a second opinion, worry that you are hurting your doctor's feelings, or feel that you are in some way betraying him or her in doing so. Ask yourself this question: "If my doctor had a sibling or parent with a new cancer diagnosis, wouldn't he or she want to get a second opinion?"

SHOULD I LOOK INTO EXPERIMENTAL TREATMENTS?

The rate of cure for any type of cancer is never 100 percent. Thus, cancer researchers are constantly trying to improve on existing therapies through the use of experimental therapies, or clinical trials. For some cancers, established, well-studied treatments exist. If you have one of these types of cancer, experimental treatments may not be an option. If, however, the treatment for your particular kind of cancer is not as well established, experimental protocols may exist. Your oncologist should know if and where such clinical trials are ongoing. He or she is your best source of advice concerning the pros and cons of becoming involved in an experimental trial. See Chap. 18 for more information about experimental therapies and clinical trials.

SHOULD I LOOK INTO ALTERNATIVE OR COMPLEMENTARY HEALTH CARE PRACTICES?

Some people find acupuncture, aromatherapy, massage, herbal agents, and other nonwestern therapies helpful, both physically and psychologically. Patients often find that practitioners of such therapies tend to be more "holistic" in their approaches because they are concerned with other aspects of their patients' lives—psychological, emotional, and spiritual—as well as their physical well-being. In a modern medical world often indicted for the high premium it places on technology, such attention to the *psyche* as well as the *soma* (or body) is much appreciated and valued.

Be sure to check with your physician(s) before embarking on any of these alternative courses of treatment, because some of them may interact adversely with treatments prescribed by your western-style practitioner. Even if you think it is unlikely that a contraindication exists, it is better to be absolutely certain than to risk an adverse outcome. See Chap. 21.

SHOULD I SEEK PROFESSIONAL COUNSELING OR PSYCHIATRIC HELP?

This depends on the extent of your support system as well as on your psychological handling of a cancer diagnosis. If you are experiencing symptoms of depression, anxiety, alcoholism or other drug addiction, or a recurrence of a previously controlled psychiatric disorder, you should mention these symptoms and conditions to your physician. If you have few people around you who can serve as sources of support, comfort, and encouragement, a professional counselor or therapist may be able to serve these functions.

SHOULD I TURN TO RELIGION?

Religion may serve the functions of support, comfort, and encouragement that family, friends, and professional counselors or therapists serve. Some people may find organized religion or an interest in the spiritual helpful in giving their suffering a sense of meaning. Finding a spiritual purpose behind physical discomfort may transform the experience into a more tolerable one. This topic is covered in more detail in Chap. 23.

DO I NEED TO GO TO A SPECIALIZED CANCER CENTER?

This probably depends on how rare your particular type of cancer is. Some cancers are encountered commonly; thus, your physician is likely to be adept at treating these. For rarer tumors, you may want to seek the services of a specialized center that likely sees more of these cases than does your local medical center. Or, you may want to get involved in a clinical trial or experimental therapy, both of which are more likely to be available at a specialized cancer center. In some cases, your own physician may even refer you to one of these tertiary centers. If he or she does not and you think it may be helpful, you can always discuss this idea with him or her.

CHAPTER 3

The Different Types of Cancer

EPHRAIM HOCHBERG, M.D.

OUTLINE

HOW DO DOCTORS THINK ABOUT DIFFERENT TYPES OF CANCER?

One of the major differences between how patients think about cancer and how oncologists (cancer doctors) do is that oncologists always classify a cancer or tumor by its site of origin—where in the body the cancer cells were originally located.

You might have heard a friend or relative say that he or she had cancer in the bones. This probably means that the cancer started somewhere else in the body and then spread to the bones, as cancer that starts in the bones is actually extremely rare. An oncologist would describe that person's cancer as, for example, lung cancer metastatic to bone (*metastatic* means that a cancer has spread to another organ).

This distinction is important, because even after a cancer has spread into the bones, in many ways it still keeps the characteristics of the organ in which it started. For example, breast cancer that has spread into the bones can sometimes be treated with hormonal therapy given as a pill, whereas lung cancer that has spread to the bones almost always requires intravenous (by vein) chemotherapy. The location where the cancer starts almost always helps your oncologist decide what kinds of treatments will make the cancer shrink, or *respond* to therapy (Fig. 3-1).

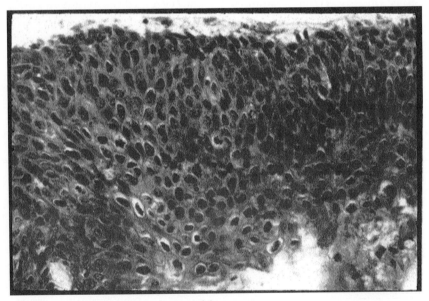

FIGURE 3-1 *Microscopic views of cancer of the uterus.*

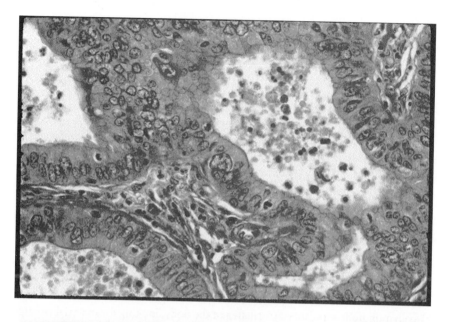

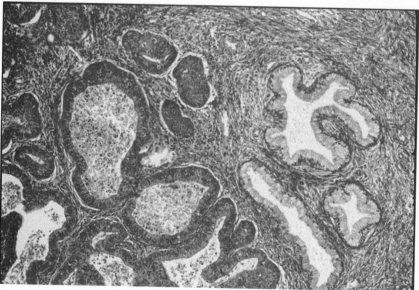

FIGURE 3-1 (continued)

WHAT DOES STAGING MEAN?

Another important factor in determining the type of therapy a tumor is most likely to respond to is the stage of the tumor. This is covered in more detail in Chap. 11. Simply stated, staging of the tumor is a fancy way of explaining how far a tumor has spread. It lets oncologists in different cities and around the world specifically define the extent of tumor spread and thus compare the effects of different therapies on similarly advanced cancers. Staging for most tumors goes from stage 1 to stage 4; stage 1 indicates a tumor with the least spread, while stage 4 indicates that a tumor has spread widely throughout the body.

Staging has three major components (Table 3-1). The first of these is the size and the location of the main tumor mass (called the *primary*). For example, in lung cancer, a tumor 1 centimeter across (about ½ inch) in the middle of the lung is staged differently than a tumor 1 centimeter across near the main airway in the lung.

The second major component to staging is the number of lymph nodes involved. Lymph nodes are small collections of cells of the immune system that are scattered all over the body. As part of the immune system, they act as a border patrol for the area of the body near them, preventing infections from "invading." Each lymph node monitors a small area of the body, looking for material (foreign bodies, bacteria, viruses) that shouldn't be there. When lymph node cells discover an invader, they become active and mobilize the immune system to fix the problem. When a cancer begins to spread, it usually starts spreading into the lymph nodes closest to the primary tumor. Therefore, knowing which lymph nodes are involved is a good way of determining how far the tumor has spread.

The last element of staging involves determining whether or not a tumor has spread to another organ (i.e., has metastasized). When a tumor has spread from a primary site (such as the breast or the lung) into the bones or brain, it is considered to have metastasized. In such a case, it is judged to be an advanced-stage cancer (even if the primary tumor is small and there is no obvious lymph node involvement).

WHAT ARE THE MAJOR GROUPINGS OF CANCERS?

All cancers come from normal tissues of the body; for every organ in the body there is a different possible cancer. Although it may seem odd, your blood and the parts

TABLE 3-1 **Major Components of Tumor Staging**

Tumor size
Tumor location
Number of lymph nodes involved
Extent of spread (i.e., metastasis) of a tumor
Depth of tumor invasion into an organ, or tumor thickness
Size of the lymph nodes (for head and neck cancers)

TABLE 3-2 Incidence of Common Tumors in the United States

Tumor Type	Number of New Cases Each Year
Breast cancer	200,000
Prostate cancer	190,000
Lung cancer	170,000
Colon cancer	107,000
Bladder cancer	56,000
Non-Hodgkin's lymphoma	55,000
Malignant melanoma	53,000
Endometrial cancer	40,000
Cancer of the kidney	32,000
Pancreatic cancer	30,000
Cancers of the liver and gallbladder	24,000
Ovarian cancer	23,000
Stomach cancer	22,000
Multiple myeloma	14,000
Esophageal cancer	13,000
Cervical cancer	13,000
Acute myeloid leukemia	10,000
Chronic lymphoid leukemia	9,000
Hodgkin's disease	7,500
Chronic myelogenous leukemia	5,000
Acute lymphoblastic leukemia	1,000

of your bones that make the blood are actually considered organs. The tumors (leukemias, myelomas, and lymphomas) that come from this system are called "liquid" tumors; they are one of the two major groupings of cancers. The other grouping (the "solid" tumors) includes every other type of cancer. Within this group, tumors are subdivided by the organ in which they arise. For example, tumors of the lung are all considered as a separate group, as are tumors of the breast (though there may be a good deal of variability among cancers within a group) (Table 3-2).

WHAT IS CANCER OF THE LUNG?

The lungs are two large organs located in the chest cavity. They extend from just under the collarbone to the bottom of the rib cage. Like any other organ, the lungs can become cancerous. Lung cancer is one of the most common cancers in the United States; it is the leading cause of cancer deaths. Approximately 170,000 new cases of lung cancer are diagnosed each year in the United States and 155,000 people die each year from lung cancer. Lung cancer is the most common cause of cancer deaths in men; in the late 1980s it became the most common cause of cancer deaths in women (passing breast cancer). Lung cancer is the only major type of cancer that has become more common in the last 30 years.

All of this is particularly poignant, because the majority of lung cancers are preventable. It is estimated that 70 to 80 percent of yearly lung cancer deaths are attributable to smoking. The risk of lung cancer extends beyond the individual who smokes cigarettes. Some studies suggest that 30 percent of cancers that develop in people who do not smoke (but who live with a smoker) are due to the effects of passive smoke inhalation. Other risk factors for lung cancer (e.g., exposure to asbestos or radon) pale in comparison to smoking when one considers the number of lung cancer cases they cause. Asbestos, a fibrous mineral, was used as an insulator until its relationship to lung cancer became known. Many older buildings are still insulated with asbestos, and precautions must be taken when asbestos is disturbed or removed. Radon is a colorless, odorless, radioactive gas that comes from deep within the earth. It can accumulate in poorly ventilated buildings and, with prolonged exposure, may cause lung cancer.

The two major types of lung cancer are small cell lung cancer (SCLC) and non-small-cell lung cancer (NSCLC). The major difference between the two types, aside from their "cells of origin" within the lungs, is that SCLC is significantly more likely to have metastasized by the time it is detected.

Unlike almost all other tumors, SCLC is divided into only two stages: limited disease and extensive disease. Limited disease is defined as SCLC that can be treated with a single beam of radiation. This usually means that the cancer resides only in the lung and in the nearby lymph nodes. Extensive SCLC has spread too far to be treated with a single beam of radiation.

NSCLC follows the usual system of staging, defined by the size and location of the tumor and whether lymph nodes or other organs are involved with cancer. Lung cancer that is still completely contained within the lung and the nearby lymph nodes (stages 1 and 2) is usually treated by surgery, although in some situations you may also receive radiation before or after the operation. When cancer has spread outside the lungs (stages 3 and 4), it is almost always treated with chemotherapy, most often in combination with radiation.

Both kinds of lung cancer can spread to the brain, and many people with lung cancer will need cranial radiation (brain radiation) either to treat the cancer that has spread or to prevent future spread. In general, lung cancer can be more difficult to treat than other solid tumors, although it is quite curable in the early stages.

One of the most interesting recent developments in lung cancer treatment is a new strategy to find lung cancers (while they are still small and more treatable) in smokers. Several ongoing large research studies of smokers are examining whether yearly computed tomography (CT) scans can find lung cancers before they grow large.

WHAT IS CANCER OF THE ESOPHAGUS?

The esophagus is a long muscular tube that carries chewed food from the mouth to the stomach. The part of the esophagus closer to the mouth has the same type of tissue lining as does the mouth, and the part closer to the stomach has a lining more similar to that of the stomach.

Cancer of the esophagus comes in two major types. Cancers that arise in the upper two-thirds of the esophagus (closer to the mouth) are called *squamous cell carcinomas* and are, like lung cancers, highly associated with smoking. They are also associated with alcohol use. Cancers that occur lower down in the esophagus, closer to the stomach, are usually cancers that arise from small glands lining this area. These cancers are called *adenocarcinomas*. There is some evidence that adenocarcinomas stem from a precancerous change (called Barrett's esophagus) in the lining of the esophagus, which probably occurs when a person's stomach acid leaks into his or her esophagus over many years—a condition commonly called heartburn or gastroesophageal reflux disease (GERD). After a long period of exposure to this acid, the esophagus changes its lining to protect itself from more damage. Unfortunately, this change makes cancer of this area slightly more likely to develop. Less frequently, squamous cell carcinomas also arise in this portion of the esophagus. Approximately 13,000 new cases of esophageal cancer are diagnosed each year in the United States.

Most people with either type of cancer of the esophagus will require some form of surgery. Unless they are extremely small, cancers of the esophagus can only be cured by surgery. Even if surgery does not cure the cancer, it can prevent blockages of the esophagus later on. These blockages can be debilitating and deleterious to a person's quality of life. In addition to surgery, many people with esophageal cancer receive a combination of chemotherapy and radiation. Particularly in adenocarcinoma of the esophagus, new types of chemotherapy may work more effectively than the older types.

WHAT IS CANCER OF THE STOMACH?

The stomach is a large muscular pouch near the bottom of the rib cage that produces acid and uses the acid and a grinding action to help digest food. It is connected to the esophagus at one end and to the small intestines at the other.

Stomach cancers, most of which are adenocarcinomas, are related closely to adenocarcinomas of the lower esophagus; the two types of cancer are treated in similar ways. Interestingly, while some of the causes of cancer of the esophagus have been determined, the causes of stomach cancer remain more mysterious. The consumption of large quantities of smoked or salted meats and fish seems to be a risk factor for gastric (stomach) cancer; why this occurs remains unclear. There also is some evidence that infection of the stomach with a certain type of bacterium (called *Helicobacter pylori*) might be a risk factor for gastric cancer. Approximately 22,000 cases of stomach cancer are diagnosed each year in the United States.

Stomach cancer is staged a little bit differently from some other cancers. The staging of stomach cancer places more emphasis on how deep the cancer extends into the wall of the stomach and slightly less emphasis on exactly which lymph nodes are involved. Most people with stomach cancer are managed with a combination of all three types of treatment: surgery, chemotherapy, and radiation. In general, the smaller the tumor and the less it invades into the wall of the stomach, the more likely it is to be treated successfully.

Another type of stomach cancer, called a MALT (mucosa-associated lymphoid tissue) lymphoma, differs from the more common type, adenocarcinoma of the stomach. MALT lymphomas arise when the immune cells that live in the stomach wall overreact to the presence of bacteria in the stomach. Scientists believe that the immune cells are so stimulated by the bacteria that, in their rush to kill it, they grow much too fast and form a tumor. The bacterium involved, already mentioned above, is again *H. pylori*. This organism is fairly common and, in most people, causes no more than irritation of the stomach. The MALT lymphoma is unusual because taking antibiotics that eradicate the bacteria can sometimes cure the cancer.

WHAT IS CANCER OF THE PANCREAS?

The pancreas is an organ about the size and shape of a bottle of hot sauce that is located in the abdomen, next to the stomach. Down the center of the organ is a small tube that carries the chemicals made by the pancreas into the small intestine. This tube, called the pancreatic duct, joins another tube, called the common biliary duct, which carries bile from the liver into the intestines. The chemicals made by the pancreas serve three important functions: they neutralize the acid produced by the stomach that has helped to digest the food; they break down the food passed from the stomach into the intestines to a form that the body can use more easily; and they help the body to store sugar—a process handled by the chemical insulin. People with a pancreas that doesn't produce insulin become diabetic.

Risk factors for developing pancreatic cancer include smoking, surgical removal of the stomach, and a condition called pernicious anemia. Cancer of the pancreas is difficult to cure; this is not because the cancer grows quickly but because it is extremely difficult to diagnose when it is still curable by surgery. Most are adenocarcinomas, the same cell type that leads to stomach cancer and to some cancers of the esophagus. The most common symptoms of pancreatic cancer are yellowing of the skin (jaundice), caused by obstruction of the common biliary duct (the tube that joins the pancreatic duct and drains the gallbladder), and a dull pain in the mid- to upper back. The pain usually is felt in the back instead of in the abdomen because the tumor often spreads toward the back. Approximately 30,000 new cases of pancreatic cancer are diagnosed each year in the United States.

The treatment for pancreatic cancer depends on the stage of the disease. As with most solid tumors, surgery, along with the possibility of radiation therapy, is used for early-stage disease, while more advanced disease can be treated with chemotherapy alone. The surgery to remove the cancerous part of the pancreas (called the *Whipple procedure*) is complicated and should be performed only at a hospital where the surgeons have significant experience with this procedure.

WHAT IS CANCER OF THE COLON?

The colon is a muscular tube about 10 feet long that connects the small intestine to the anus. It starts along the right-hand side of the body (near the right hip) and travels up the right side to the rib cage. This part of the colon is called the *ascending colon*. The colon continues as the *transverse colon*, crossing the body from the right-hand side to the left. The *descending colon* starts at the left rib cage and travels down the left-hand side of the body to the left hip. It then extends down into the pelvis as the sigmoid (S-shaped) colon, where it becomes the rectum.

Cancer of the colon is extremely common. It is the third most common cancer of both men and women, and approximately 107,000 new cases are diagnosed in the United States each year. It is thought that most colon cancers arise from polyps of the colon. Polyps are small bunches of tissue that grow on the colon's walls. Although they are not themselves cancerous, they are also not considered normal tissue, as they grow faster than normal tissue.

This raises one of the most important issues surrounding colon cancer. Screening for these polyps can detect them before cancers develop; then, they can be removed. Particularly in the setting of a family history of colon cancer or of inflammatory bowel disease (especially ulcerative colitis and Crohn's disease), it is important to be screened regularly with a full colonoscopy. Unfortunately, the screening process is not perfect, and some colon cancers form in the absence of polyps. There is also a good deal of debate as to whether a diet high in fat, low in folate, or low in fiber is a risk factor for colon cancer; this issue has not yet been resolved. A more detailed discussion of screening for cancer is provided in Chap. 5.

Once colon cancer has developed, it is staged primarily by the degree to which it has invaded the wall of the normal colon and spread to lymph nodes or other organs. Surgery is commonly used when early-stage colon cancer is detected. Depending on the depth of the primary tumor and the number of cancerous lymph nodes found at surgery, some people also will receive chemotherapy. In almost all cases, colon cancer will spread initially to the liver, and it is important that the liver be evaluated (using radiologic scans) before surgery is performed. Once colon cancer has spread to more than three sites in the liver or to other parts of the body (such as the lungs), it is generally not curable by surgery; in such instances, chemotherapy is the primary treatment.

WHAT ARE CANCERS OF THE LIVER AND GALLBLADDER?

The liver is a large organ located under the right-hand side of the rib cage and shaped something like a football. It sits directly under the right diaphragm, the large muscle that helps the lungs to breathe. Inside the liver is an enormous sponge-like network of small blood vessels called *sinusoids*. The cells that line these sinusoids break down the toxins and drugs in the bloodstream. These cells take the toxins that they have broken down and send them as sludge (bile) down a series of tubes called the *biliary ducts*. The bile flows out of the liver and into a holding chamber called the *gallbladder*. When you eat a heavy meal, the gallbladder pushes the bile out into the intestines to aid in the digestion of your food.

Cancers of the gallbladder and liver are relatively rare in the United States. These do not include cancers that have started in another organ (such as the colon) and spread (metastasized) to the liver. Approximately 24,000 new diagnoses of gallbladder and liver cancer are made each year in the United States, but these cancers are much more common in other parts of the world. In all likelihood, cancers of the liver and gallbladder are caused by factors in the environment that are more prevalent in other countries. For example, aflatoxin is a powerful natural chemical that causes liver cancer. It is produced by a mold called *Aspergillus flavus*. In parts of the world where grain gets moldy before it is used, the rates of liver cancer are up to 150 times higher than in the United States. In addition to chemicals such as aflatoxin, liver cancer is strongly associated with viruses that attack the liver. In particular, hepatitis B and hepatitis C viruses both seem to be risk factors for liver cancer.

The staging for liver cancer depends on the size of the primary (main) cancer mass as well as on the amount of the liver that is involved with tumor. For example, a person with multiple nodules of tumor in one small part of the liver has a better prognosis than one having the same number of tumor nodules spread throughout the entire liver.

Many liver cancers also make a protein (a tumor marker) called *alpha-fetoprotein* (AFP). Changes in the level of this protein can be used by your doctor to assess whether or not the treatment is working.

The mainstay of therapy for cancers of the liver and gallbladder is surgery. Almost all people in whom the tumor has not spread outside the liver will have an operation to remove as much of the tumor as possible. When it is not possible to remove the entire tumor or when a person is too sick to have surgery, therapy might involve chemicals that are injected directly into the tumor via the bloodstream. In some cases, a probe can be inserted via the blood vessels into the center of the tumor. The probe can then be made extremely cold to kill the tumor (*cryotherapy*), or radio waves can be emitted by the probe to kill the tumor around the probe (*radiofrequency ablation*). Radiation is used relatively rarely for liver tumors because the normal liver is easily damaged by radiation, and damage to the normal liver cells outweighs the benefits of killing cancerous cells.

Cancer of the gallbladder is staged somewhat like cancer of the colon, with one important addition. As with colon cancer, the extent to which the cancer has invaded the wall of the gallbladder is an important staging factor. In addition to the degree of penetration into the wall, the shape and characteristics of the individual cells in the tumor are important. Tumor cells that retain most of the characteristics of the normal cells of the gallbladder are much easier to treat than tumor cells that have developed abnormal shapes and features. This aspect of describing tumor cells is called the *histologic grade* of the tumor.

As with cancer of the liver, the treatment of cancer of the gallbladder revolves around surgery. In early cancers, it is sometimes possible to just remove the entire gallbladder. Usually, a significant portion of the liver edge on which the gallbladder rests has to be removed as well. Chemotherapy sometimes is used for gallbladder cancer that has spread beyond the immediate area around the gallbladder.

WHAT ARE CANCERS OF THE HEAD AND NECK?

Cancers of the head and neck are a large group of tumors with some common features. The first common feature is the cell of origin—the cell that becomes cancerous. Most head and neck cancers, regardless of exactly which structure they arise in, come from the cells that line the mouth, nose, sinuses, and throat. These cells are called *squamous cells*, and the cancers that arise from them are called *squamous cell carcinomas*.

Another feature common to these cancers is *field cancerization*. An easy way to think about field cancerization is to compare it to painting a car. The first step in painting a car is to lay down a coat of primer. This is a gray paint that helps the brighter paint stick to the metal of the car. In head and neck cancers, a large area of the mouth can develop invisible genetic changes that make it easier for cancer to start in that area later on, akin to a "primer" that allows the cancer to "stick" in that area of the throat. This concept is important, because many people who have been treated for head and neck cancer in one part of the mouth are at risk for another cancer occurring in another part of the field of cancerization.

A final common feature of these cancers is the role of tobacco and alcohol. The use of these two substances over long periods may lead to field cancerization, which eventually leads to full-blown cancer.

The staging of head and neck cancers is complicated and is different for every part of the mouth, nose, throat, and sinuses. The only common features in the staging systems include the size of the primary tumor and the size of the lymph nodes. This is one of the only tumor types in which the size of the lymph nodes makes a difference in determining the cancer stage.

Treatment of tumors of the head and neck usually requires all three modes of therapy: surgery, radiation therapy, and sometimes chemotherapy. Depending on the size and location of the primary (main) tumor, some people will have better outcomes with chemotherapy and radiation therapy prior to surgery. In other cases, surgery will be performed first, followed by radiation therapy. Chemotherapy will be used only if the disease has spread. In some centers, this care is coordinated in a multidisciplinary clinic in which a surgeon, a radiation oncologist, and a medical oncologist work together to develop a treatment plan for each person.

WHAT IS CANCER OF THE BLADDER?

The bladder is an organ in the pelvis that is shaped like a triangular balloon. Tubes called *ureters* enter the bladder on either side, carrying urine down from each of the kidneys. At the bottom of the bladder triangle, another tube called the *urethra* empties urine from the bladder. The bladder's only job is to store urine. Urine can sit in the bladder for many hours at a time, exposing the bladder surface to any carcinogens (cancer-causing agents) present in the urine. This is how cancers of the bladder develop.

The most common cause of bladder cancer is cigarette smoking. Tobacco smoke contains many known carcinogens that are eliminated from the body through the bladder. In the United States, up to half of all cases of bladder cancer are felt to be due to smoking. Quitting smoking has been shown to reduce the risk of bladder cancer rapidly. Bladder cancer accounts for about 4 percent of all cancers in the United States, for a total of 56,000 new diagnoses of bladder cancer every year. Most cases occur in people over 65 years of age.

Almost all cases of bladder cancer arise from the cells that line the bladder. These are called *transitional cells*, and the cancer arising from them is called a *transitional cell carcinoma*. Most people with bladder cancer will be diagnosed because they have blood in their urine (the amount of blood may be very little and thus discovered only by a urine test), prompting a doctor to order tests to evaluate the bladder even further. Few people will actually have symptoms, such as pain. The test that usually is ordered is a cytoscopy, in which a fiberoptic catheter is placed through the urethra into the bladder to look for a tumor.

The treatment of bladder cancer depends on the stage at which it is found and on the grade of the tumor (a measure of the cancer's aggressiveness). At the time of diagnosis, one-third of bladder cancers will be at an early stage, called *in situ*. This implies that the tumor is sitting on top of the bladder lining and has not penetrated into the bladder wall. These tumors can usually be treated by a surgical procedure called a *transurethral resection*. In this procedure, a fiberoptic probe inserted via the urethra removes the tumor. In some cases, intravesicular therapy (medications infused into the bladder) may also be used.

More advanced stages of bladder cancer require more intensive therapy. In people with bladder cancer in whom the cancer has invaded the muscle wall only slightly, it is sometimes possible to use a combination of chemotherapy and radiation in order to avoid bladder-removal surgery (cystectomy). When the tumor has invaded further into the wall of the bladder, a cystectomy is necessary. In people in whom the tumor is more advanced, radiation therapy may be used prior to surgery. Many different chemotherapy regimens have been used when the tumor has spread outside the bladder wall, and some newer combinations are much less toxic than older regimens.

WHAT IS CANCER OF THE PROSTATE?

The prostate is a gland about the size of a walnut located at the base of the penis, below the bladder and in front of the rectum. It surrounds part of the urethra, the tube that carries urine from the bladder to the outside of the body. Functionally, the prostate gland makes fluid that becomes part of the semen. Cancer of these fluid-producing cells is called an *adenocarcinoma*.

Prostate cancer is the most common cancer in men. There are expected to be almost 190,000 new diagnoses in the United States this year. People who have a strong family history of prostate cancer clearly are at an increased risk of getting this cancer, and people of African descent are at a slightly increased risk.

Most prostate cancers are found by screening (see Chap. 5). The recommendations for screening for prostate cancer vary widely, but most experts agree that men over the age of 50 should get a yearly rectal examination, during which the size and texture of the prostate gland can be palpated. Some doctors also use a blood test that measures prostate-specific antigen (PSA) and is known as the PSA test. PSA is a chemical made by the prostate and secreted into the bloodstream. The normal prostate produces a small amount of PSA, but a cancerous prostate can produce much more. When the PSA is above a certain level or a mass is detected during rectal exam, a series of biopsies (tissue sampling) is recommended. The PSA level in the blood of a person with known prostate cancer also provides a rough measure of a therapy's effectiveness. If the therapy is working, the PSA level will decrease or remain stable. If the therapy is ineffective, the PSA will continue to rise.

Once cancer has been diagnosed by a prostate biopsy, men with prostate cancer will be presented with a wide variety of options for therapy. These include radiation therapy given from outside the body (external-beam radiotherapy); radiation given by implanting radioactive pellets inside the prostate (brachytherapy); surgical removal of the prostate; and/or hormonal therapy. Despite the large number of people with prostate cancer, there is still no agreement on which of these therapies is the most effective. Each has certain advantages and disadvantages in terms of side effects, particularly regarding the rates of sexual dysfunction and incontinence. These potential side effects should be discussed in great detail with your doctor.

In contemplating treatment for prostate cancer, you should keep in mind that this type of cancer sometimes grows extremely slowly, and the side effects of treatment must always be considered in relation to your overall health and the likelihood that you will become ill from the cancer. Some oncologists say that more people die *with* prostate cancer than die *from* prostate cancer. For example, if a slow-growing prostate cancer is diagnosed in an 85-year-old man who also has heart disease, it is likely that the prostate cancer will not be the cause of significant illness for this man. For a person in this situation, it might not make sense to consider surgical removal of the prostate, because the side effects of the surgery will outweigh the long-term benefit.

After cancer has spread outside the prostate, hormonal therapy and chemotherapy are the major modes of treatment. In some cases, radiation therapy can be used to treat small masses of prostate cancer in the bones that are causing pain or are placing a person at risk of fracture.

Hormonal therapy is the name for a group of treatments that target those hormones, such as testosterone, that promote the growth of prostate cancer. One type of hormonal therapy is *androgen ablation*, which involves either a combination of two drugs (rendering a man functionally castrated) or the removal of the testicles. Another type of therapy, called *secondary hormonal therapy*, includes some herbal remedies that appear to be effective (such as PC SPES; *PC* stands for "prostate cancer" and *spes* is Latin for "hope"). Chemotherapy can also be used for prostate cancer, but there is no consensus on the most effective regimen.

WHAT IS CANCER OF THE KIDNEY?

The kidneys are a pair of organs located in the back of the abdomen, near the bottom of the rib cage. They help regulate the amount of water in the body and remove some toxins and medications from the circulation. Up to 40 percent of the blood that the heart pumps with each beat travels to the kidneys so that it can be filtered and urine can be produced. This urine passes through tubes called ureters into the bladder and then out of the body through the urethra.

The medical name for the most common cancer of the kidneys is *renal cell carcinoma* (RCC). In children, the most common tumor is *Wilms' tumor* of the kidneys. This tumor is extremely rare in adults; therefore the discussion here is limited to a discussion of RCC. There are approximately 30,000 cases of RCC each year in the United States. The risk factors for the development of RCC are not well defined, but there appears to be an association with cigarette smoking and with exposure to heavy metals, such as cadmium. There is a familial syndrome called von Hippel-Lindau syndrome, in which RCCs are much more common.

The staging of renal cancers follows the usual pattern (see Chap. 11), with the size of the main tumor, its extension into nearby organs, and the location of the lymph nodes to which it has spread determining the overall stage. One twist to the staging unique to RCC is that it incorporates tumor growth into the main vein that drains the kidney and from there into the inferior vena cava (the large vein that drains the lower half of the body).

Surgery is the primary therapy for cancer of the kidneys. Even if the disease has spread beyond the kidneys to one other location, removal of the metastatic cancer (the cancer that has spread elsewhere) and the original (primary) tumor is often recommended. Some urologists even recommend removing the kidney when the disease has spread to many other sites.

The other treatments for RCC are based on the concept of immunotherapy. Immunotherapy tries to activate the body's immune system to fight off the cancer—a notion stemming from the observation that somewhere between 0.5 and 1 percent of people with RCC experience a spontaneous disappearance of their cancer—without therapy! This probably occurs because the immune system successfully fights off the tumor; the observation of this phenomenon has given rise to the idea that activating the immune system with certain drugs might be especially effective in RCC. Unfortunately, this idea has not proven to be completely successful. Even the best immunotherapy medicines, drugs called *interferons* and *interleukins*, work only modestly well. One new, promising avenue is bone marrow transplantation. The first small study to investigate this type of therapy was performed at the National Institutes of Health (NIH) and had promising results.

Once RCC has spread into the bones, radiation therapy can be used to treat those areas that cause pain as well as to prevent fractures.

WHAT IS CANCER OF THE OVARIES?

The ovaries are a pair of organs that make up part of the female reproductive system. Each ovary is about the size of a small walnut. They are located in the pelvis, one on each side of the uterus. The ovaries have two major functions: they produce eggs once a month, and they produce certain female hormones.

More than 90 percent of cancers of the ovaries are of a subtype called *epithelial carcinoma*. The other subtypes are much more rare and are not discussed here. There are approximately 25,000 new diagnoses of ovarian cancer each year in the United States. The only well-understood risk factors for ovarian cancer are the cancer genes *BRCA1* and *BRCA2*, a family history of ovarian cancer, and the use of fertility drugs (which conveys a slightly increased risk).

The evaluation and therapy of ovarian cancer begins with a determination of the stage of the disease. The stage of ovarian cancer is not determined by the size of the main tumor, as it is with many other tumors, but rather by the pattern of spread of the tumor. Early-stage ovarian cancer is defined as any cancer that remains entirely within the pelvic cavity and has not spread into the abdomen. Oncologists define the pelvis as essentially the entire area enclosed by the hip bones. Unfortunately, most women with ovarian cancer are diagnosed at a fairly advanced stage, when the tumor has spread beyond the ovaries and pelvis and into the larger abdominal cavity.

The therapy for ovarian cancer consists of (1) primary surgical removal of the ovaries and of any cancerous growth that has spread throughout the pelvis and abdomen (often called surgical *debulking*) and (2) chemotherapy. Both of these treatment modalities may have to be repeated if the cancer recurs.

WHAT IS MELANOMA?

Melanoma, also known as malignant melanoma, is a tumor of the skin. It is not the most common skin tumor but is by far the most dangerous. Melanomas arise in cells of the skin called *melanocytes*. These cells protect the deeper layers of the body from damage caused by ultraviolet (UV) radiation—(i.e., damage from the sun). Over time, however, this UV radiation damages the melanocytes and can cause them to become cancerous.

Melanoma is a relatively common cancer. This year, 53,000 Americans are expected to be diagnosed with melanoma. It is the sixth most common cancer in men and the seventh most common in women. The risk factors for developing a malignant melanoma include fair skin, blond or red hair, blue eyes, lots of freckles, excessive sun exposure, and a history of blistering sunburns in childhood. A family history of either melanoma or nonmelanoma skin cancer is also a risk factor, as is the diagnosis of any one of a number of precancerous skin lesions (including dysplastic nevi, lentigo maligna, and congenital moles). As with many of the other cancers, there is a familial syndrome in which melanoma is more common. This syndrome causes family members to develop many dysplastic nevi that, in turn, can develop into melanomas.

The diagnosis of melanoma is made by the *ABCD* rule. This acronym stands for **a**symmetry (one side of the melanoma is not a mirror image of the other), **b**order irregularity (a melanoma does not have a perfectly round circumference), **c**olor variegation (color diversification that includes a dark black color); and **d**iameter greater than 0.6 cm (the size of a pencil eraser). Each of these signs makes a skin lesion more likely to be a melanoma (Table 3-3).

The staging of melanoma is unique in the field of oncology. In 1967, a doctor named Clark observed that the likelihood that a melanoma would return after being surgically removed was directly proportional to the thickness of the melanoma. In other words, thin melanomas were easy to cure, but thick ones were difficult. The staging system for melanoma is now based mostly on the thickness of the tumor. Tumors less than 1.5 millimeters deep are stage I. Tumors between 1.5 and 4 millimeters thick are stage II. Beyond stage II, the presence of tumor in the local lymph nodes becomes important. As can occur with other cancers, melanomas can spread to nearby lymph nodes. If only one area of the lymph nodes is involved, the tumor is stage III. Any other involvement makes the tumor stage 4.

Most people with stage I or II melanoma will have sentinel lymph node mapping performed to determine the exact location of the involved lymph nodes. This procedure, which is now being used with breast cancer as well, can be explained by the following concept: underlying the skin of every part of the body is a network of small ducts called *lymph ducts*. These are responsible for collecting fluid from the cells in that part of the skin and transferring the fluid to a local collect-

TABLE 3-3 **Features Suggestive of a Diagnosis of Malignant Melanoma: The ABCD Rule**

Asymmetry (one side of the skin lesion is not a mirror image of the other side)
Border irregularity (melanomas do not have perfectly round circumferences)
Color variegation (color diversification that includes a dark black color)
Diameter greater than 0.6 cm (the size of a pencil eraser)

ing station, the lymph node. When a melanoma begins to spread, it will almost always follow the path of the closest duct and invade the local lymph node into which the duct drains. By injecting a blue dye into the melanoma and then looking to see in which lymph nodes the dye becomes concentrated, a surgeon can determine which lymph node is most likely to be the first one involved with melanoma. If there is no cancer in that node, it is unlikely that the tumor has spread to other lymph nodes or elsewhere.

The primary therapy for melanoma is surgery. For early-stage disease (stages I and II), the surgeon will remove the tumor and a small area of normal skin around the tumor. Stage III melanomas will usually require a larger surgery, and most people will be offered chemotherapy as well.

Interferon is the most common chemotherapy drug used. In one large clinical trial, people who had stage III melanomas and who received interferon lived longer than those who did not receive the drug. Another common type of therapy offered to people with melanoma is vaccine therapy. Theoretically, these vaccines can make the immune system more aware of melanoma and prevent it from coming back. For people who have metastatic (widespread) melanoma, many chemotherapy and biochemotherapy agents can cause a response (shrinkage of the tumor), but there is as yet no standard therapy.

WHAT IS CANCER OF THE BONE MARROW (LEUKEMIA)?

Leukemias, along with lymphomas and multiple myeloma, are sometimes referred to as *liquid tumors*. Leukemias are the prototypical liquid tumors because, unlike lung cancer or breast cancer, leukemias are located primarily in the bloodstream and thus have almost always spread throughout the body at the time of diagnosis.

Many of the bones of your body have two functions. Bones have a strong outside shell (called the *cortex*) that supports the weight of the body and the pull of your muscles. Inside this shell is a spongy compartment (the *marrow*) made of specks of bone, some fat, and the specialized cells that generate your blood and your immune system—the red blood cells, which provide oxygen to tissues; the platelets, which help stop bleeding; and the white blood cells, which fight infection. The bone marrow is the factory in which the blood cells and immune cells are made. It is located in the bones of the spine and hips as well as in the shoulders, ribs, sternum, and upper legs.

Every cell in the bloodstream and the immune system starts out in the bone marrow as a stem cell. This cell is called a *stem* cell because it is literally the stem from which all the other cells branch out—the "grandfather" or "grandmother" cell that produces all future generations of blood cells. The stem cell first divides into either a myeloid or lymphoid stem cell. The lymphoid stem cell then divides and becomes either a T lymphocyte or a B lymphocyte. T lymphocytes help kill cells in the body that are infected by viruses, and B lymphocytes make antibodies that help defend the body against certain types of bacteria. The myeloid stem cell

TABLE 3-4 Types of Leukemia

Acute lymphoblastic leukemia (ALL)
Acute myeloid leukemia (AML)
Chronic lymphoid leukemia (CLL)
Chronic myeloid leukemia (CML)

divides and can grow to become one of five different types of cells. These include red blood cells (which carry oxygen from the lungs to the rest of the body), platelets (which help close up cuts and stop bleeding), granulocytes (white blood cells that capture bacteria and destroy them), eosinophils (white blood cells that protect against parasites), and basophils (white blood cells that help regulate allergic responses).

Leukemia occurs when a problem arises in one of the stem cells. There are actually four kinds of leukemia that occur in adults, and they are quite different from each other. The same leukemias occur in children, but at extremely different rates, and they are often treated differently than what will be described here. The four leukemias are acute lymphoblastic leukemia (ALL), acute myeloid leukemia (AML), chronic lymphoid leukemia (CLL), and chronic myeloid leukemia (CML) (Table 3-4).

Acute Lymphoblastic Leukemia

ALL is the rarest leukemia (with only about 1000 cases per year in adults). There are few known risk factors for ALL. Some evidence suggests that Down's syndrome can predispose a person to contracting ALL and that chemotherapy for other cancers can cause ALL. Weaker evidence reports that smoking, living near a paper mill, and using a permanent hair dye on multiple occasions are linked to the development of ALL.

ALL occurs when a mutation in the lymphoid stem cell causes this immature cell to divide endlessly instead of developing into mature B and T lymphocytes. These cancerous stem cells serve no useful purpose, as they have not matured enough to fight infections. Over time, these immature cells can take up all the space in the bone marrow and replace most of the healthy, nonleukemia stem cells.

ALL has three subtypes, called L1, L2, and L3. The therapy of L1 and L2 is divided into three phases. In the first phase, called *induction* therapy, high doses of multiple chemotherapy agents are used to destroy most of the leukemia cells. The second phase is known as either *consolidation* or *intensification* therapy. Some cancer centers prefer to use a slightly lower dose of chemotherapy for the second phase (consolidation) and some prefer to use a higher dose for this phase (intensification). The third phase is called *maintenance* therapy. In this final phase, lower doses of chemotherapeutic drugs are given every 1 to 4 weeks for up to 3 years. All patients with ALL should also receive some special therapy to prevent the leukemia from coming back (relapsing) in the brain. L3 ALL, also called mature

B-cell ALL or Burkitt's lymphoma, is considered to be a slightly different disease and is usually treated with alternating types of chemotherapy for a slightly shorter period.

Acute Myeloid Leukemia

AML is much more common than ALL. Roughly 10,000 new AML diagnoses are made each year in the United States. As with ALL, there are few known risk factors. The major ones appear to be increased age, exposure to certain chemotherapy agents for other cancers, exposure to radiation, and certain hereditary diseases (such as Fanconi's anemia and Down's syndrome). With AML, the myeloid stem cell stops growing and dividing normally and just makes copies of itself (similar to what occurs with the lymphoid stem cells in ALL). These immature cells are incapable of fighting infections and take up space in the bone marrow, thus replacing normal cells.

Because the normal myeloid stem cell can divide into five different types of cells, it makes sense that AML, the myeloid leukemia, also has multiple subtypes. In fact, there are eight subtypes, designated M0 to M7. They are typically treated identically, except for M3.

The standard therapy for AML is divided into two phases. The first phase is called *induction therapy;* the goal of this phase is to *induce* remission through the use of high-dose chemotherapy, which kills most of the leukemia cells. The usual induction therapy consists of two drugs given over a week in the hospital. People with AML are usually fairly sick during induction therapy and must typically stay in the hospital for a month or longer. The second phase is called *postremission, consolidation,* or *intensification* therapy, which usually consists of similar drugs to those given during induction therapy, though they are given over only 2 to 5 days. With M3, or acute promyelocytic leukemia, an additional drug, called *all-trans retinoic acid* (ATRA) is given, and sometimes also the drug arsenic trioxide.

Chronic Lymphoid Leukemia

The two chronic leukemias are called *chronic lymphoid leukemia* (CLL) and *chronic myeloid leukemia* (CML). CLL is the second most common adult leukemia, with about 9000 cases diagnosed each year in the United States. It is quite different from AML and ALL in that the cell type that produces the cancer is a mature B lymphocyte, the cell that usually makes antibodies to defend the body against bacteria. Because the lymphocyte is already a more mature cell than the stem cell that gives rise to ALL, this leukemia grows much more slowly than do the acute leukemias.

Most people with CLL are diagnosed by a routine blood test; few have symptoms from their disease. Interestingly, there are no known risk factors for this leukemia. The earliest stage of CLL is diagnosed when too many lymphocytes appear in the blood. Later stages are typified by enlarged lymph nodes and by an enlarged spleen. At the most advanced stages, people with CLL develop low blood cell counts. Because people with early-stage CLL can live for many years without therapy, sometimes even decades, the first treatment-related decision in this disease is whether to treat it at all. For example, if we imagine a situation in which a man in his eighties is diagnosed with early-stage CLL, it might make sense to leave the disease alone. In all likelihood, he will pass away from another cause before the CLL becomes problematic. In younger people or in those with more advanced disease, some chemotherapy, usually a single drug, may be necessary. If this is unsuccessful, other chemotherapeutic agents or biotherapies can be used.

Chronic Myelogenous Leukemia

CML is a relatively uncommon disease, with about 5000 cases diagnosed each year. The only known risk factor for CML is radiation exposure. This cancer is particularly important because it was the first in which the exact genetic change that causes cancer was determined. CML is a disease of the earliest stem cell that gives rise to all other cells in the blood and the immune system. This stem cell becomes cancerous when a small piece of one of the chromosomes, which carry DNA (the determinant of one's heredity or genetic code), changes places with a piece of another chromosome. This chromosomal *translocation* puts two different pieces of DNA next to each other—a new juxtaposition that makes the cell cancerous. The genes placed next to each other are called *bcr* and *abl*.

The treatment of CML changed dramatically in the year 2000. Before then, the major treatment of CML was a bone marrow transplant (see Chap. 20). This procedure uses high doses of chemotherapy and often radiation to try to eliminate most of the stem cells in an individual's bone marrow. The patient is given an infusion of new stem cells from another person. The new stem cells fill up the crevices in the bone marrow and start to make new blood and a new immune system. Because the immune system that grows up is completely new, it can sometimes finish the job of killing off any residual leukemia. The new treatment that changed the therapy of CML is a drug called imatinib mesylate (Gleevec.) This drug is the first of its kind, in that it specifically stops the new cancer-promoting DNA translocation (*bcr-abl*) from working. Without *bcr-abl*, there can be no CML. It is hoped that Gleevec will be a long-term answer for people with CML, though the drug has been in existence for too short a time to be sure of that yet.

WHAT IS MULTIPLE MYELOMA?

Multiple myeloma is another liquid tumor, along with lymphomas and the leukemias. It occurs both in the bone marrow and in collections of cells, called *plasmacytomas*, outside the bone marrow. The cells that become cancerous in multiple myeloma are called B cells; they are an important part of the immune system. Their usual role is to make the antibodies that protect the body from infections, and they also play an important role in responding to vaccines, thereby protecting the body from future infections. When a person is given a vaccine, a certain

B cell recognizes the vaccine and begins to make antibodies. This special B cell (a memory B cell) can live a long time; when a person is exposed to the bacteria from which the vaccine was made, even years later, the B cell is ready to respond and to protect the body.

One of the ways in which the B cell protects the body is to divide rapidly when it "sees" the bacteria again. Each of the copies of the original memory B cell can make thousands of units of the antibodies. In this way, the body can make millions of the antibodies in a short time. B cells making a particular type of antibody that keep dividing without a reason become multiple myeloma cells. Problems arise from the enormous amounts of antibodies that are made by the B cells and from the large clusters of B cells in the bone marrow that absorb the bone and take over space from the normal bone marrow. The antibodies can collect in the kidneys and cause kidney failure, and they can prevent the body from reacting normally to infections. The clusters of cells in the bone marrow can cause the bones to become so fragile that they break from minor trauma, sometimes from just getting out of bed. The only clear risk factor for multiple myeloma is exposure to ionizing radiation. About 14,000 cases of multiple myeloma are diagnosed each year in the United States, and the diagnosis is confirmed with a bone marrow biopsy.

There are many staging systems for multiple myeloma. Because myeloma is a liquid tumor, meaning that the cells of the tumor are found mainly in the bloodstream, the usual system of tumor size (T), number of lymph nodes (N), and presence of metastases (M) cannot be used. Instead, the disease is staged by measuring its effects on the bones and on the three types of blood cells (red blood cells, white blood cells, and platelets).

One of the most commonly used staging systems is called the Durie-Salmon Staging System, after the two oncologists who devised it. In their system, stage I patients have normal red blood cell counts, normal levels of two types of antibodies in the blood and urine, normal calcium levels (calcium is released from the bones when multiple myeloma is active), and no holes in the bones as seen on x-rays. Stage II is defined as a state that fits neither stage I or III. Stage III patients have any one of the following abnormalities: low red blood cell counts, large amounts of antibodies in the blood or urine, a high calcium level, or many holes in the bones. This staging system also divides patients on the basis of their kidney function. Patients with normal kidney function are stage A, and those with abnormal kidney function are stage B. For example, a person with multiple myeloma who has a high calcium level and kidney damage along with some evidence of multiple myeloma in a bone marrow biopsy would be classified as stage IIIB.

The treatment of multiple myeloma depends on the stage of the tumor and on an individual's ability to tolerate different treatment regimens. For the rare person with multiple myeloma who has only a cluster of multiple myeloma cells in one location (a plasmacytoma), radiation alone might be used. For the majority of people with stage III disease, chemotherapy is usually offered.

Many different chemotherapy agents are used to treat multiple myeloma. Two of the most common are called VAD [a combination of vincristine, doxorubicin

(Adriamycin) and dexamethasone] and MP (melphalan and prednisone). Some people in particularly good physical condition and below a certain age (which varies from medical center to medical center) can undergo bone marrow transplantation (BMT) for the disease. One fairly large French trial showed that those receiving a BMT lived longer than those who received standard chemotherapy. Other promising new therapies for multiple myeloma include the drug *thalidomide* and a new type of BMT. Thalidomide has been thought to work by blocking the formation of tiny blood vessels that the myeloma cells need in order to grow. Another important therapy for almost every patient with multiple myeloma are the drugs zoledronate and pamidronate. This drug strengthens bones and has been shown to reduce the number of bone fractures in people with multiple myeloma.

WHAT IS CANCER OF THE LYMPH NODES (LYMPHOMA)?

The third type of liquid cancer is called *lymphoma*. The lymphomas are a large group of cancers that include both slow-growing tumors as well as one of the quickest-growing tumors known. The first major division in the grouping of lymphomas is the distinction between Hodgkin's disease (HD) and the other lymphomas, which are called the non-Hodgkin's lymphomas (NHLs).

Hodgkin's Disease

Hodgkin's disease is classified separately from the other lymphomas for four major reasons. First, from a purely historical perspective, HD was described by Dr. Thomas Hodgkin in 1832 before almost every other type of cancer was known and before standardized classification schemes were developed. Second, it is a clearly distinct type of cancer as opposed to some of the NHLs, which will be discussed later. Third, the actual cancerous cells seem to make up only a small part of the disease (more about this further on). Finally and most importantly, HD is an easily treatable and often curable disease.

Hodgkin's disease occurs most commonly in two age groups: 20- to 25-year-olds and people above age 75. About 7500 cases are diagnosed every year in the United States. HD itself has four pathologic subtypes, the most common being nodular sclerosing Hodgkin's disease. Like multiple myeloma, it is a disease of the type of white blood cells called B cells, which usually produce antibodies that protect the body from infections. Unlike myeloma, however, the B cell from which Hodgkin's disease arises is immature and doesn't make any of the antibodies that cause so many of the problems in multiple myeloma.

In addition, unlike multiple myeloma and almost every other type of cancer, the actual tumor cells that define HD can be hard to find. Although people with the disease usually have large, swollen lymph nodes (glands) in the neck or armpits, these nodes might contain only one or two thousand cancer cells mixed in with millions of inflammatory cells, which make up the rest of the mass. The few cancer cells that appear in the lymph node produce cytokines, special chemicals that are thought to attract the inflammatory cells, thus causing the swollen nodes. These cytokines also make all of the other lymph node cells grow and divide. The same cytokines cause the symptoms that typify Hodgkin's disease: usually fevers, weight loss, and night sweats.

The staging system for Hodgkin's disease is called the Ann Arbor system, developed in Ann Arbor, Michigan. Stage 1 disease is a single area of lymph nodes that are affected by the tumor (for example, one large group of lymph nodes in the neck or a single group in the armpit). Stages 2 and 3 are defined by the location of the lymph nodes relative to the diaphragm. The diaphragm is the large muscle that powers the lungs; it is located at the bottom of your rib cage. A person having multiple cancerous lymph nodes all on one side of the diaphragm (either above or below) has stage 2 HD; a person having nodes on both sides of the diaphragm has stage 3 disease. So a group of lymph nodes in your neck and one in your armpit would give you stage 2 disease, but involvement of neck nodes and groin nodes would give you stage 3 disease. Stage 4 Hodgkin's disease is widespread disease and indicates that either the liver or bone marrow is involved with lymphoma or that there are multiple sites of disease outside of the lymph nodes.

Another element of staging for Hodgkin's disease is defined by whether a person has fever, weight loss, or night sweats. A person with these symptoms has "B" disease and a person without them has "A" disease. The final part of staging for Hodgkin's disease is whether there is a single lymph node mass that is larger than 10 cm in diameter (about 4 inches). A person with a tumor this large is staged as an "X". As an example of this staging, take the case of a 40-year-old man with fevers every night who comes to the hospital with a very large lymph node in his neck (6 inches across), another in his groin, and an x-ray that reveals smaller masses in his lungs. He would have stage 4BX Hodgkin's disease.

The treatment for Hodgkin's disease is divided by the stage of disease and somewhat by the subtype. Stage 1A patients can sometimes be treated with radiation alone. All other patients will likely receive some chemotherapy in their treatment or a combination of chemotherapy and radiation. Patients with stages 3 and 4 disease will almost always receive only chemotherapy to treat their disease unless they have a large tumor mass, designated X in the staging. Almost all patients with X-stage disease will receive some radiation therapy, most commonly to the area of the large mass. The most common type of chemotherapy used is called ABVD, for doxorubicin (Adriamycin), bleomycin, vinblastine, and dacarbazine. See Chap. 14 for more information about this therapy.

Hodgkin's disease is extremely curable. Over 90 percent of people with stages 1 and 2 disease will be completely cured. Even those with stages 3 and 4 disease will be cured more often than not. Because the cure rate for this tumor is so high, doctors are paying careful attention to the amount and type of chemotherapy and radiation used in treatment. Many current research efforts are focusing on minimizing long-lasting side effects and, in some cases, on placing patients at a lower risk for developing another type of cancer.

Non-Hodgkin's Lymphoma

The other major grouping of lymphomas besides Hodgkin's disease are the non-Hodgkin's lymphomas (NHL). These lymphomas comprise a diverse group of diseases that range from aggressive, fast-growing subtypes to indolent, slow-growing ones. Overall, about 55,000 NHL are diagnosed every year in the United States, making it the sixth most common cancer diagnosis for men and women. The most common subtypes of lymphoma are diffuse large B-cell lymphomas (DLBCL), which account for about one-third of all cases, and follicular lymphoma (FL), which accounts for about 20 percent of cases. The numerous other types of lymphoma are rare, accounting for fewer than 5000 cases each. The two major types are discussed in some detail below.

There are several important general issues that must be considered with lymphomas. The first of these is the need for a surgical biopsy (a removal of tissue). For an accurate lymphoma diagnosis to be made, a sizable piece of tissue, often an entire lymph node, should be obtained, rather than just a small needle biopsy. In many cases distinctions among the different types of lymphomas can greatly influence treatment, but these cannot be made from small pieces of tissue.

In addition, with certain types of lymphoma, the dividing line between leukemia and lymphoma may be unclear. Leukemia literally means that an excess of white blood cells is present in the bloodstream, whereas lymphoma implies that a cluster of white blood cells is gathered together, often in a lymph node. In some cases, these two events can occur simultaneously. The same type of tumor can both float in the bloodstream and gather in clusters. Thus, occasionally a diagnosis cannot be made until a series of special tests have been completed to distinguish between lymphoma and leukemia.

The third important factor to consider with an NHL diagnosis is called the *International Prognostic Index* (IPI). This is a group of clinical signs that can help doctors predict whether a lymphoma will come back after treatment. The five signs, each of which make the lymphoma more likely to come back, include patient age greater than 60 years, stage 3 or 4 lymphoma, lymphoma that occurs outside of lymph nodes, poor patient performance status (the ability to attend to the activities of daily living and self-care), and an elevated lactate dehydrogenase (LDH) blood test.

The last factor common to most but not all lymphomas is the staging system. This system is the same as that described above for Hodgkin's disease.

Diffuse large B-cell lymphoma is the most common lymphoma, representing about 30 percent of all of the non-Hodgkin's lymphomas. It usually occurs in people in their sixth decade of life. Like multiple myeloma and Hodgkin's disease, it is a disease of the B-cell subtype of white blood cells, although it doesn't produce the antibodies that myeloma produces. It most commonly becomes manifest as a lump in the neck, which in actuality is a cluster of enlarged lymph nodes. Most people with diffuse large B-cell lymphoma will have widespread disease at diagnosis, either stage III or IV.

The treatment of this lymphoma depends on the stage at diagnosis. People with early-stage disease who have a small amount of lymphoma in one location can either be treated with a shorter course of chemotherapy as well as radiation therapy to the involved lymph nodes or with a longer course of chemotherapy alone. People with advanced-stage disease are treated exclusively with chemotherapy. The recommendations for the most effective type of chemotherapy are changing rapidly, but the most current recommendations are for CHOP (cyclophosphamide, hydroxydoxorubicin, Oncovin, and prednisone) chemotherapy for six cycles, often given in combination with an antibody called rituximab (Rituxan). Antibodies are special proteins, made by the body, that have the ability to attach themselves tightly to one specific protein located on the outside of cells, as if they were recognizing a bar code. Other cells can then detect the antibody stuck to the protein and can remove both the antibody and the cell to which it is bound.

An analogy that might make this more clear is to think about a pretty tree-lined street in your neighborhood. There is a local city official who is responsible for making sure that all of the trees are healthy. When a tree is unhealthy, the official spray paints a large red symbol on the tree and sooner or later a crew comes along in a truck, sees the red paint, and removes the tree. The antibody that is given for this lymphoma is called rituximab. It specifically binds to a protein on the lymphoma cells and targets them for destruction, just as the city official paints a red mark only on those trees that are dead and must be removed. Sooner or later a special cell in the bloodstream (called a *monocyte*) floats by the cell with the antibody stuck to it and kills and removes the lymphoma cell. These antibodies are among the most exciting developments in lymphoma therapy. They have far fewer side effects than most traditional chemotherapy agents and allow oncologists to use the body's own immune defense mechanisms to kill off the cancer cells.

The newest development in antibody therapy is called a *conjugated antibody*. These are still in clinical trials, but the concept is easy to understand. Imagine if the city official in charge of getting rid of those dead trees had a special paint that could destroy the tree all by itself. The official could just walk down the street, find a dead tree, and spray a special tree-removal chemical on the tree. The spray then would dissolve the tree without any need to wait for the guys in the truck to remove it. Conjugated antibodies find the lymphoma cells in the same way that regular antibodies do, but they also carry around a tiny bit of a radioactive element. When the antibodies stick to the cancer cell, the radioactive element can emit enough radiation to kill that cell. Then the body's usual processes for getting rid of dead cells can take over. In early clinical trials, these conjugated antibodies seem to do a good job getting rid of the lymphoma, though there are still some long-term safety issues to be dealt with about the effects of that radiation on surrounding normal cells.

The other major subgroup of non-Hodgkin's lymphomas is called *follicular lymphoma*. Follicular lymphoma is the second most common lymphoma, making up about 20 percent of all cases of lymphoma. Like diffuse large B-cell lymphoma, it most commonly occurs in people approximately 60 years of age, although it does appear to be slightly more common in women than in men. It usually becomes manifest as a painless lymph node in the neck, armpit, or groin that has been present for quite some time. Most people will have widespread disease at the time of diagnosis. An interesting point about follicular lymphomas is that about 5 to 10 percent will turn into diffuse large B-cell lymphomas, spontaneously, every year.

Follicular lymphoma can be one of the slowest-growing tumors. In many cases, people can survive for many years without any therapy at all. This can make deciding on the right kind of therapy difficult. For example, if this lymphoma is detected in an 80-year-old man who has had a stroke and is taken care of in a nursing home, it might not make sense to remove him from his comfortable environment and bring him to a hospital to receive chemotherapy, which could make him sick. In this scenario, the man is more likely to die from some other cause (for example, another stroke) than from his lymphoma, so treating the lymphoma will not prolong his life. On the other hand, if this lymphoma is found in a 55-year-old woman who is otherwise perfectly active and healthy but has symptoms from the lymphoma, it makes sense to treat her lymphoma aggressively, with chemotherapy.

The decision to treat a person with follicular lymphoma must take these factors into account. In many cases, the preferred therapy when the disease is detected is simply to follow the condition closely. At some point, most people will require therapy for the tumor, and it doesn't seem to make a difference in terms of overall survival when this treatment is given—whether at diagnosis or years later. There are many treatment options available for a follicular lymphoma that has grown to a size requiring therapy. These include radiation therapy to specific areas of disease (such as a lymph node in the groin), single chemotherapy agents such as fludarabine or cyclophosphamide, a regimen of multiple chemotherapy agents such as CHOP or CVP (cyclophosphamide, vincristine, and prednisone), or the addition of antibody-based therapies such as rituximab to any of the above. The choice of a particular therapy is often dictated by the individual's needs during therapy.

WHAT IS UTERINE (ENDOMETRIAL AND CERVICAL) CANCER?

The uterus is an organ of the female reproductive system. It is about the size and shape of a large upside down pear and is located in the center of the pelvis. It is connected to the vagina on one side (via the cervix) and to the ovaries on the other (via the fallopian tubes). The uterus's major function is to support a growing fetus. There are two important layers of the uterus that assist with this. The innermost layer is called the *endometrium* and is mainly composed of a network of small blood vessels. A hormone called *estrogen* causes this layer to grow and thicken each month to prepare for pregnancy. If pregnancy does not occur, the endometrial lining sloughs off and is discharged in the process of menstruation. The other layer is a thick band of muscle called the *myometrium*. This layer helps slough off the endometrium each month and also helps mobilize the child at the time of delivery.

There are two major types of uterine cancer. The first arises from the endometrial layer, or the main body of the uterus, and is commonly called endometrial cancer. The continual growth and shedding of the endometrial layer under the influence of estrogen seems to make it particularly vulnerable to the development of cancer. Uterine endometrial cancer is the fourth most common female cancer, accounting for about 6 percent of cases. In all, approximately 40,000 new cases of endometrial cancer are expected to be diagnosed this year in the United States.

Because of the relationship between estrogen and the endometrium, any situation that increases a woman's exposure to estrogen or estrogen-like agents will increase the risk of endometrial cancer. On the other hand, exposure to the hormone progesterone will decrease the risk of endometrial cancer. As a woman ages, her uterus is exposed to estrogen over a long period of time; thus, increasing age is a risk factor for endometrial cancer, as is menopause after the age of 55 years. Therapy with oral contraceptives that contain only estrogen, particularly over a long time period, is another clear risk factor for the same reason. On the other hand, therapy with combination oral contraceptives that contain both estrogen and progesterone actually decreases the risk of endometrial cancer as compared to the risk in untreated women. Because being pregnant decreases the number of times the uterus is exposed to estrogen, having remained childless is another risk factor for endometrial cancer. On the other hand, women who have had many children have a decreased risk. Finally, fat tissue can generate excess estrogen: thus, obesity contributes to endometrial cancer risk.

Other less well understood risk factors include diabetes, hypertension, a high-fat diet, and a genetic cause called *hereditary nonpolyposis colon cancer syndrome*. One important risk factor that has generated a lot of controversy is use of the drug *tamoxifen*. Tamoxifen is an effective drug for breast cancer; it has the side effect of increasing the risk of endometrial cancer by acting a little bit like estrogen. In several large studies it has been shown that women still benefit from the anti–breast cancer effects of the drug more than they increase their risk of endometrial cancer. This question is also becoming less relevant as other drugs without the cancer risk, such as raloxifene, replace tamoxifen.

The most common symptom of endometrial cancer is abnormal uterine bleeding. This can either represent the onset of new bleeding after menopause or unusual bleeding between menstrual cycles. Once bleeding is noted, an accurate evaluation of the risk of endometrial cancer will include an endometrial biopsy (a sampling of endometrial tissue) via either an office procedure called endometrial sampling or a small operation called dilatation and curettage (D&C).

Once the presence of endometrial cancer is confirmed by a biopsy, therapy will depend on the stage of the tumor. The evaluation and therapy of endometrial cancer begins with a determination of the stage of the disease, which depends on the pattern of spread of the tumor at the time of surgery. The surgery that usually is performed consists of removal of the entire uterus, both ovaries, and both fallopian tubes (a total abdominal hysterectomy and bilateral salpingo-oophorectomy, or TAH/BSO). The uterus then is examined quickly and, if indicated, further surgery, such as lymph node removal, is performed before the operation is completed.

Early-stage endometrial cancer is defined as any cancer that remains entirely within the uterus and has not spread into the abdomen. Once the tumor has spread into the bladder, bowels, or elsewhere outside the uterus, it usually is considered to be advanced disease. Another factor that determines treatment choices is the grade of the tumor. Tumor cells that appear to be extremely abnormal under the microscope are considered to be of a higher grade and sometimes call for a change in therapy.

Women with limited disease who have low-grade tumors can sometimes be cured with surgery alone. Interestingly, some research indicates that in women who were too ill to undergo surgery and who therefore received radiation therapy alone, the long-term outcomes were not much worse than for those who received surgery. Rarely, women with extremely early disease who still wish to have children can be treated with the hormone progesterone alone, although these women will require close follow-up.

Many women who have limited cancer (cancer that has not spread extensively) will be offered radiation therapy after surgery. Women with more advanced disease should receive radiation therapy after surgery. The addition of chemotherapy after surgery is also offered in some settings. Women with metastatic (widespread) disease are treated with either hormonal therapy or chemotherapy. As mentioned above, progesterones can be used in selected women with early disease. Similarly, progesterones can be used to slow tumor growth once the cancer has spread. Standard types of chemotherapy including cisplatin and carboplatin may also be used.

The second major type of uterine cancer arises in the cervix and is commonly called *cervical cancer*. Approximately 13,000 new cases of cervical cancer are expected to be diagnosed in the United States this year. The variations in the incidence of this cancer and the mortality rates arising from it in different parts of the world are striking. In developed countries, there has been a 75 percent decrease in the occurrence of cervical cancer over the last 50 years. However, in developing countries, cervical cancer is the second most common tumor, and half of all women who develop cervical cancer in these countries die of the disease. This difference is almost entirely due to the widespread use of cervical cancer screening programs in developed countries. The most common screening procedure is a regular Pap smear.

A unique aspect of cervical cancer is that the cause of the disease is fairly well understood. A virus called human papillomavirus (HPV) is found in 95 percent of cases of cervical cancer, although not all people infected with HPV get cervical cancer. HPV is a sexually transmitted disease, and the risk factors for cervical cancer reflect this. The major risk factors include sexual activity starting at a young age, multiple sexual partners, a high-risk sexual partner, and a history of sexually transmitted diseases. Two less well understood risk factors are smoking and a low socioeconomic status.

Most cases of cervical cancer are found by Pap smear in women who are screened regularly. Cases discovered in women who have never been screened tend to be much more difficult to treat and tend to be more advanced. When a Pap smear reveals the presence of cervical cancer, women undergo a procedure called a *colposcopy*. This allows the gynecologist to get a better view of the cervix. Biopsies are frequently taken at this time to confirm or disprove the diagnosis made on Pap smear.

The staging of cervical cancer (using the International Federation of Gynecology and Obstetrics, or FIGO, system) is based on physical examination and clinical evaluation. Stage 1 disease is confined to the cervix (there are substages of stage 1 depending on the tumor's size and visibility). Stage 2 cancer extends beyond the uterus itself but not into the pelvic wall or into the lower third of the vagina. Stage 3 extends to the pelvic wall and can involve the kidneys. Stage 4 extends beyond the pelvis to other sites.

As with most cancers, the appropriate treatment depends on the tumor's stage. Early-stage tumors can sometimes be treated simply by removal of a portion of the cervix; however, most tumors up to late stage 2 are treated with removal of the entire uterus. Many centers will also remove pelvic lymph nodes at the time of surgery.

Depending on what is discovered during this surgery, different treatment options will be recommended, including radiation therapy and/or chemotherapy. In some cases, radiation therapy or a combination of chemotherapy and radiation therapy can be given alone, without surgery, for early-stage cancers. There is some disagreement about the most appropriate therapy for women who have large tumors at the time of diagnosis. Some centers use radiation and chemotherapy followed by surgery and some reverse the order. Tumors that are greater than early stage 2 are usually treated with combined chemotherapy and radiation. If a tumor comes back after this initial therapy, several chemotherapy agents may provide a benefit, either alone or in combination.

WHAT IS CANCER OF THE BREAST?

The breasts are glands located on the chest wall whose primary purpose is to produce milk. The area of the chest covered by breast is rectangular, bordered by the sternum (breastplate) in the middle; the clavicle (collarbone) at the top; a line extending straight down from the center of the armpit at the side; and the "bra line" at the bottom.

Breast cancer is the most frequently diagnosed cancer in American women and the second most frequent cause of cancer death (behind lung cancer). Approximately 200,000 new cases of breast cancer are diagnosed each year in the United States and 41,000 people die each year from breast cancer. Almost all breast cancers are adenocarcinomas. There are two subtypes of adenocarcinomatous breast cancer, ductal carcinoma and lobular carcinoma.

The risk factors for breast cancer include both environmental and genetic factors. Both sets of factors work together, so a person with a genetic risk for developing breast cancer will have an even greater risk when exposed to specific environmental influences. Specific risk factors that are associated with breast cancer include increasing age (as a woman ages, her likelihood of developing breast cancer also increases); benign breast disease (i.e., women who undergo biopsies of breast lumps that are negative for cancer—this does not mean, of course, that performing the biopsy *causes* breast cancer); radiation exposure (particularly in people treated with radiation therapy early in life); and alcohol consumption (which promotes estrogen production in the body, and thus breast tissue cell growth). Other factors that increase the risk of breast cancer include early age of menarche (the age a woman has her first period); late age of menopause; and not having any children.

These last three risk factors are related to the total amount of time that a woman's breast tissue is exposed to estrogen. Estrogen stimulates breast tissue growth. The question of whether long-term use of oral contraceptives can place a woman at higher risk for breast cancer is still somewhat controversial. However, the great body of data from numerous studies over the years seems to indicate that the use of oral contraceptives does not place women at a higher risk of breast cancer. The use of hormone replacement therapy in postmenopausal women, however, does appear to be associated with a higher breast cancer risk.

The most important risk factor for the development of breast cancer is a family history of breast cancer. A woman's chance of being diagnosed with breast cancer increases by 1.5 to 3 times if a mother or sibling has the disease. Breast cancer that runs in families may be related to one of two genetic mutations identified over the past few years: *BRCA1* and *BRCA2* (see Chap. 8 for more details about genetic mutations and cancer risk). *BRCA1* and *BRCA2* account for 6 to 10 percent of all breast and ovarian cancers in the general population in the United States and only 3 percent of all breast cancer cases.

Breast cancers are divided into carcinoma in situ and invasive cancers. Carcinoma in situ refers to small collections of cancerous cells that are still confined to the small part of the breast in which they originated. Ductal carcinoma in situ (DCIS) originates in the very small ducts within the breast. Most cancers of this type are detected by mammography. On a mammogram, DCIS appears as tiny calcifications (microcalcifications), or white dots against the black background of the rest of the breast. Lobular carcinoma in situ (LCIS) originates in and is confined to the lobules of the breast. It usually is discovered by accident, in the process of obtaining a biopsy of the breast for another indication, such as a biopsy to remove fluid from a cyst. It is rarely associated with microcalcifications and thus is usually not identifiable on mammography.

Invasive cancers are distinguished from the carcinomas in situ because they grow beyond the local tissues in which they arose. DCIS remains in the breast ducts, but invasive ductal carcinoma spreads to surrounding breast tissues and blood vessels and even beyond to other body structures. The same holds true for invasive lobular carcinoma. Invasive carcinomas usually come to a person's attention as a lump or mass (though they also can be discovered through mammography), while in situ tumors do not. Although a distinction is made microscopically between invasive ductal carcinoma and lobular carcinoma, the two are treated in much the same way clinically and carry similar prognoses.

Most breast cancers are first diagnosed by women themselves, who feel a lump on a monthly self-exam; by doctors who feel a lump on a yearly breast exam as part of the yearly physical exam; or on mammography. Once a breast cancer is suspected, either on a mammogram or on physical examination, the next step is to biopsy (take a piece of tissue from) the area. This can be done either by using a thin needle to pull cells out of the lump, by taking a larger needle and getting a core of the lump, or by cutting the entire lump out.

Once cancer has been diagnosed by a biopsy, a woman with breast cancer will undergo a few more tests to assess her stage accurately. The exception is for women with breast cancer (either ductal carcinoma or lobular carcinoma) in situ, in whom the biopsy itself may be curative and further staging studies therefore unnecessary. In other cases, a woman who has had a breast biopsy will undergo a lumpectomy or mastectomy to remove the entire tumor. At the same time, some of the lymph nodes in the armpit on the same side as the cancer will be removed to determine whether the cancer has spread into these nodes.

The stage of the cancer is determined in three parts: the size of the tumor; whether lymph nodes are involved with cancer (and if so which ones), and whether the cancer has spread to another part of the body.

The last important part of the workup before treatment is to determine whether the tumor cells have certain characteristics. To do this, a pathologist will look for the presence or absence of hormone receptors, including estrogen and progesterone receptors, and whether the cancer contains the HER-2/neu gene. Hormone receptors indicate that, just as the cancer's growth can be accelerated by estrogen and progesterone, so too can its growth be suppressed by antihormonal agents, such as leuprolide (Lupron) or tamoxifen. The presence of the HER-2/neu gene indicates that the cancer may shrink better in response to certain types of chemotherapy.

The treatment of breast cancer is a complicated topic that is best subdivided by the stage of the disease. There are three types of medical therapy that can be used for early-stage breast cancer: radiation therapy, chemotherapy, and hormonal therapy. In some cases all are used, and in others only one or two are employed.

For most people, the first step of therapy is a surgical procedure called a *modified radical mastectomy* (MRM) or another procedure called a *lumpectomy*. An MRM involves removal of the entire breast tissue, while a lumpectomy, as the name implies, removes only the section of the breast that is involved with tumor. Women who receive a lumpectomy alone without radiation therapy have an unacceptably high risk of the cancer's return, so the standard choices include either an MRM or a lumpectomy *and* radiation therapy. Several large trials have shown that the outcome from these two options is the same.

The primary surgical procedure also allows assessment of the lymph nodes, to determine whether the cancer has spread from the breast. Lymph nodes are small collections of cells located throughout the body. Fluid from body tissues or from areas of skin surrounding the node are brought to the node through lymph ducts. Slightly larger ducts connect the nodes to each other. While the main purpose of lymph nodes is to detect infections, this system of ducts and nodes can also function as a pathway through which cancer can spread. The lymph nodes that sample fluid from the breast are in the armpit. Even with small cancers, it is possible that some of the cancer cells have already spread to these nodes in the armpits. In order to detect this cancer in the lymph nodes, either the entire group of lymph nodes must be removed and examined under a microscope by a pathologist or the primary (also called the *sentinel*) lymph node, thought to be closest to the breast, must be removed. It has been shown that if there is no cancer in the sentinel lymph node, it is much less likely that the tumor had spread to other lymph nodes or elsewhere in the body.

Once the main cancer has been surgically treated by either MRM or lumpectomy/radiation therapy and the lymph nodes have been examined, it is possible to determine whether giving a woman hormonal therapy or chemotherapy would be helpful.

Whether hormonal therapy is appropriate therapy is determined by three factors: (1) Are you post-menopausal? (2) Does the tumor specimen have the hormone receptors ER (estrogen receptor) and PR (progesterone receptor)? (3) Are you at high risk for a return of your tumor (for example, do your lymph nodes have tumor in them)? The general recommendations are that almost all women who have tumors with the ER and/or PR hormone receptors should receive hormonal therapy for 5 years. Hormonal therapy can consist of either tamoxifen or other drugs called aromatase inhibitors, but the exact therapy choices are beyond the scope of this chapter. It is unclear whether there are any women whose tumors do not have the hormone receptors but who should nevertheless receive hormonal therapy.

The use of chemotherapy in women with early breast cancer is also complicated. In general, women with cancer in their lymph nodes should receive chemotherapy after surgery and radiation, although the exact type of chemotherapy used is again beyond the scope of this chapter. There are some subgroups of patients without tumor in their lymph nodes who should also be offered chemotherapy, although these subgroups are not as clearly defined. Similarly, there are subgroups of women with cancer in their lymph nodes for whom chemotherapy may not be appropriate.

In addition to traditional chemotherapy, an antibody called trastuzumab (or Herceptin) is sometimes used. Trastuzumab targets a protein called Her2/neu (or, *c-erb2*), found in about 30 percent of breast cancers. In women whose cancers express this protein, the antibody offers an additional choice in therapy.

In women who have breast cancer that has spread beyond the breast, the treatment choices are complicated. Many times, older treatment regimens of drug combinations such as CMF and AC are being replaced by newer drugs of the same types as well as by drugs from the taxane family (see Chap. 14 for more information about these drugs). The exact treatment schedule, dose, and order in which these drugs should be used are still unclear.

CHAPTER 4

Delivering the News

ANNA C. MURIEL, M.D., M.P.H.
PAULA K. RAUCH, M.D.

OUTLINE

WHY SHOULD I TELL OTHERS ABOUT THE DIAGNOSIS?

The initial shock of a cancer diagnosis can be overwhelming. Being diagnosed and treated for cancer will change your life inside and out. Those around you will be affected on an emotional and a practical level. You will need support to cope, as well as help with the day-to-day activities of your life and your health care. Your closest family and friends will need each other to create a network that will help everyone get through what may be a long period of treatment for you. People with cancer sometimes face social isolation; this can be a significant source of distress and may have an impact on your recovery and quality of life. Letting others know about your diagnosis will give you a chance to address your feelings and relationships as well as to help others to provide the assistance you will need.

Your personality and coping style will dictate with whom you talk, how much you reveal, and when you tell people about your diagnosis. The reactions of others to the news of your illness may be supportive and reassuring. Having those around you know what you are struggling with will help them understand any changes in your emotions and behavior. Sharing information about your condition may make it unnecessary for you to put up a front when you are having a bad day. Also, you may be able to ask for help more readily with specific practical issues.

On the other hand, others' reactions may be confusing, disappointing, or overwhelming to you. Their responses to your news may have to do with their own personalities, their relationship with you, or their own experiences. Nevertheless, open communication about your illness will help provide you with the emotional and practical resources you will need to cope with your diagnosis and treatment. Letting others in on your situation also conveys a measure of respect; they will likely see this as an indication of trust in them and in their capacity for being available and helpful (Table 4-1).

WHOM SHOULD I TELL?

Whom you tell about your cancer will depend on many factors, including your general style of coping and your usual needs for privacy or for sharing your experience with others. Your spouse or other close family members may be involved immediately at the time of your diagnosis, but in all likelihood you will need additional support and help. Anyone involved in your daily life will notice changes

TABLE 4-1 **Factors That Affect Your Decision to Tell Others about a Cancer Diagnosis**

Your general style of coping
Your need for privacy
The coping abilities of others you might wish to tell
Your relationships with others (e.g., coworkers, employers, friends, family members)

in your emotional or physical state as well as in the time and transportation demands of diagnostic procedures and treatments. People closely involved in your life probably will overhear a conversation or wonder about changes in your behavior or schedule. It may be worse for them to find out about your cancer inadvertently than for you to decide when, how, and what they will know. Sometimes people hesitate to discuss their diagnosis with their children, but even young children must be included and supported through the experience of your illness. Chap. 10 covers this in more detail.

Friends and extended family may be needed to provide both emotional support and practical help. Social isolation can be a significant problem for individuals with cancer, and your ability to cope with and to fight your illness likely will be enhanced by having a strong support network. While it may be awkward for you to talk about your cancer with your friends, they will want to help; moreover, they can do so only if you tell them about your needs and share information about your illness. Their responses will vary, and they may need your help to guide them toward what you need from them. Not knowing how to help may keep friends and family distant, while specific requests may give you the assistance you need and may help others to feel involved in a useful way.

How much you discuss your illness with your employer or coworkers will depend on your relationships with them as well as on the nature of your work or school demands. Your illness and treatment may change your ability to function, or you may need short or long absences from work. Having employers or coworkers know what is happening will help them understand your limitations and prevent misunderstandings if you are not able to do your job in the same way as you have in the past. You may also want to have a close colleague help you with the flow of information as your treatment progresses, so that you are not burdened with having to respond to multiple inquiries about your health status. Sometimes people are reluctant to tell employers about their illness for fear of discrimination or of losing their job. There are laws in each state to protect the rights of cancer patients. If the need arises, your health care or social service providers should be able to direct you to legal resources in your area.

If you are a member of a religious community, clergy members or members of the congregation may be important sources of support, guidance, and practical help. This also may be a way to find others who have struggled with cancer and to help you feel less alone with your experience.

There may be other people with whom you feel compelled to talk about your illness but with whom you face specific challenges. These may include estranged loved ones or individuals with whom you have had a conflicted relationship. Sometimes people find illness to be a time for reconciliation, and they make efforts to resolve old hurts or conflicts. On the other hand, stirring up these issues, especially in the early emotional stages of diagnosis and treatment, may distract or drain you in the face of everything else with which you are grappling. Close family or friends can help you get some perspective on these issues and help you decide how and when to talk with these other individuals. Struggling with a potentially life-threatening illness can be a time to repair relationships, but it takes some thought to decide how this is to be done.

WHEN SHOULD I TELL OTHERS ABOUT THE CANCER?

Some people have impulses to tell those around them about the diagnosis immediately, while others will have trouble bringing themselves to discuss their condition with family, friends, and coworkers. The timing of your discussions with people may be determined by your initial reactions to the diagnosis, by your relationships with them, and by the nature of your illness and treatment course as well as by the kinds of practical help you need (Table 4-2).

The time between your diagnosis and either surgery or the beginning of treatment is known to be the most emotionally stressful. There may be waves of timed discussions, initially only with your closest family and friends, then with more distant coworkers or friends. You will need to gauge your and their comfort level with your illness as well as the impact that your illness and treatment may have on your interactions with them. Also, you may want to consider what it would be like if they found out by accident or from a source that you do not trust. You may want to inform some people about your cancer in stages because it could be overwhelming for you or them all at once. They may not be able to take in the details of your treatment or prognosis and when they are dealing with the shock or emotions of the diagnosis itself, you may have trouble deciding how you would like them to help. There might be other people in your circle of family, friends, and acquaintances who will be affected but with whom you may not feel like sharing the details of your cancer. You may want to tell them only that you are struggling with some health issues right now but aren't quite ready to discuss them.

HOW CAN I TELL OTHERS ABOUT THE DIAGNOSIS AND THE PROGNOSIS?

When you do decide to let others know, you will want to be thoughtful and honest as well as prepared for a range of reactions. The amount of information you share with others will depend on your relationships with them and on your hopes

TABLE 4-2 **Factors That Influence the Timing of Your Decision to Tell Others about Your Diagnosis**

Your initial reaction to the diagnosis and the treatment
The types of practical help you need
Your comfort level with your diagnosis
The anticipated effect your news will have on your relationships with others
The impact of your news being learned about by others by accident

for how they might be supportive. Talking with your children about your diagnosis raises specific issues that are addressed in Chap. 10.

There is no easy way to tell people that you have cancer. Choose a quiet place and time that will allow you to say what you need to say and to answer the questions you may be asked to the best of your ability. Tell them the name of the cancer you have and as much about the prognosis or plan for treatment as you feel is appropriate. They may have questions that you cannot answer or that you may find overwhelming to discuss. Sometimes others' past experiences with cancer will affect their reactions. You may want to have a spouse or other family member present—someone who can offer support or take over for you if it becomes too difficult. You also may decide to have a discussion about prognosis, treatment plans, or ways that others can help you and your family in subsequent meetings (Table 4-3).

WHAT SHOULD I TELL OTHERS?

The amount of information that you share with others will vary depending on your relationships with them, their capacity to process and understand what you tell them, and their level of involvement in your life and illness. Those closest to you need to know the name of your illness. Euphemisms or generalities may seem to spare people pain, but the reality of your illness will not be tempered by not saying the word *cancer*. Initially, you may need to use whatever terminology is comfortable for you, but most people find that *cancer* will become another word in their vocabulary. The specific name for your cancer may sound unfamiliar or scary, but using it will at least get everyone "on the same page." The general term *cancer* can raise associations to experiences that people have had or have heard about and to other people's cancers; these associations can keep them from responding specifically to you and to your illness and prognosis.

The question of death often is on people's minds. They may not know how to ask and you may not know how to address this with them. Sometimes this issue goes unspoken because it is too painful to discuss or because you just don't know what to expect. Your loved ones (children especially) may at first need to hear something as simple as a recognition that while people sometimes die from cancer, you and your treatment team are doing their best to fight it, and that you expect to try and live each day as fully as possible (Table 4-4).

TABLE 4-3 **How Should You Tell Others about a Cancer Diagnosis?**

Choose a quiet place and time
Decide what you need to say
Be thoughtful and honest
Answer the questions others may have to the best of your ability
Consider whether you want to have a family member or friend available for support

TABLE 4-4 **What Should You Tell Others about Your Cancer Diagnosis?**

The amount of information that you share depends on your relationship with others, with their capacity to process and to understand what you tell them, and on the level of involvement they have with your life and your illness.

Those closest to you should know the name of your illness; euphemisms and generalities rarely temper the pain of cancer.

Let others know that you and your treatment team are doing the best to fight the illness, and that you expect to try and live each day as fully as possible.

The information about your specific diagnosis and treatment will unfold over time and will change according to your course and response to treatment. You will need to decide to what extent you want to keep others informed of your progress. Some of this will depend on how much you rely on them for day-to-day help with household duties, child care, work responsibilities, transportation, or emotional support. Some people allow a spokesperson to disseminate information, while others prefer to do so themselves, either in person, by phone, or via e-mail.

HOW CAN I PREPARE MYSELF TO HEAR GOOD OR BAD NEWS FROM MY DOCTOR?

Medical information about your diagnosis, treatment, and prognosis will come in stages and will depend on the results of tests and diagnostic procedures as well as on the natural course of your cancer. Your doctors and health care providers should be updating you regularly throughout this process; unfortunately, they may not always be able to give you clear-cut answers, and this uncertainty is difficult to bear. When good or bad news is presented to you, however, having supportive, open communication with family and friends frequently helps buffer its impact.

Anticipating a meeting with your doctor regarding the effectiveness of treatment or the result of a diagnostic test might include preparing a list of questions or contingencies about treatment choices. Having a list in advance of a meeting can help you manage the emotional responses to good or bad news. You also may want to have a trusted family member or friend come with you to remind you about your concerns regarding symptom control or pain management. Advance preparation can ensure that these concerns are brought to the attention of your health care team even when other events become distractions.

Taking in information about your illness can call up a range of emotional responses, including joy, relief, gratitude, fear, anger, sadness, and despair. Allowing yourself to experience these emotions without censure from yourself or from your loved ones is a part of coming to terms with your illness and of making sense of your experience. Finding ways to express these feelings safely may help you to cope more effectively with the next phase of your illness. Sometimes, coping will come in the form of concrete actions, while at other times it will come in the form of increased reflection and acceptance.

HOW SHOULD I EXPECT MY DOCTOR TO DELIVER GOOD OR BAD NEWS TO ME?

Part of your doctor's job is to communicate effectively with you about your illness, treatment, and prognosis. Regardless of the news being delivered, you should expect to have a respectful, succinct, honest discussion that provides you with information in a manner you can understand and allows you to ask questions and to clarify choices. Whenever possible, you should expect your doctor to sit down with you in a private setting for these discussions. You may need to express preferences about whether you would like to receive information on the phone or through other family members. Historically, doctors have informed family members about diagnosis or prognosis without discussing the facts with the patient. These days, this practice is largely discouraged, and you should expect to hear directly from your doctor about these matters. In addition, your family members should not expect to receive information before you are informed.

Because news about your health may be overwhelming and may have an emotional impact that can prevent the absorption of important information or effective decision making, your doctor may present information to you in a series of meetings rather than in a single visit. Based on your own style of managing emotions and information, you may want to let your doctor know how you are best able to handle this. While there are practical limits to how physicians can respond, you might want to request additional meetings to discuss or review treatment options after you and your family have had a chance to process the news you have received. There may also be medical issues that will affect the speed with which decisions or medical interventions must be made.

As you receive bad news, you may have specific concerns about treatment choices, pain control, personal dignity, survival time, finances, or issues related to communication of the news to others. Hopefully, your doctor will be able to listen to these concerns and provide you with guidance and reassurance based on his or her experience with other patients and families. Although it may be difficult for your physician to deliver news about the progression of disease and the limitations of treatment, you should at the very least expect to be informed with honesty and not given false hope. At best, your physician should be able to support your own hope and drive to fight the illness as well as to help you and your family prepare for the possibility of death in practical and experiential terms. While the practice of medicine strives for clarity and scientific surety, uncertainty and emotion are part of the reality. As with your family and friends, honest, compassionate communication with your doctor can go a long way toward alleviating any suffering you may experience in having a life-threatening illness.

CHAPTER 5

Early Detection of Cancer: The Implications of Screening Tests

TIMOTHY GILLIGAN, M.D.

OUTLINE

WHAT IS CANCER SCREENING?

Cancer screening refers to the testing procedures performed for people who have no symptoms of cancer and have not already been diagnosed with the cancer for which they are being tested. In other words, medical evaluations are performed on people who appear to be healthy to determine whether they have an unsuspected cancer. With screening, doctors attempt to diagnose cancer at the earliest possible stage, before it causes symptoms and, one hopes, before cancer cells have started to break away from the original tumor and travel throughout the body (i.e., before the cancer metastasizes). The goal of screening is to diagnose cancer while it is still curable and thus prevent the cancer from causing suffering and death. The tools used to screen for cancer range from a basic physical examination to blood tests and even imaging studies such as x-rays, computed tomography (CT) scans, and ultrasounds.

At its best, cancer screening saves lives by detecting cancers while they are still curable. By identifying early-stage cancers, screening also makes possible less drastic treatments that have fewer complications and milder side effects. Screening tests for breast, colon, and cervical cancer are widely recommended to the general population because there is persuasive evidence that they prolong lives.

Unfortunately, there are no good screening tests for most cancers. The development of effective and affordable screening tests for all cancers represents one of the most important goals of cancer research. But this is easier said than done. The rationale for cancer screening is quite straightforward, and medical imaging technologies [such as CT and magnetic resonance imaging (MRI) scans] have advanced tremendously over the past two decades; it may seem odd, then, that it has been difficult to develop effective screening tests and that some tests of this kind are highly controversial. The goal of this chapter is to explain the complexities of cancer screening so that you can make a more informed decision about whether to undergo such testing.

WHAT IS THE GOAL OF CANCER SCREENING?

In thinking about cancer screening tests, it is essential to remember their ultimate goal is to reduce suffering and extend lives. In general, cancers cause symptoms only when they have grown quite large or have spread to other organs. Therefore, if we wait until people have symptoms before we start testing them for cancer, most of the cancers we find will be too far advanced to be cured. By testing people for cancer when they have no symptoms, doctors hope to detect cancers while they are still small and contained within the original organ. The purpose of screening is thus to detect cancers that can be cured either with surgery or, less often, radiation and/or chemotherapy. If this strategy is effective and people with early-stage cancer are cured without suffering too many complications from diagnostic tests and treatment, screening can enable people to live longer and suffer less from their cancer.

If people don't live longer or suffer less, however, the screening test has not accomplished its goal. In other words, it is not enough to demonstrate that a screening test detects cancers before a person becomes symptomatic or to demonstrate that people who are screened are diagnosed with smaller tumors than people who are not screened. It isn't even enough to demonstrate that people who are screened are less likely to have cancers that have spread throughout the body.

A person diagnosed with a smaller, localized cancer benefits from that early discovery only if it translates into a longer life or at least less suffering from the disease. What would be the point of undergoing a cancer screening test that might lead to additional medical procedures, including surgery, if there were no clear evidence that people screened with that test enjoyed either longer lives or a higher quality of life? If undergoing a screening test doesn't result in people living longer and/or suffering less, then there is probably no justification for the inconvenience, anxiety, discomfort, and cost associated with the test. A screening test must offer a benefit that has value to the person undergoing the test. Unfortunately, studies that evaluate whether screening tests save lives require thousands of patients and many years to complete. Thus, for some screening tests, the question of whether those tests save lives has not yet been answered.

WHAT MAKES A TEST A GOOD CANCER SCREENING TEST?

While keeping in mind the main goals of screening discussed in the preceding paragraphs, it may be helpful to examine the essential elements of a good screening test from a different perspective. A good cancer screening test must meet the requirements shown in Table 5-1.

Safety

Remember that a cancer screening test is used on a large population of healthy people and that in almost all cases only a small percentage of those people will be found to have cancer. In other words, a screening test assesses many people but benefits only a small proportion of them. The test thus must be safe; otherwise it could easily harm more people than it benefits.

TABLE 5-1 **Characteristics of a Good Cancer Screening Test**

It must be safe
It must be accurate
It must be able to detect cancers at an early stage
It must be affordable and widely available
It must test for diseases for which there is effective treatment at early stages

Accuracy

A screening test can be inaccurate in two ways: it can appear to find a cancer when in fact none exists, or it can fail to find a cancer that does exist. The first scenario is referred to as a *false-positive* result (in medicine, a result is said to be "positive" when an abnormality is discovered); the second scenario is referred to as a *false-negative* result (a result is said to be "negative" when no abnormality is discovered). If a test produces an abundance of false-positive results, many people who do not have cancer will be told that maybe they do. They will then have to undergo additional diagnostic tests, such as radiology tests or even surgical biopsies, in order to find out whether the screening test may have been wrong. On the other hand, if a test produces a lot of false-negative results, the screening process will fail to diagnose many people who do in fact have cancer, and the cancers will have more time to grow, possibly to an incurable stage, before being diagnosed.

There are many ways of measuring the accuracy of a medical test; these are described below. While you don't need to memorize these terms, it is important to recognize that they all represent attempts to characterize, in different ways, the likelihood that a test's result is correct. All medical tests have some potential to yield incorrect results, and it is important to be aware of this limitation of medical science. If you undergo a screening test, you may wish to ask your physician what the likelihood is that the test results will be incorrect (Table 5-2).

The term *accuracy* refers to the proportion of a test's results that correctly identify the tested individual as either having or not having the relevant cancer.

The term *sensitivity* refers to the proportion of people who actually have cancer in whom a given test would have correctly identified them as having the cancer. In other words, if 100 people with cancer are tested for that cancer and the test indicates that only 80 of them have the cancer (and, incorrectly, that 20 do not), then the sensitivity of the test would be 80 percent.

Specificity refers to the proportion of people who do not have the cancer who are correctly identified by a given test as not having the cancer. If 100 people known

TABLE 5-2 **Test Characteristics (Expressed in Percentages)**

Accuracy	The proportion of a test's results that correctly identify the tested individual as either having or not having the relevant cancer
Sensitivity	The proportion of people who actually have cancer in whom a given test would have correctly identified them as having the cancer
Specificity	The proportion of people who do not have the cancer who are correctly identified by a given test as not having the cancer
Positive predictive value	The probability that a positive test result correctly identifies the presence of cancer in the person tested
Negative predictive value	The probability that a negative test result correctly identifies the absence of cancer in the person tested

to be cancer-free are tested for cancer and the test indicates that 80 of those people do not have cancer but, incorrectly, that 20 do, the test's specificity would be 80 percent.

A *positive predictive value* refers to the probability that a positive test result correctly identifies the presence of cancer in the person tested (i.e., the probability that a positive test result means that the tested person does in fact have the cancer).

A *negative predictive value* refers to the probability that a negative test result correctly identifies the absence of cancer in the person tested (i.e., the probability that a negative test result means that the tested person does not in fact have the cancer).

Detecting the Cancer at an Early Stage

Cancer screening tests must detect cancers at an early stage (when the cancers are smaller, are confined to one organ, and have not spread to lymph nodes or to other areas of the body); otherwise, the tests are unlikely to have a meaningful impact on the disease. If a screening test for lung cancer could detect the presence only of those lung cancers that were at an advanced stage and thus incurable, the test would not accomplish its goal of saving lives by detecting curable cancers. Chest x-rays, for instance, are not recommended for screening for lung cancer because it appears that they do not detect enough cancers early enough to have a measurable benefit. Because CT scans detect smaller tumors than regular chest x-rays (and thus discover lung cancer at an earlier stage), it is hoped that CT scans will be a more effective screening test for lung cancer. Mammography is a good test in part because it detects breast cancers when they are small and at an early, curable stage.

Currently, the vast majority of cancers are curable only if they are detected while they are still contained within the organ in which they first developed or within the lymph nodes to which that organ drains (referred to as *regional nodes*).* If the cancer has spread more distantly or if it has grown too much to be completely removed by surgery, there is usually little chance of cure (although there are some important exceptions to this generalization). In many cases, even if the cancer has spread only to regional nodes, the chance of cure falls substantially.

Thus, if a lung cancer is detected when it is small and before it has spread to any lymph nodes, surgery will probably cure the disease. On the other hand, if the tumor has spread to lymph nodes or if it is big or has grown through the edges of the lung itself and invaded other organs or structures, achieving a cure becomes

---

*Lymph nodes are tiny organs scattered throughout the body that participate in the immune system. When blood flows into organs and tissues, water and some chemicals leak out of the blood vessels. The excess fluid that does not return immediately to the bloodstream is called *lymph* and flows through channels called *lymph vessels*. These lymph vessels carry the lymph to the lymph nodes, where the lymph circulates through cells of the immune system, which are on the lookout for bacteria, viruses, and other infectious agents. The lymph then travels through a chain of lymph nodes before ultimately being channeled back into the bloodstream. When cancer cells leave the original tumor and spread throughout the body, they usually travel either through the lymph vessels or through the bloodstream.

more difficult. A cancer that has spread to more distant sites or has grown to the extent that it cannot be removed surgically is considered incurable (again, there may be rare exceptions to this generalization). The same is true of breast cancer, colon cancer, stomach cancer, and almost all other solid tumors. Cancers of the blood cells (liquid tumors–leukemia, lymphoma, and multiple myeloma) are more complicated, as blood cells normally circulate through the body and thus are almost always widely spread throughout the bone marrow and the bloodstream at the time of diagnosis. Nonetheless, even for blood cancers, it appears that achieving a cure is more likely if the disease is detected at an early stage in its development.

This is the rationale for screening. If most cancers are curable only if they are diagnosed when they are small and localized, then a test that can detect cancers earlier than they otherwise would be detected ought to result in more cancers being cured. That is to say, if we aren't curing more cancers because we're diagnosing them too late, then diagnosing them earlier ought to solve at least part of the problem.

In order for a screening test to accomplish the goal of extending life and/or reducing suffering, however, it must detect cancers early enough to either cure the individual or at least to slow the progression of the cancer by allowing earlier treatment. Mammography, for instance, is widely accepted because it has been shown to extend women's lives by detecting cancers at a curable stage. The age at which to start screening and the regularity of screening are controversial. Most agree, mammograms save lives. On the other hand, screening for lung cancer by taking chest x-rays of smokers has not resulted in longer lives for those undergoing screening; thus, screening for lung cancer is not recommended. It is not clear that periodic x-rays detect lung cancer at an early enough stage to change the course of the disease.

Cost and Availability

Screening tests must be affordable and widely available, as they are designed to be used in large populations. Whether screening is focused on the general population or only on individuals at high risk for developing a cancer, almost all screening tests are used in large numbers of people, most of whom will not have cancer. Even a relatively inexpensive test, such as a chest x-ray, becomes extremely expensive to society if it is used on large numbers of people on a regular basis.

For example, if a chest x-ray costs $50 and is used to screen everyone in the United States over the age of 50 years (approximately 75 million people), the total expense per year would be $3.75 billion! On the other hand, an expensive test that is used only infrequently on a few high-risk individuals will not be especially costly to the nation. A CT scan of the chest, which costs approximately $400, could be used to screen for lung cancer in heavy smokers in the United States, let's say 1 million people, for a total cost of $400 million, or less than one-ninth the cost of chest x-ray screening in a less select population.

Evaluating the cost of a test takes into account the number of people who will be tested, how frequently they will be tested, how many people will be diagnosed with the cancer, whether any cost savings result from diagnosing people earlier, and how much additional cost will be generated as a result of further evaluating people who have abnormalities (real or false) detected by the screening test. Realistically, as a society, we have a limited number of health care dollars to spend, and we should spend them wisely. Tests must be made widely available in order to be useful to the society as a whole. A great screening test that is only available in Baton Rouge, Louisiana, will be unlikely to have a significant impact on the nation's health.

Screening Tests Must Detect Diseases That Are Treatable

An old saying in medicine warns that it is difficult to make a person who has no symptoms feel better. In other words, if there is no clear problem that a medical intervention can solve, any intervention runs the risk of doing more harm than good. If all we accomplish with a screening test is to diagnose more people with incurable cancers, we only increase these people's mental anguish. If a screening test is affordable, widely available, and highly accurate but detects only incurable diseases for which there is no effective treatment, the test has little value.

This is one way in which screening tests differ from other medical tests. If someone feels or appears sick, most physicians and patients would agree that it is perfectly appropriate to perform diagnostic medical tests to determine what's wrong, even if the tests are likely to reveal an incurable disease. If a disease is causing a person to feel sick or is causing an obvious deterioration in his or her health, then we know that the disease is harmful. One hopes that by making an accurate diagnosis, treatments that will lessen the symptoms from which the person is suffering can be instituted, even if a cure is not possible. On the other hand, in performing screening tests on people who look and feel well, there is no ongoing suffering to reduce, so a screening test is unlikely to be of benefit unless it detects diseases for which there is an effective treatment. Thus, we screen for skin cancer because there are effective, curative treatments for it. We would not screen for asymptomatic, inoperable brain tumors, however.

WHAT CANCERS HAVE GOOD SCREENING TESTS?

Several cancer screening tests are widely accepted as being useful and effective. These include tests for breast cancer, colorectal cancer, and cervical cancer. Other cancer screening tests, such as those for prostate cancer and lung cancer, are highly controversial. Many sources recommend skin cancer screening for people at high risk of this disease, but the effectiveness of screening has never been established clearly; thus it is not recommended for the entire population. A number of other

TABLE 5-3 Which Cancers Have Good Screening Tests?

Type of Cancer	Screening Test
Breast cancer	Mammography Physician- or self-examination of the breasts
Colorectal cancer	Testing bowel movements for blood Sigmoidoscopy Colonoscopy
Cervical cancer	Pap (Papanicolaou) smears
Skin cancer	Visual inspection of the skin

cancers are too rarely fatal for health policy professionals and doctors to feel that the high cost of screening the whole population would be justified (Table 5-3).

Screening tests for breast cancer include mammography (x-rays of the breasts), examination of the breasts by a health care provider, and self-examination of the breasts. Screening for breast cancer with mammography is widely accepted because research has shown that women who undergo mammography live longer than women who do not (Fig. 5-1).

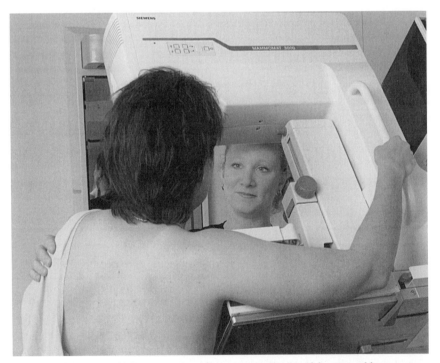

FIGURE 5-1 Screening for breast cancer with mammography is widely accepted because research has shown that women who undergo mammography live longer than those who do not.

Screening tests for colorectal cancer include (1) digital rectal examination (in which a health care provider inserts a gloved finger into the rectum); (2) testing bowel movements for blood (also called stool guaiac or Hemoccult testing); (3) sigmoidoscopy; and (4) colonoscopy. Sigmoidoscopy and colonoscopy involve inspecting the rectum and colon visually by inserting a device through the rectum into the colon (the colon is the large intestine, also referred to as the large bowel). Screening for colorectal cancer has been shown to reduce deaths from this disease and to extend lives.

Similarly, screening for cervical cancer by performing Pap (short for Papanicolaou) smears on women (in which the cervix is scraped and a sample of the tissue is examined under a microscope for evidence of precancerous or cancerous cells) has resulted in a sharp decline in the number of deaths from cervical cancer. Skin cancer screening simply involves a visual inspection of the skin, looking for any area suspicious for skin cancer. This type of cancer screening is recommended despite the lack of strong evidence of its effectiveness because a skin exam poses little risk to you and cancers detected at an early stage can be cured easily.

WHAT ARE PREMALIGNANT CONDITIONS?

Screening for breast cancer, colon cancer, and cervical cancer detects cancers at early stages before they have spread and can even diagnose abnormal tissue growths before they have had time to transform themselves into cancers. Such abnormal growths are called *premalignant conditions* because they are thought to represent cells that have a high likelihood of becoming cancerous over time.

Diagnosing a premalignant condition before it has become an actual cancer is advantageous because the treatment of premalignancies is usually less aggressive than the treatment of full-blown cancer. A colonoscopy, for example, may detect a polyp that appears to be precancerous. Such polyps can generally be removed during the colonoscopy itself without the need for surgery, whereas a true cancer requires the surgical removal of a section of the colon or rectum. Similarly, Pap smears often detect premalignant conditions that can be treated by removing a superficial section of the cervix, whereas treatment of cervical cancer generally requires the removal of the entire uterus.

HOW IS THE IMPACT OF SCREENING TESTS ASSESSED?

Assessing the impact of screening tests on how long people live is more complicated than one might suspect. The only way to clearly measure this impact is to take a large group of people and divide them into two halves. One half of the group should be given the screening test and the other half should not be screened but should continue to receive usual medical care. After a number of years have passed, the two halves would be compared to see whether the people who were screened lived longer than the people who were not screened. One could look for other differences as well, such as which group spent more time in the hospital, which group had higher health-care costs, and which group experienced more pain and suffering. This is called a *randomized control trial*. Such a study is expensive and takes many years to complete, but it is difficult if not impossible to accurately measure the impact of a screening test without conducting such a study.

An easier way to study the impact of a screening test might be to compare patients whose cancers are diagnosed as a result of screening to patients whose cancers are diagnosed without the help of screening tests. However, this is not a fair comparison. There may be important differences between people who get screened and people who do not get screened; these differences, rather than the screening itself, may result in differences in survival.

For instance, people who live healthy lifestyles may be more likely to go to the doctor regularly and to undergo screening tests. People who live unhealthy lifestyles may be less likely to go to the doctor unless they're feeling sick. These differences in lifestyle may result in the healthy-lifestyle people living longer even if they develop cancer. If you compare healthy-lifestyle people who get screened to unhealthy-lifestyle people who do not get screened, there is no way to know whether any differences in how long they live are due to the lifestyle differences or to the screening test. Therefore, in measuring the effectiveness of screening, it is essential that the people being screened are similar to the people who are not screened. The only way to ensure this similarity is to have the study determine whether or not people get screened.

WHAT ARE LEAD-TIME BIAS AND LENGTH-TIME BIAS?

The second problem with comparing cancers diagnosed as a result of screening to cancers diagnosed without screening involves lead-time bias and length-time bias.

The following example explains lead-time bias. Imagine that two women of the same age both develop lung cancer at the same time. Let's say that their cancers become big enough to be detected on an x-ray at the time of their fiftieth birthdays and that both women die of the cancer at age 54. Now suppose that one woman undergoes screening and the other woman does not. The screened woman goes to her doctor when she is 50 years old, has a screening x-ray, and the cancer is discovered. She goes through treatments but the cancer can't be cured and she dies at age 54, as stated above. She survived for 4 years after she was screened and was given her diagnosis. The second woman doesn't go through screening but develops a cough that won't go away when she is 53. She goes to see her doctor about her cough and he orders an x-ray to see if she has some disease in her lungs. The cancer is discovered but cannot be cured and she dies at age 54. She survived only 1 year after her x-ray and diagnosis.

If we judged the effectiveness of screening by comparing the survival of these two women, we would conclude that screening resulted in 3 extra years of life because the screened woman survived for 4 years and the other woman survived for only 1 year. And yet they lived exactly the same overall length of time. In this example, the only clear effect of the screening was that the screened woman spent more years of her life knowing that she had cancer. The woman who wasn't screened may actually have been better off, as she enjoyed more years of her life without the burden of knowing she had lung cancer. Those extra years of survival that don't represent more years of life but instead represent more years of knowing that one has cancer are referred to as lead-time. Lead-time can also be thought of as the time period between the point at which a cancer becomes detectable by screening and the point at which it becomes symptomatic.

This scenario would be very different if the screening chest x-ray that the first woman obtained had resulted in the detection of the cancer at a stage when it was curable. She then might have undergone a surgical removal of the cancer and perhaps have lived to age 70. In that scenario, the screening would have resulted in a true benefit: an extra 16 years of life (from age 54 to age 70). Studies that focus on how long people survive after they are diagnosed with cancer thus are not very helpful in evaluating screening tests as they may be prone to lead-time bias.

Length-time bias refers to the possibility that the kinds of cancer that are detected by screening are different from the kinds of cancers that are detected after a person develops cancer-related symptoms. Let's say that there are two different kinds of cancer: cancers that grow extremely slowly and only rarely cause any significant health problems and cancers that grow quickly and spread throughout the body, killing a person within 2 years. The slow-growing cancers would usually not come to a doctor's attention unless screening tests were conducted or the cancer happened to be detected by a medical test evaluating an entirely unrelated problem. On the other hand, fast-growing cancers make people sick. These people would go to their doctor to find out what was the matter, and the cancers would be discovered when diagnostic tests were ordered.

If you conducted a screening program in one town but not in another, you would expect to find the following differences: in the screened town, you would diagnose a mixture of slow- and fast-growing cancers. Even if all the people with fast-growing cancers died of their disease, the people with slow-growing cancers would be expected to live many years. In addition, the people with fast-growing cancers would be likely to develop symptoms before they were screened and thus might be diagnosed as a result of *diagnostic* tests ordered to evaluate symptoms rather than as a result of the *screening* tests. In the screened town, the survival of cancer patients would be about the average of the groups. In the town without screening, the slow-growing cancers would remain largely undetected and the majority of the cancers diagnosed would be the fast-growing kind. The survival of cancer patients in this town would be close to the survival of the those with fast-growing cancers.

Survival thus would be longer in the screened town, and it would appear that the screening resulted in longer survival, even if it in fact had no impact on how long people lived. In this scenario, the cancers detected by screening are fundamentally different than the cancers detected as a result of symptoms. This kind of error is referred to as length-time bias, or the tendency of screening tests to detect slow-growing cancers. Again, the way to avoid this bias is to evaluate how many people are dying of cancer and at what ages and to ignore how long people survive after their diagnosis.

HOW DO YOU BALANCE THE BENEFITS AND HARMS OF SCREENING TESTS?

Even if a screening test can detect cancers at an early enough stage to result in more people being cured, it still isn't necessarily a good test. To understand why not, you have to recognize that screening tests have the potential not only to benefit individuals but also to harm them. Think about what happens to you after a screening test is performed. If the result is normal, you receive the benefit of peace of mind and no additional tests are needed until the next routine screening test is due. If the screening test is abnormal, more tests and procedures may be recommended. However, an abnormal screening test result does not mean that you have cancer. It is possible that the test is simply wrong: the test may appear to reveal an abnormality that isn't really there (a false-positive test result, as described above).

Second, the test may reveal a real abnormality but one that isn't cancer. For instance, mammograms frequently identify breast abnormalities that turn out to be benign (noncancerous) when a biopsy (a surgical removal of tissue) is performed. Third, the test may reveal a cancer that is extremely slow-growing and that is never destined to cause a person any harm (length-time bias, as described in the previous section). Finally, the abnormality detected by the screening test may actually be a dangerous cancer that needs treatment. In this fourth scenario, the cancer may have been detected at a curable stage or at an incurable stage.

Now imagine that you fall into one of the first two categories above: that is, you go to have a screening test performed and it reveals an abnormality that appears to be cancer but isn't. Because of this abnormality, your doctor recommends a surgical biopsy. The biopsy is performed and it reveals no cancer. When you get the final result, you will most likely be relieved. But the process of learning that the test result was abnormal and then waiting for the biopsy, undergoing the biopsy, and waiting for the result often generates a significant degree of anxiety and distress. In such a scenario, the screening test may seem to do more harm than good by subjecting a person to unnecessary procedures and generating unnecessary distress.

Moreover, if the abnormality detected on the screening test leads to a more aggressive procedure than a biopsy, significant medical complications may ensue. For instance, if a benign lung nodule or mass looks like cancer on a chest x-ray, your doctor may recommend that the nodule be surgically removed. In this hypothetical example, we know that the nodule doesn't need to be treated; in real life, though, there's no way to know that until after it has been removed and carefully examined under a microscope by a pathologist. If you suffer a serious complication as a result of the surgery, that complication was entirely unnecessary as well. In such an example, you would have suffered harm as a result of undergoing a screening test that, in retrospect, didn't need to be done. The only way you could have avoided the harm would have been to not undergo the screening test in the first place.

Let's frame this clearly before proceeding further: screening tests can set off a cascade of subsequent medical tests and procedures that have the potential to cause harm. This harm may be in the form of psychological distress that results from thinking you may have cancer when in fact you don't or in the form of injury from medical procedures. Once the cascade has begun, stopping it is difficult. Some potential benefit to the screening test must offset the risk of harm. If, on average, the screening test results in people living longer, the risk of harm may well be justified.

Let's now look at another potential problem with cancer screening tests. When we discussed the potential meanings of an abnormal screening test result, one possibility included the detection of cancers that pose little risk to the individual. Although this is a controversial subject, it appears that some cancers grow slowly and spread only late in their course if ever.

For instance, previously undiagnosed prostate cancers are often discovered when autopsies are performed on elderly men who have died of other causes. These men had prostate cancer while alive but never knew it and probably never suffered from these undetected cancers. They never received treatment for prostate cancer and were never subjected to the anxiety that would almost certainly have accompanied the knowledge that they had cancer. If someone had decided to screen these men for prostate cancer while they were alive, they almost certainly would have worried about suffering and perhaps dying from the disease; they might even have chosen to undergo treatments that had unpleasant side effects. In other words, they were almost certainly better off not knowing about their disease, as they were destined to die of another, unrelated cause (such as a heart attack).

The subject of slow-growing tumors emphasizes that screening tests acquire a substantial amount of information that otherwise would not be available. Some of this information may be valuable, but some may be meaningless or even lead to unintentionally harmful actions. Clearly, some screening tests (such as mammograms and Pap smears) save lives, and for most (and society as a whole), the benefits far outweigh the risks. Still, even for these tests, and particularly for screening tests that are not as well validated, it is important to think about what you would do with the information provided by the test.

PSA AND PROSTATE CANCER: A SPECIFIC EXAMPLE OF A SCREENING TEST DILEMMA

Screening for prostate cancer by measuring the level of prostate-specific antigen (PSA) in the blood is one of the most controversial cancer-screening tests. The controversy illustrates the many issues discussed above and demonstrates the problems that arise when a screening test is popularized before it has been proven to prolong lives.

PSA is a protein made by both healthy and cancerous prostate cells. When men develop prostate cancer or when they have certain other abnormalities of the prostate gland (such as benign enlargement of the gland, also called benign prostatic hypertrophy or BPH), their blood levels of PSA usually become elevated. Often, an elevated PSA is the only early evidence of prostate cancer. Like other solid tumors, prostate cancer is curable only when it is diagnosed before it has spread throughout the body. By the time prostate cancer becomes symptomatic (for example, by causing difficulties with urination or back pain if it has spread to the spine), it is frequently too late to bring about a cure. Thus, a test that accurately detects the disease at an early stage should be able to decrease the number of men who die of prostate cancer.

PSA testing has been clearly shown to provide a diagnosis of prostate cancer at an earlier stage, but it has never been shown to result in more men being cured or in men living longer or suffering less. Logically, PSA testing *should* result in more men being cured, but there is no persuasive evidence at this time that it does in fact accomplish that goal. As the discussion below illustrates, the absence of compelling evidence that prostate cancer screening either prolongs life or reduces suffering makes decision making about prostate cancer screening difficult.

Should a man undergo PSA screening at this point in time? The answer to this question depends on how a man weighs the risks and benefits of PSA testing. Prostate cancer is the most common cancer among men in the United States and the second leading cause of cancer death among men. Each year, roughly 190,000 men in the United States are diagnosed with prostate cancer, and over 30,000 die of the disease. Deaths from prostate cancer are often painful. Thus, there are excellent reasons for wanting to diagnose prostate cancer while it is still contained within the prostate gland and can still be cured. However, before undergoing PSA testing, it is essential for a man to think through what he's going to do with the information he acquires as a result of screening.

If a man has his PSA measured, it will come back either normal or elevated. In addition to looking at the PSA at just one point in time, his doctor may also consider whether the PSA is increasing and, if so, how quickly. If the PSA is considered to be abnormal (the cutoff value is generally 4 ng/mL, but that normal value increases with increasing age) or to be rising too quickly, the physician probably will recommend a biopsy of the prostate. However, many men with elevated PSAs do not have cancer. For instance, if the PSA is only slightly elevated, at 6 ng/mL, there would be less than a 50 percent chance of finding cancer: most biopsies in that setting would be unnecessary. Moreover, in a man with prostate cancer whose PSA is 6, there's a good chance that even if biopsies were taken, they would miss the cancer and be falsely reassuring. This is the first problem with PSA screening: it leads to many prostate biopsies in men who don't have cancer, and many of the biopsies that are performed as a result of a slightly elevated PSA miss cancers that are present.

Let's say that the man in our example has his PSA checked, it comes back elevated, and he decides not to have a biopsy. In this scenario, it's not clear why he had the PSA checked in the first place; without the biopsies, he probably will just worry about his elevated PSA and whether or not he has cancer. So let's suppose that instead he does have the biopsy performed and cancer is not detected. The normal biopsy result does not prove that he doesn't have cancer; he'll probably need repeat biopsies in the future to increase the proportion of the prostate that has been examined. He has thus begun what may be a long series of tests that are of no proven benefit.

So let's change the scenario again and suppose that this man's prostate biopsies reveal cancer, but there is no evidence that the cancer has spread outside the gland. He now has to decide whether he wants to undergo treatment for the cancer. He has four major options: (1) watchful waiting, in which no active treatment is given but he is monitored regularly by his physician for evidence of progressive disease; (2) radical prostatectomy, in which the prostate is removed surgically; (3) external beam radiation therapy, in which the prostate is irradiated with the goal of killing all the cancer cells; or (4) radioactive seed therapy, in which radiation is administered by inserting radioactive pellets through the skin into the prostate gland.

Unfortunately, no one knows whether any one of these radically different treatment options is better or worse than any of the others. We don't know if surgery or radiation leads to longer or shorter lives. We do know, however, that these treatments have side effects. Half or more of all men who undergo surgery are left impotent and a small but significant number are left with an inability to keep their urine from leaking—in other words, with some degree of incontinence. About half of all men who undergo radiation therapy are also left impotent and may develop a chronic irritation of the rectum. Watchful waiting doesn't have side effects per se, but many men feel anxious knowing that they have cancer and aren't doing anything about it. One could argue that if our man knew ahead of time that he would decide to not receive treatment if diagnosed with prostate cancer, he would be better off not going through the screening process in the first place. That is, if you're not going to choose treatment, why undergo screening? It may be better not to know. On the other hand, many men feel uncomfortable going without active treatment once they hear the word *cancer*, even if the available treatments carry with them substantial side effects and may not prolong survival. As a result, radical prostatectomies and radiation therapies are extremely common in the United States.

To further complicate matters, there is strong evidence that some prostate cancers don't need to be treated, though we don't know how to distinguish these cancers reliably from the more dangerous prostate cancers that do require therapy. As discussed earlier, we believe that relatively benign (nonaggressive) prostate cancers exist, because over one-third of men who live past the age of 80 years and had never been diagnosed with prostate cancer are found to have prostate cancer if an autopsy is performed after their death. In other words, it appears that a lot of elderly men are walking around with prostate cancer without any apparent harm due to the cancer. As a result, there is widespread concern that PSA screening diagnoses many cancers that don't merit treatment. If we return to our hypothetical man who underwent PSA screening and subsequent prostate biopsies that revealed cancer, we have no reliable way of telling him whether his cancer is life-threatening. If he undergoes surgery or radiation therapy, he may be cured of prostate cancer or he may not. We can't even tell him whether treatment will affect the likelihood that he will live another 10 years or the likelihood that he will die of prostate cancer.

These then are the problems with PSA screening:

It is not a highly accurate test.

There are high levels of uncertainty about the need to treat some of the cancers that are detected as a result of screening: PSA screening thus may result in the detection of many cancers that aren't dangerous.

There are high levels of uncertainty about the ability of surgery and radiation therapy to prolong lives.

All of these problems would be less troubling if we had clear evidence that PSA screening had the overall effect of making men live longer. If it is ever shown that the benefits of PSA screening outweigh the risks, then the controversy over this subject will start to subside. Ongoing studies have randomly assigned men to either undergo prostate cancer screening or simply to receive routine health care. If the group undergoing screening lives longer, then we will have a powerful argument in favor of PSA screening.

To summarize, PSA screening is not necessarily a bad idea. Weighing the risks and benefits of PSA screening, however, is complicated, and the decision as to whether or not to undergo prostate cancer screening is a personal one. Many men die from prostate cancer and many more suffer from pain caused by this cancer. It is perfectly reasonable for a man to decide that he wants to minimize the chance of dying of prostate cancer and that he therefore wants to undergo prostate cancer screening and to have surgery or radiation therapy if any cancer is detected. But this man must recognize that we don't actually know whether PSA screening has the power to reduce his chance of dying of prostate cancer. If he decides that the potential benefit of screening outweighs the potential risk, he should be screened after *being informed of these potential risks and benefits*. At this point in time, prostate cancer screening represents something of a leap of faith, and each man must decide for himself (preferably with the aid of his physician's counsel) whether or not to take that leap.

CHAPTER 6

Epidemiology of Cancer— You Are Not Alone

GEOFFREY LIU, M.D.

OUTLINE

HOW COMMON IS CANCER?

In the year 2000, some 2.5 million Americans developed cancer; of those, approximately 1.3 million developed the two most common types of skin cancers (basal cell carcinoma and squamous cell carcinoma). These skin cancers are generally excluded from most cancer statistics because they (unlike melanoma) rarely cause significant illness or death. Overall, more than half a million Americans die each year from cancer—this means that more than 1500 people die as a result of cancer daily. Cancer is the second leading cause of death (behind heart diseases), and it accounts for one-quarter of all causes of death in the United States. Approximately 8.5 million people currently living in the United States have had cancer at some time in their lives (that is, they are cancer survivors).

WHO GETS CANCER AND WHY?

Cancer affects individuals of all ages. In young infants and children, genetic abnormalities are often the underlying cause of cancer. Certain cancers (such as retinoblastoma and neuroblastoma) are seen most commonly in small children. Specific leukemias and lymphomas are seen commonly in young adults. However, individuals aged 55 years or older account for more than 80 percent of all diagnosed cancers. In adults, both genetic and environmental factors play a role.

The American Cancer Society estimates that nutrition and lifestyle factors (collectively known as *environmental factors*) account for up to one-third of the cancer deaths in the United States. Two major modifiable lifestyle factors are cigarette smoking and use of alcohol. Taken together, up to 200,000 cancer deaths each year in the United States can be attributed to these two risk factors. The association is particularly striking in the case of lung cancer, the most common cause of cancer deaths in both men and women: 90 percent of people who develop lung cancers are current or former smokers.

Scientific evidence is mounting that viral infections are also associated with a sizable number of cancers. For example, infection with hepatitis B and/or C can lead to liver cancer, while infection with human papillomavirus (HPV) is a risk factor for cervical cancer. Human immunodeficiency virus (HIV) and HTLV-1 are both associated with cancer development. Lifestyle and behavioral modification can prevent some of these infections: each of the viruses listed as examples can be transmitted through blood or other bodily fluids. Thus, sexual practices and the use of shared needles (in the setting of intravenous drug use) are potentially modifiable behaviors.

Other examples include exposure to certain environmental substances (such as asbestos) or chemicals (such as arsenic) associated with specific cancers. Sun exposure and damage is directly related to the most common skin cancers. High fruit and vegetable intake, lower red meat intake, and a whole host of other nutritional factors have all been cited as being protective against cancer development, in particular the development of colon cancer. Obesity also has been linked to a number of cancers, including cancer of the breast, colon, and prostate. In addition, lack of physical activity has been associated with breast and colon cancer.

The proportion of risk that can be attributed to each of these factors is still not known; nor is it clear which of these components is key to cancer development. Nonetheless, the preponderance of evidence supports a healthy diet, physical activity, avoidance of heavy alcohol use, and avoidance of smoking and second-hand smoke in the prevention of cancer.

Our understanding of the genetic contribution to cancer development in adults is limited. Certain cancers (including breast cancer, ovarian cancer, and many others) are more common in individuals with a family history of these cancers. The risk of developing breast and ovarian cancer may be related to genes called *BRCA1* and *BRCA2*. It has been estimated that between 5 and 10 percent of cancers are clearly hereditary. However, a sizable proportion of cancer develops as a result of the complex interplay between genes and the environment. Thus, cancer development may involve damage to genes during our lifetimes or the way we digest (or process) nutrients, hormones, and toxins in our bodies in addition to external (or environmental) factors (such as diet, sunlight, heavy use of tobacco and alcohol, or viral infections).

CAN CANCERS BE PREVENTED?

Cancers (such as lung cancer and cancers of the head and neck) that are largely attributed to smoking and drinking heavily can be prevented. A healthy diet and physical activity also reduce one's risk of cancer. Regular screening examinations (i.e., tests that look for cancer in perfectly healthy individuals) will not necessarily prevent cancer, but they are crucial for the detection of some cancers at an early stage. Currently, screening by a health professional is recommended for the detection of cancer of the breast, cervix, prostate, skin, and colorectal area; these cancers, taken together, account for half of all cancers diagnosed in the United States. See Chap. 5 for more information on this topic.

WHAT DO THE TERMS OVERALL SURVIVAL AND DISEASE-FREE SURVIVAL MEAN TO ONCOLOGISTS?

It is only natural that a person with a new diagnosis of cancer will want to know what his or her chances of survival are. There are a number of ways that a doctor can provide a forecast of the probable outcome of a disease (that is, the prognosis for an individual patient). Unlike fortune-tellers who use crystal balls or Tarot cards to discern the future, doctors must use the accumulated scientific information available to them to provide a realistic scenario to people with cancer and their families. Usually, this information derives from the experience of other individuals affected by the same type of cancer whose disease has spread to a similar extent.

"What are my chances?" is a natural question to ask when a person has just been given a cancer diagnosis. There is no single scientific way to measure your chances for cure. However, doctors will discuss either the *overall survival* or the *disease-free survival*. These terms are similar but not identical. The *cure rate* is what people with cancer ultimately want to know; this term describes the chances that you will be free of cancer for the rest of your life. Yet, doctors cannot predict specifically how long any given individual will live. In order to be more accurate, doctors will tell patients what the chances are that they will be alive at a specific time (usually measured in months or years) after diagnosis. This is known as overall survival. *Overall survival* simply indicates the proportion of patients remaining alive after a given number of months or years following a cancer diagnosis.

However, overall survival doesn't take into account whether a person is actually cancer-free a given number of months or years following a diagnosis. In other words, overall survival is simply a head count of the number of living cancer patients without regard to whether the cancer has disappeared or still exists. Clearly, doctors must have another way to answer this question. In fact, they will use another term to describe prognosis—*disease-free survival*—which describes the proportion of people whose cancer has never returned at a specific time after diagnosis. This term is closer to the meaning of *cure rate*.

Why, then, don't doctors consistently use the concept of disease-free survival instead of overall survival? This is a more complex question. Anyone who has ever completed a census survey can understand that conducting a head count of who in the country is alive is easier than asking every person in the country specific questions about his or her medical background and then checking whether those who have died had cancer at the time of their demise. Thus, many believe that the statistics used to determine overall survival are more accurate than those for disease-free survival. However, recent medical studies have done a much better job of ensuring that measurements of disease-free survival are just as accurate as those of overall survival. Both are legitimate and are used to provide an estimate of the chance for cure. Generally, if only the word *survival* is used, it usually (but not always) means overall survival.

HOW SHOULD I INTERPRET THE SURVIVAL STATISTICS GIVEN TO ME BY MY ONCOLOGIST?

Now that your doctor has estimated your overall or disease-free survival rate (for your situation and with your stage of disease), what should this mean to you? What does it really mean when, for instance, your doctor tells you that your overall survival is 30 percent at 5 years? If you've ever bought a lottery ticket, you will understand the concept of chance.

In any game of chance, there are optimists and there are pessimists. An optimist will consider an overall survival of 30 percent at 5 years to mean that a person has a 3 in 10 chance of being alive at 5 years. The pessimist will say that the same person has a 7 in 10 chance of dying. It becomes quite clear that a person cannot be three-tenths alive and seven-tenths dead. So, in this manner, overall and disease-free survival should be interpreted with caution. If you are the lucky individual who is alive at 5 years, would you care if your original chance was as low as 0.0001 percent? Similarly, how lucky would you feel if your cancer came back even though your chances were 99.9999 percent for cure? Thus, asking your doctor, "What are my chances" is a double-edged sword. These chances can serve as rough guides; they are not absolute truths gleaned from a crystal ball.

DOES TIME FACTOR INTO DISCUSSIONS OF "OVERALL SURVIVAL" OR "DISEASE-FREE SURVIVAL"?

An important concept in interpreting both overall survival and disease-free survival is the time frame. A doctor may quote an overall survival of 30 percent *at a specific time after diagnosis.* In most cases, if a cancer is going to recur, it will do so within a specific time frame. For instance, if you have colon cancer and are cancer-free after 5 years, the chance that your cancer will spread to other parts of the body is low. That is to say, you may still develop a new colon cancer, but your original cancer is essentially cured. Thus, quoting an overall or disease-free survival rate for colon cancer at 5 years is very appropriate (i.e., it closely resembles the true cure rate). Quoting a survival rate for colon cancer at 1 year may not accurately reflect reality.

In the case of breast cancer, some individuals have slow-growing tumors and can still develop cancer that spreads after 20 years. The proportion of people with breast cancer who have this experience, though, is small. In this circumstance, quoting an overall or disease-free survival rate after two periods, say at 10 and 20 years, may provide a more complete picture of a person's prognosis. Most doctors will now quote overall and disease-free survival to patients along with the time frame they are using. The key to interpreting this information is to understand whether the time frame being provided is reasonable compared to the typical time frame for cancer recurrence in a specific disease.

HOW CAN INFORMATION REGARDING OVERALL SURVIVAL AND DISEASE-FREE SURVIVAL HELP ME MAKE TREATMENT DECISIONS?

Doctors also use the terms *overall survival* and *disease-free survival* to compare the efficacy of different treatments and to compare the outcomes of patients who receive a given treatment with that of patients who elect not to be treated. For example, a fictitious chemotherapy called "Cancerkill" may improve the average disease-free survival in a group of people with lung cancer by 30 percent over a 5-year period

compared with another fictitious chemotherapy called "Cancergrow," or by com- ·
parison with no therapy at all. The goal of using these terms in these situations is to
help a person with cancer decide whether a treatment is worth undertaking.

The key to any decision is knowing what is at stake. For both overall survival
and disease-free survival, the stakes are high: for overall survival, the stakes are being alive, and for disease-free survival, the stakes are being alive without disease.

How a doctor frames the chances has an effect on how a person thinks about a
treatment. If you were told that a treatment works 5 percent of the time, you might
not be enthusiastic about receiving that treatment. However, if you were told that
your chance for being alive at 5 years was increased by 5 percent if you received a
given treatment, you might express more enthusiasm. When these questions were
posed to a group of women with breast cancer, most of them considered even a 1
to 3 percent chance of increased survival worth the risk of significant side effects
of chemotherapy.

WHAT IS A "REMISSION"?

The strict definition of *remission* refers to the improvement (i.e., the shrinkage or
disappearance) of a cancer. This improvement may be complete or partial and may
last permanently (the ultimate sign of being cured) or only temporarily. Usually,
remissions are strictly defined within each cancer; a 50 percent shrinkage in the
tumor diameter may indicate a partial remission in one type of cancer but not another. When a doctor speaks of a remission, he or she should specify how much of
an improvement has occurred and for how long that improvement will last.

In many instances, however, remissions are described to people in more general terms. Fortunately, most oncologists apply the "reasonable man" approach to
the concept of remission. This is similar to the legal concept of the reasonable man.
In medicine, if a reasonable man (or woman) would agree that the amount of improvement in a cancer for a specific length of time was meaningful, then it would
be considered a remission. Of course, using this approach is subjective, so appropriate adjectives and terms are added to provide a more objective estimate of remission.

Like the concept of survival, the concept of remission rests on two basic foundations: (1) the chance a person with cancer will attain a remission and (2) a time
factor (that is, how long the remission will last). The meaning of a remission depends on whether the cancer is potentially curable and is discussed separately.

HOW DO ONCOLOGISTS THINK ABOUT REMISSIONS IN POTENTIALLY CURABLE CANCERS?

In potentially curable cancers (usually cancers that are less advanced), the ultimate measure of success is either overall survival or disease-free survival. How-

ever, two other concepts are important: complete remission and relapse rate. A *complete remission* is defined as the total disappearance of cancer from all parts of a person's body *that can be detected by x-rays or other special tests.* This last phrase is important, as it is possible that a person with cancer may be thought to be in complete remission, yet in truth the cancer is not completely eradicated, just not detectable. *Relapse rate* is defined as the chance that a cancer that has been in complete remission will come back. Sometimes, relapse rate is also known as *recurrence rate.* Both a complete remission and lack of recurrence are necessary to produce a cure.

Placing these concepts in a time frame, complete remission is a short-term goal for a person undergoing treatment of his or her cancer. It can serve as a benchmark as a person with cancer looks ahead toward overall and disease-free survival. Once treatment is completed and a complete remission has been achieved, the focus shifts to the chances for recurrence (or relapse). Thus, each of these concepts provides a specific viewpoint that is useful at different times in the treatment and follow-up of a person with cancer.

HOW DO ONCOLOGISTS THINK ABOUT REMISSIONS IN INCURABLE CANCERS?

An incurable cancer is one that cannot reasonably be expected to disappear, even with the best therapy available. However, a person with an incurable cancer can attain a complete remission; by definition, incurability means that the relapse rate in these individuals is 100 percent over time (and their cancer will recur).

Incurability does not imply that rapid death or rapid growth of a cancer will occur. In many circumstances, people who have incurable cancers have a chronic disease that can be controlled for months, years, and, in rare circumstances, decades.

HOW DO ONCOLOGISTS CONVEY PROGNOSIS MEANINGFULLY TO A PERSON WITH AN INCURABLE CANCER?

Four terms are used to provide more specific information about the prognosis of a person with an incurable cancer who is receiving therapy: *partial remission, total response rate, stable disease,* and *time to progression.*

Partial remission refers to a significant shrinkage of the tumor. Often, this is arbitrarily set at 50 percent shrinkage of the diameter (which is measured in two dimensions) of a specific cancer nodule. This standard was originally adopted for research purposes but has spread into common usage.

The *total response rate* is the proportion of people who have experienced either a partial or complete remission (or response) to a specific therapy.

The definition of *stable disease* is self-evident: it is the proportion of people whose cancers have not substantially increased or decreased in size. Having stable disease is particularly important for a person who experienced few or no effects from the cancer; as long as the cancer does not continue to grow, the person may continue to feel well. Because oncologists and patients are most concerned about cancer growth, sometimes the definition of *total response* is expanded to include individuals with stable disease in addition to those with either a complete or partial remission. Stable disease may also indicate that a cancer is responding to treatment; while the treatment may not be shrinking the tumor, it is preventing the cancer from growing.

While the concepts of partial remission, response rate, and stable disease are important in describing how a cancer responds to therapy, none of these terms incorporates any sense of time. *Time to progression*, on the other hand, is the amount of time a cancer does not grow (i.e., the time during which it remains stable or responds to therapy).

One of the ultimate goals of treatment for a person with an incurable cancer is to enable him or her to live longer. Unfortunately, not all treatments can produce this result. In some cases, the goals of treatment are to prevent or alleviate symptoms of the cancer. Often, doctors assume that if a cancer does not grow or if it shrinks, symptoms can be prevented or alleviated. That is why both response rate (which considers complete and partial responses as well as perhaps stable disease) and time to progression are important concepts in describing the treatment course of people with incurable cancers.

WHAT IS "QUALITY OF LIFE"?

Ironically, none of the traditional indicators of how well a treatment works (i.e., response rate, remission rate, recurrence rate, time to progression) mentions or incorporates a measure of how well a person actually feels during or after treatment or in the absence of treatment! Oncologists carefully follow each person's symptoms, assess how that person is functioning, and ask how well he or she feels; these factors generally define the term *quality of life*. Yet finding some way of comparing how well specific groups of cancer patients are feeling during, after, or in lieu of treatment is also important, particularly if the treatment is being given in the setting of incurable cancer.

Quality of life (QOL) studies compare patients receiving different therapies or who are in different situations. Formal studies involve interviews and/or questionnaires given to people with cancer. Although it is reasonable to assume that a cancer that is responding to treatment should produce fewer symptoms and allow people to feel better, this assumption does not always hold true. In the past decade, major strides have been made to incorporate QOL measures into many of the clinical research studies of cancer treatment. That is why oncologists can now tell their patients that some treatments not only have a certain chance of shrinking their tumors for a certain period of time but can also make them feel better.

WHEN IS A DISCUSSION OF QUALITY OF LIFE IMPORTANT?

It is always important to bear quality of life (QOL) in mind. However, there are times when improved short-term QOL may *not* be the ultimate goal of therapy. Implicit in any treatment decision a person makes is the trade-off between the potential benefits gained from the treatment (e.g., a delayed time to progression or an improved overall survival) and the chances of developing side effects from the treatment. Most people will tolerate feeling poorly temporarily during treatment if their chances of cure are improved. In contrast, QOL becomes paramount in discussing palliation of incurable disease. Discussing QOL is useful because it emphasizes the goals of many treatments; curing a cancer or palliating a cancer both have as their ultimate purpose enabling people to feel better for a longer time.

WHY DO ONCOLOGISTS USE SO MANY TERMS TO DESCRIBE PROGNOSIS?

The goal of an oncologist is to provide an overall perspective about the potential benefits and drawbacks of each treatment (or nontreatment), so that a person with

TABLE 6-1 **Definitions of Epidemiology Terms**

Overall survival	The proportion of patients who are alive after a given number of months or years following a cancer diagnosis.
Disease-free survival	The proportion of people whose cancer has never returned at a specific time after diagnosis.
Remission	The improvement (i.e., the shrinkage or disappearance) of a cancer.
Complete remission	The total disappearance of cancer from all parts of a person's body that can be detected by x-rays or other special tests.
Partial remission	A significant shrinkage of the tumor. Often, this is arbitrarily set at 50 percent shrinkage.
Relapse rate	The chance that a cancer that has been in complete remission will come back.
Total response rate	The proportion of people who have experienced either a partial or complete remission (or response) to a specific therapy.
Stable disease	Disease in which the cancer has not substantially increased or decreased in size.
Time to progression	The amount of time a cancer does not grow (i.e., the time during which it remains stable or responds to therapy).
Quality of life	A measure of how a person feels and functions and of his or her symptoms.

TABLE 6-2 The Relationship between the Goals of Treatment for Cancer and the Indicators of Effective Treatment

If the primary goal of treatment is:	The usual measures of how effective a treatment are:	Comments
Cure	Overall survival (OS) Disease-free survival (DFS) Complete remission/response Recurrence/relapse rate	Both overall survival and disease-free survival reflect the long-term outcomes of therapy. The first goal of therapy is to achieve a complete remission, and the second goal is to prevent a relapse or recurrence. The combination of these two goals is reflected in OS and DFS.

To treat or prevent symptoms but not to cure	Overall survival
	Disease-free survival
	Total response rate
	  –Complete remission/response
	  –Partial remission/response (PR)
	  –Stable disease (SD)
	Time to progression (TTP)
	Quality of life (QOL)
		Both improved overall survival or disease-free survival are compelling reasons to consider treatment. However, because a cure is not expected, other goals may be important in deciding if a treatment is appropriate.
		
		QOL is an important goal in this circumstance, but accurate information on QOL may be limited for many treatments.
		The (total) response rate includes complete remission and partial remission and sometimes includes stable disease. It can give a sense of how effective a treatment is, along with time to progression (which provides a sense of how long a treatment may work).

cancer can make an informed decision. There really is no single correct measure of a therapy's potential benefit that applies to all patients. Thus, different terms are used in different circumstances. Unfortunately, the barrage of new terms and data can be overwhelming during an initial visit, particularly considering the stress and shock associated with receiving bad news. Tables 6-1 and 6-2 summarize the information presented in this chapter.

CHAPTER 7

The Impact of Cancer on the Family

Erika Ryst, M.D.

OUTLINE

HOW DO FAMILIES TYPICALLY RESPOND TO A FAMILY MEMBER WHO HAS CANCER?

Each family's experience with cancer is as unique as the family itself. The response of families and people with cancer to the cancer diagnosis is based on a multitude of variables. These include religion, personal and family belief systems, education, finances, socioeconomic status, employment status, current age, and gender. Other factors that play a role are the quality and availability of medical care, the ability to communicate with treating physicians, the overall health status of the family, and how the affected family has coped with similar life events in the past.

In addition, a family's or an individual's response depends on the availability of community supports; the age at diagnosis and initial treatment; the tumor type, stage, and prognosis; one's marital status and sexuality; one's culture; and the developmental stage of the family. It also depends on the knowledge and understanding of the family about the diagnosis and the family's interpretation of the meaning of illness. Yet, despite the differences among families, a common thread runs through all of their cancer experience: cancer evokes significant stress. The ways in which a family appraises, responds, copes, and calls on supports determines the ultimate outcome for all involved (Table 7-1).

Research suggests that families respond to cancer similarly, in certain patterns. First, spouses and families, like the person with a cancer diagnosis, react negatively to the diagnosis, and studies that measure the level of distress of families and the individual with cancer find that they are correlated. That is, cancer patients and their families share in their initial shock and grief. For spouses and family mem-

TABLE 7-1 Influences on a Family's Reaction to Cancer*

Religion
Personal and family belief systems
Educational background
Financial status
Employment status
Current age
Gender
Quality and availability of medical care
Ability to communicate with treating physicians
Overall health status of the family
Coping ability of family members
Availability of community supports
Age at initial diagnosis and treatment
Tumor type, stage, and prognosis
Marital status and sexuality
Culture
Developmental stage of the family
Knowledge about and understanding of the diagnosis

*List adapted from variables outlined in an article by M.A. Weitzner and R. Knutzen, "The impact of pituitary disease on the family caregiver and overall family functioning."

bers, this can mean the development of insomnia, an appetite disturbance (eating too much or too little), and problems at work.

One study that polled the surviving family members of deceased ovarian cancer patients identified similarities in their experience. According to respondents, the most common reaction at the time of diagnosis was typified by the question, "What went wrong?" The worst part of treatment for them was continued chemotherapy. They treasured most the ability to travel and the amount of time they had with the person diagnosed with cancer following his or her diagnosis. During the battle with cancer, the worst part for family members was feeling helpless and watching their loved one suffer. Finally, the effects of their experience were long-lasting; even after their loved one's death, family members remained unrealistically fearful that someone else in the family would be diagnosed with ovarian cancer.

The impact of a cancer diagnosis over time is less clear; it probably depends on how well families cope. Family members commonly worry about how they can help the person with cancer cope with his or her illness and how they will manage the inevitable disruptions caused by cancer. Because family members also fear cancer recurrence, they may react with anger, uncertainty, and anxiety if the cancer does return.

IN WHAT WAYS DO FAMILIES COPE WITH CANCER?

Coping, in general, refers to conscious (voluntary or chosen) strategies that decrease the distress associated with a life event. Families cope in a variety of ways, and their coping mechanisms may or may not be helpful. Strategies such as information seeking, problem solving, or active participation in treatment tend to be more helpful. In contrast, avoidant strategies—such as not talking about the cancer or refusing to participate in treatment—can be more problematic. Other possible modes of coping with cancer include acceptance (facing the reality realistically), cognitive reframing (looking at the "silver lining" of the experience), and rationalization (trying to explain why the cancer happened).

Coping with cancer evolves over time. Family members' initial reactions may be different from their responses over the long term. In the beginning, families may rally with support; however, they may become more fatigued, burdened, or resentful over time. Later, coping can become more difficult because of the family's pressing need to get back to life's ongoing tasks as well the relatively decreased social support they may be able to provide compared to what they could provide during the period surrounding the diagnosis.

Families use coping strategies that they know and have used in the past. For example, if a grandfather coped with cancer by reframing (e.g., using the cancer diagnosis as a call to enjoy life), his descendants who face cancer may also try to value each day.

Finally, the developmental stage of the family influences how the members will deal with and respond to stress. Families, like individuals, go through a process of maturation as they age together. Research on family functioning suggests six separate family life-cycle stages: (1) for the unattached adult, differentiation of self, development of peer relations, and establishment of work is required; (2) for the newly married couple, realignment of relationships (to include the spouse) with extended families and friends is required; (3) for the family with young children, parenting roles must be dealt with; (4) for the family with adolescents, parent-child relationships must shift; (5) for the family with children launched (to college or to their own adult lives), renegotiations of the marital system as a dyad, and formation of adult relationships with grown children is appropriate; and (6) for the family in later life, room must be made for the middle generation while still valuing the wisdom of elders. From this theoretical perspective, it is possible to hypothesize how cancer might threaten (more at some stages than others) the integrity of families. According to this model, a sick young adult who is a first-time parent may feel more stressed by the need to regress from a "caring" to "a cared for" role, whereas the role of being cared for is more natural to an ill, elderly adult. Evidence suggests that cancer is more disruptive to the psychosocial adjustment of younger than that of older adults.

WHAT ARE WAYS IN WHICH MY FAMILY MIGHT CHANGE AS A RESULT OF DEALING WITH CANCER?

Normal, healthy families are dynamic systems that change and accommodate to new demands. You may find that over time, as your family adapts to the cancer, new ways of relating emerge (see Table 7-2).

WHAT ARE SOME INDICATORS THAT SOMEONE IN MY FAMILY IS NOT DEALING WELL WITH THE DIAGNOSIS?

As already discussed, partners may experience depression, sleep disturbance, anxiety, and helplessness. As many as 20 to 30 percent of partners suffer from psy-

TABLE 7-2 **Cancer-Induced Changes in Family Function***

New patterns of communication may arise, such as increased discussion about feelings and reactions related to the cancer.

New self-concepts by family members may develop (for example, a partner may take on a new identity as caretaker).

Roles for multiple family members may change. Adolescents might take on more responsibilities around the household, or the well partner might take on tasks formerly performed by the sick partner.

Status or social structure may shift. Illness of a family member could take on meaning within a larger social system, such as within a church community.

Basic patterns and daily routines may be altered. Necessary practical aspects of treatment (such as transportation) may need to be incorporated into the daily routine.

*Based upon material in the article, "The crisis of cancer: Psychological impact on family caregivers," by C. Blanchard, T. Albrecht, and J. Ruckdeschel.

chological impairment or mood disturbance as a result of the spouse's cancer. Levels of distress in the cancer patient and in his or her spouse are usually correlated. People with cancer and their partners may simultaneously experience high levels of distress. This may result from situational factors (such as disease severity), individual factors (such as depression of one partner that can affect the mood state of the other), or family system factors (such as lack of mutual support, leading to poor coping by both).

Factors that may predict high levels of spousal distress include advanced disease stage, poor emotional adjustment of the person with cancer, female gender, younger age, decreased marital satisfaction or adjustment, and impaired family functioning. According to one author, Christina Blanchard, both illness-related variables and contextual variables may predict the distress of family members (Table 7-3).

WHAT ARE SOME SIGNS THAT MY FAMILY AS A WHOLE IS NOT COPING WELL WITH THE DIAGNOSIS?

Overall, most families cope quite well with cancer. Prior coping with other stressors tends to predict how a family will cope with the new stress of a cancer diagnosis. If your family has weathered other storms, chances are that the same coping mechanisms that were previously effective will again take effect. Those families that have had more difficulty are not likely to cope as well with a new cancer diagnosis.

Researchers have attempted to identify those characteristics of family systems that contribute to less adaptive functioning. Olson and associates have developed a "Circumplex model of family functioning," which looks at a family's "cohesion" and "adaptability." *Cohesion* refers to closeness and emotional bonding within a family. A family's cohesion can vary between the extremes of disengagement (no cohesion) and enmeshment (too much cohesion, to the point that individual members lose identity). Similarly, the variable of *adaptability*, which represents a family's ability to change and to cope as needed, can vary between rigid (with no ability to change) and chaotic (too much change, which results in confusion.)

TABLE 7-3 **Factors Associated with Familial Distress and Inadequate Coping Associated with Cancer**

Advanced forms of cancer
Female gender of the partner
Young age of the partner
Numerous life stressors (e.g., low socioeconomic status, poor health of other family
  members)
Inadequate supports for the partner
Poor communication within the family
Rigid styles and/or chaos within the family

A family copes best when its response is balanced. That is, a healthy family will have a medium amount of cohesion, which allows members to feel supported but not smothered. It will also have a medium amount of adaptability, which allows for change as needed within an established and predictable structure.

Problematic family coping may reveal itself when family members challenge medical staff, answer for the person with cancer, focus on insignificant matters, interfere with treatment procedures, seem disinterested, or are highly emotionally reactive (i.e., they respond as though every situation were a crisis). If your doctor notices that your family seems to be struggling, he or she may suggest pursuing professional help. Even if your family has used more disengaged, enmeshed, rigid, or chaotic ways of coping in the past, that doesn't mean that these patterns are etched in stone. Family therapists can be helpful in introducing new skills and improved ways of relating.

HOW MIGHT MY OWN COPING BE INFLUENCED BY MY FAMILY?

As you might expect, the emotional support of families profoundly affects how a person copes. People who enjoy this support do better than those who don't. Yet sometimes the spouse or partner or family members of a person with cancer are unable to provide this kind of support, for reasons already discussed. The partner may criticize or give unwanted advice, may harp too much on the scary parts of the diagnosis, or may discourage the person with cancer from talking about it because of his or her own discomfort. One research study suggested that in these situations, people with cancer feel less confident about their own ability to cope. Perhaps because they are unable to vent or to get positive feedback, people with cancer retreat into the less helpful strategy of avoiding their medical condition and, as a result, feel more distressed.

WHY DO FAMILY AND FRIENDS NEED SUPPORT?

Early research on cancer and coping focused on the individual's struggle with cancer. More recently (starting in the 1970s), we have realized that families share in the suffering of the person with cancer. Now cancer is considered more of a "family disease" than an individual's problem. Families experience the same level of distress as do people with cancer. Since they suffer too, they should be included in the treatment process. Moreover, families can do a better job of supporting the person with cancer when they, too, receive sufficient support.

IS IT WRONG FOR A FAMILY MEMBER TO RESENT ME OR MY CANCER?

Families are affected by cancer in a variety of ways. Inevitably, a cancer diagnosis generates secondary stressors (such as financial strain, employment strain, role strain, and disruption of the daily routine). A 1994 study of people with chronic illnesses (including cancer) concluded that 31 percent of families reported loss of most or all of their family savings. Some 20 percent of families needed a family member to quit work in order to care for the person with a chronic illness, and 34 percent of people required considerable assistance from a caregiver. Because of cancer, a family member's job within the family may also change. Others may need to step in to take on the roles formerly performed by the caretaker or the person with cancer. This alters how everyone structures his or her day-to-day schedule. Additional secondary stressors include less time for recreation or leisure, a change in the relationship with the spouse and other family members, and a decrease in sexual activity.

Given all of these secondary stressors, family members can often develop depression and poor health; in addition, they may generate, anger, resentment, a sense of being overwhelmed, helplessness, stress, fatigue, social isolation, guilt, and anxiety. Such effects understandably stem from the huge stress associated with cancer. To prevent or reverse these potential negative effects, health care providers and families should try to promote healthy coping.

WHAT CAN MY FAMILY DO TO DEAL MORE EFFECTIVELY WITH A CANCER DIAGNOSIS?

First, identify any family member who displays signs of poor adjustment or depression (including the person with cancer) and refer that person for professional help. Generalized anxiety and uncertainty can be decreased by actively seeking information about the disease. Material on expected outcome, available treatments, the equipment being used for treatment, the time course of treatment, and expected side effects are some areas worth looking into. Evidence reveals that family members who take an active part in treatment maintain their own social support networks better. Open communication to avoid the "conspiracy of silence" (which develops when no one talks about the cancer) also is recommended.

A variety of family supports are available in the community. It is important to ensure that families have adequate support, because with either decreased support (actual or perceived), levels of depression rise. Research on stress and coping suggests that the way a person interprets stress may be more important than the actual stressor. For this reason, many existing programs help families and people with cancer increase their support network and reframe their appraisal of their disease.

Specific programs include support groups, information programs, individual therapy, couples or family therapy, respite care, chaplaincy services, telephone-based counseling, sex therapy, and family weekend retreats. Because of the demonstrated positive effects of support groups for cancer patients, interest in this type of intervention for families has risen. Family members who participate in support groups often feel comforted by the knowledge that others share their problems; in addition, they gain valuable information about the disease itself. Group interventions based on specific skills (for example, anger management or self-care) also exist. Hopefully, in the near future we will gain a better understanding of the most appropriate target families, timing, and types of interventions needed.

WHAT CAN MY DOCTOR DO TO HELP MY FAMILY DEAL MORE EFFECTIVELY WITH A CANCER DIAGNOSIS?

Medical staff can help families cope. In the initial period following the diagnosis, the family should be included early in discussions about the cancer and its treatment. Many families appreciate being included in regular family meetings with the primary doctor. When people with cancer are hospitalized for protracted treatment or for the treatment of complications, the medical staff should call family members at home if the patient's condition changes significantly. Knowing that they will be contacted when a medical condition becomes serious gives family members the peace of mind to enjoy needed respite time. Similarly, families should be updated on any scheduled transfers to other hospitals or to rehabilitation facilities, so that they can make plans accordingly. If the family needs additional information, support, or a mental health referral, medical staff should be ready to provide this assistance. Finally, family members look to nurses and to doctors for reassurance. Even in the terminal stages of illness, assurance that the dying family member is being given every possible comfort can be of great help (Table 7-4).

ARE THERE SUPPORT GROUPS FOR FAMILY MEMBERS?

"Support groups," as the name implies, are regularly scheduled, confidential group meetings designed to provide support around a particular topic. Support groups come in several types and sizes. Some groups are limited to certain types of members: for example, people of a certain age, gender, or cancer diagnosis. Some groups cater to people with a cancer diagnosis, while others serve the families and friends of cancer patients. Different types of leaders, ranging from mental health professionals to people with cancer, exist for groups. The purpose of these groups varies; groups may be organized around a theme (such as practical problem solv-

TABLE 7-4 Strategies Associated with More Effective Coping in Families Facing a Cancer Diagnosis

---

Identify any family member who displays signs of poor adjustment or depression and refer that person for professional help.

Seek information (e.g., on expected outcome, available treatments, the equipment used for treatment, the time course of treatment, and expected side effects of treatment).

Take an active part in treatment.

Maintain social supports.

Open communication to avoid the "conspiracy of silence."

Participate in a support group.

Work with the physician and his or her staff.

---

ing), or they may be more loosely structured as a forum for members to discuss and to share feelings. Family members frequently find that groups help to decrease their sense of being alone and provide an opportunity to learn and to share information.

HOW DO I GET MORE INFORMATION ABOUT SERVICES THAT CAN HELP?

The best resource about available services will likely be your medical team. Doctors, nurses, and social workers in oncology clinics frequently refer their patients to local support programs. Often, the clinic where a person with cancer receives treatment offers its own support groups and other services. Other sites where information about programs may be available include local churches, hospital social service departments, and the health supplements of newspapers. National organizations that can facilitate referrals locally include the National Cancer Institute's Cancer Information Service (1-800-422-6237; TTY: 1-800-332-8615; available in Spanish or English); the American Cancer Society (1-800-227-2345); and CancerCare, Inc., a nonprofit social services agency that helps people with cancer (1-800-813-HOPE).

The Internet is also becoming increasingly more accessible as an information resource. Multiple websites are available that provide medical information, list resources, and provide chat rooms and e-mail support services. Many valuable Internet links can be accessed through the website of the Association of Cancer Online Resources, Inc. (http://www.acor.org). Two particularly helpful National Cancer Institute face sheets can be accessed through this website: "Questions and Answers about Finding Cancer Support Groups" and "National Organizations That Offer Services to People with Cancer." The fact sheet regarding national organizations provides a listing of groups (such as the "I Can Cope" patient education program sponsored by the American Cancer Society and the Cancer Hope Network, which matches patients and families with trained volunteers who have undergone similar cancer experiences). "The Group Room" cancer radio talk show is another useful resource. Other websites that may be of help include the primary National Cancer Institute website (http://www.nci.nih.gov), the American Cancer Society website (http://www.cancer.org), and another NCI website (http://cancer-net.nci.nih.gov), which has a free link to the CANCERLIT database. This topic is covered in greater detail in Chap. 12.

CHAPTER 8

Genetic Risk for Cancer

Kristen Mahoney Shannon, M.S., C.G.C.
Kristin Baker Niendorf, M.S., C.G.C.
Paula D. Ryan, M.D., Ph.D.
Richard T. Penson, M.D.

OUTLINE

IS MY RISK FOR CANCER INHERITED?

The vast majority of cancers are *not* primarily due to an inherited gene that is passed from generation to generation. Inherited genes are responsible for only a small percentage (approximately 5 to 10 percent) of cancer cases (Fig. 8-1).

WHAT DOES INHERITED MEAN?

"Inherited" traits are passed from one generation of a family to the next. These traits, such as eye color or hair texture, are carried by *genes*. Genes are located on structures called *chromosomes* (Fig. 8-2). They can be thought of as the "blue-prints" for cell growth, reproduction, function, and in each cell for the balance between life and death. There are 46 chromosomes in every cell of the human body, and they come in pairs. The chromosome pairs are numbered 1 through 23. The 23rd pair is composed of the sex chromosomes: XX for female; XY for male. One copy of each chromosome pair comes from the mother and the other comes from the father. Similarly, one copy of each chromosome pair is passed on to the child.

5% - 10%

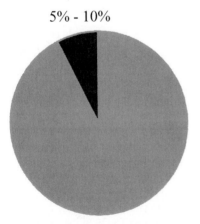

FIGURE 8-1 *Proportion of cancer that is inherited.*

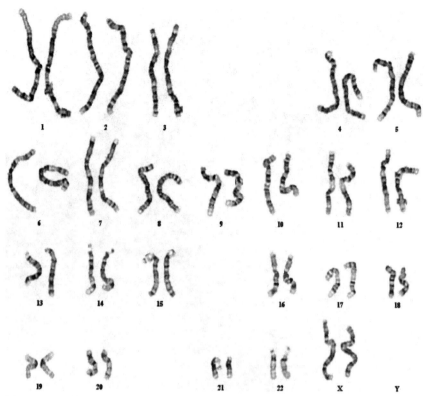

FIGURE 8-2 Chromosomes. (With permission from the cytogenetic laboratory at Mayo Clinic.)

Each chromosome contains many hundreds or thousands of genes (there are roughly 30,000 genes divided among the 23 pairs of chromosomes). Because we have two copies of each chromosome, we have two copies of each gene. Each gene is made up of deoxyribonucleic acid (DNA), which stores the information that codes for a particular trait or condition. The sequence of DNA is extremely specific; a change or mistake (called a *mutation*) in the DNA pattern in any gene may cause the gene to function improperly. Alterations in certain genes can lead to a higher susceptibility to specific diseases. A gene that could lead to a higher susceptibility to cancer is called a *cancer susceptibility gene*.

What does it mean when a cancer susceptibility gene is "altered"? If you envision each gene as being a long book, you can then think of the DNA that makes up the gene as the letters that go into making the words and sentences in the book. When a gene is altered, it simply means that there is a typographical error (typo) in the book. This typo can be as large as an entire chapter that is missing from the book or as small as a single letter change within a word (such as cat versus rat).

HOW DO INHERITED GENES CAUSE CANCER?

Every cancer results from genetic mutations, meaning that genetic changes (alterations in the DNA) in a "normal" cell cause that cell to turn into a cancer cell. Remember that all people have two copies of every gene—including cancer susceptibility genes. Most cancer susceptibility genes are called *tumor suppressor genes*, meaning that these genes normally keep a cell healthy and prevent it from becoming cancerous and producing a tumor. In other words, we all want to have these genes, and we want them to function normally.

For many complicated reasons, tumor suppressor genes (like any other gene in our body) can become altered and may stop functioning properly during an individual's lifetime. If one copy of a gene pair in a cell becomes altered, that cell will remain healthy and not become a cancer cell because there is one copy of the gene pair that is still working properly (Fig. 8-3)—a fortunate safeguard. However, as that cell ages or as a person is exposed to cancer-causing agents (*carcinogens* such as cigarette smoke or radiation), the working copy of the gene pair may become altered as well. If this occurs, the cell would no longer have any tumor suppressor gene that is working properly and could develop into a cancer cell that grows into a tumor. This is the way most cancers develop: a person is born with two working copies of a gene, and both need to be altered in order for the cell to become cancerous. This development leads to what is called a "sporadic" cancer (Fig. 8-3), although you can see that this cancer is ultimately due to "genetic" changes in an individual cell.

Inherited cancers occur in people who are born with one altered copy of a cancer susceptibility gene. These people have only one working copy of the gene in each of their cells to start with and thus only one copy in a cell has to be altered for that cell to become cancerous (Fig. 8-3). Because only one alteration (instead of two) is needed to develop cancer, it takes less for cancer to develop and, in general, such cancers are more common in this population. This also explains why most *but not all* individuals with inherited alterations develop cancer.

HOW DO I KNOW IF MY FAMILY HAS AN INHERITED RISK FOR CANCER?

One in every three individuals will develop cancer at some point in his or her lifetime. When more than one out of every three people in a family develop cancer, it is possible that the family has an inherited risk for cancer. Families that have an inherited risk for cancer usually have certain *unique* features (Table 8-1). Often, the cancer in the family is the same type (e.g., many family members will have colon cancer) or a particular combination of cancers (as in colon and uterine cancer or breast and ovarian cancer).

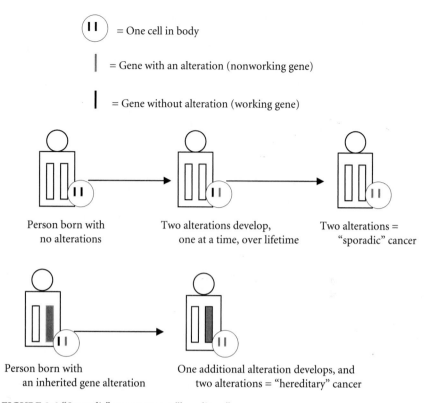

FIGURE 8-3 *"Sporadic" cancer versus "hereditary" cancer.*

Some cancers are "related"—meaning that an altered cancer susceptibility gene predisposes a person to develop more than one type of cancer (as with colon cancer and uterine cancer). Table 8-2 provides a partial list of cancers that are related because of an underlying cancer susceptibility gene. When an inherited risk for cancer exists, cancer is usually present in more than one generation and it appears to be passed on from generation to generation. Affected individuals tend to develop cancers at a younger age (often called "early-onset" cancer). For example, breast cancer is considered to be of early-onset in a woman who develops it be-

TABLE 8-1 Features of an Inherited Susceptibility to Cancer

Multiple family members are affected with the same (or other possibly related) cancers.
The onset for the cancers occurs at a younger age.
Individuals in the family may have multiple cancers.
Cancer occurs in multiple generations.

TABLE 8-2 Examples of Cancer Predisposition Genes and Their Related Cancers (Not Complete)

Cancer Type	Gene(s)	Genetic Syndrome
Breast cancer, ovarian cancer	BRCA1, BRCA2	Hereditary breast/ovarian cancer syndrome
Colon cancer, uterine cancer, bladder cancer	MLH1, MSH2, MSH6, PMS1, PMS2	Hereditary nonpolyposis colo-rectal cancer (HNPCC)
Breast cancer, sarcoma, leu-kemia, brain tumors	TP53	Li-Fraumeni syndrome (LFS)
Breast cancer, thyroid cancer	PTEN	Cowden syndrome
Colon cancer, ampullary cancer	APC	Familial adenomatous polyposis
Melanoma, pancreatic cancer	p16	Familial melanoma
Medullary thyroid cancer	RET	Multiple endocrine neoplasia (MEN)

fore the age of 45 years. Finally, there can be individuals in the family who have developed many separate cancers. If a family has some, most, or all of these four features, it is possible that an inherited cancer susceptibility gene is present in that family.

WHICH TYPES OF CANCER ARE ASSOCIATED WITH AN INHERITED RISK FOR CANCER?

Most cancers *can* be associated with an inherited cancer predisposition gene. Scientists first discovered inherited predisposition genes in families in whom rare types of cancer were overrepresented. However, we now know that inherited predisposition genes are responsible for more common types of cancer (e.g., breast and colon cancer).

Cancer also can be more common in a family because of a shared exposure to an environmental carcinogen (e.g., a cancer-causing chemical). For example, it is common for a family of smokers to have many members with lung cancer. If a known carcinogen is not present and a family has some of the features listed in Table 8-1 (regardless of cancer type), it is possible that the cancer is due to an inherited cancer susceptibility gene.

SHOULD I DISCUSS GENETIC TESTING WITH MY DOCTOR?

If your family has some of the features listed in Table 8-1, you should seek genetic counseling and cancer risk assessment. Most often, this will involve meeting with a genetic counselor and/or a physician, both of whom specialize in inherited cancers. The National Cancer Institute (www.nih.nci.gov) and the National Society of Genetic Counselors (www.nsgc.org) have listings that can help you find a cancer risk-assessment program in your area.

Cancer genetic counseling and risk assessments are essential steps in considering genetic testing. Even when someone does not want genetic testing, a genetic counseling consultation can be helpful. People in high-risk families are often anxious about cancer, and simply talking about the risks may be helpful and can reduce anxiety.

A typical genetic counseling consultation (Table 8-3) will begin by developing a detailed family history, or pedigree. The genetic counselor will ask questions about all of your relatives and will want to know each relative's current age or how old he or she was at the time of death. For relatives with cancer, the counselor will ask detailed questions about the type of cancer and the age at which the person was diagnosed with that cancer. Often, a genetic counselor will work with a family to obtain medical records and pathology reports on those individuals diagnosed with cancer to confirm the type of cancer—not because he or she doesn't trust the information, but because sometimes specifics of cancer diagnoses can be confusing. For example, occasionally a woman will learn that her grandmother, who was thought to have a stomach cancer, really had ovarian cancer. It is also quite common for a man to find out that his father, who was thought

---

TABLE 8-3 **Information Involved in a Typical Genetic Counseling Consultation**

- Introduction
  - ○ A chance to ask questions and to meet your genetic counseling caregiver(s)
- Family history taken to determine your likelihood of an inherited cancer predisposition: questions asked usually include the following:
  - ○ Who has cancer?
    - ▪ What kind?
    - ▪ How old were they when they were diagnosed?
    - ▪ Did they have bilateral disease (cancer on both sides of the body) or two separate primaries (two different types of cancer)?
  - ○ Who doesn't have cancer?
    - ▪ How old are they (how old were they when they died)?
  - ○ Have you confirmed the cancers by getting medical records?
- Risk assessment
  - ○ How likely is it that the family has an altered cancer susceptibility gene?
  - ○ Have you used statistical tools to estimate risk?
- Genetics and cancer education
  - ○ Have you obtained information about the causes of cancer and the inheritance of cancer genes?
- Discussion of genetic testing
  - ○ Do you know the pros and cons of genetic testing, and how to make a decision?
- Cancer management issues
  - ○ Have management strategies been established (including possible measures to reduce risk and screen for cancer), given the risks and the needs of the family?

to have both colon cancer and lung cancer, had only colon cancer that spread to his lungs.

The genetic counselor will then provide a great deal of information about genetics and inherited cancer. The genetic counselor will assess the family history and determine how likely it is (if at all) that the cancer(s) in the family is due to an inherited cancer susceptibility gene. If it seems possible that an inherited cancer susceptibility gene is present, the counselor will discuss genetic testing for these genes.

Because the genetic testing process can take some time, the genetic counseling consultation will usually conclude with a discussion of cancer screening recommendations. In families with an inherited susceptibility to cancer, cancer screening is often started at an earlier age and is done more frequently than usual.

IF SOMEONE IN MY FAMILY HAS CANCER, WILL I GET IT?

The short answer is probably not. Remember that most cancers (90 to 95 percent) are "sporadic," or due to random genetic changes caused by a variety of factors over a person's lifetime, and are usually not due to inherited causes. While the first-degree relatives (siblings, children, and parents) of a person with cancer tend to have a slightly higher chance of developing cancer, this probably is due to their living together in the same place, eating the same types of foods, and being exposed to the same environment. In other words, if something in a person's environment causes the first "hit" in the development of cancer, it is not unusual for his or her brother or sister to get that first "hit" as well.

In the rare instance that a family has an inherited susceptibility to cancer, it is even more likely that a person in that family will develop cancer; however, it is not a certainty. Even if a parent has an altered cancer susceptibility gene, it is not "written in stone" that his or her children will have that same altered gene.

Recall that each of us has two copies of every gene. If a person is identified as having an altered cancer susceptibility gene, we assume that the other copy of the gene is working (because it is extremely unlikely that an individual would be born with both copies of a gene altered). Remember also that we pass on only one copy of each gene to each of our children. There is a 50 percent (or 1 in 2) chance that each child will inherit an altered gene and a 50 percent chance that each will inherit a working gene (Fig. 8-4). This type of inheritance is called *autosomal dominant inheritance.*

Most inherited cancer susceptibility genes are inherited in this fashion (autosomal dominant). There are rare exceptions, however, when susceptibility to cancer is inherited in an *autosomal recessive* manner. This means that both parents must pass on a nonworking gene to their child, which occurs only 25 percent of the time if both parents are "carriers" of one copy of the gene. However, that child then (because he or she has two nonworking genes) has a high chance of developing cancer.

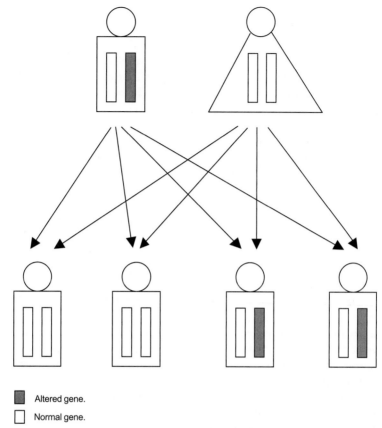

■ Altered gene.

☐ Normal gene.

FIGURE 8-4 Autosomal dominant inheritance, indicating a one-in-two or 50 percent chance for each child to inherit an altered gene.

CAN I TAKE A TEST TO FIND OUT IF I HAVE AN ALTERED CANCER SUSCEPTIBILITY GENE?

Alterations in inherited cancer susceptibility genes are rare, and genetic testing is usually reserved for individuals who have a reasonable chance of having an altered cancer susceptibility gene. For families suspected of having such a gene (based on their genetic counseling and risk assessment), it is possible to test an individual member of that family for an inherited alteration in that cancer susceptibility gene. Genetic tests currently available for these genes are listed in Table 8-2. Genetic testing is performed by taking a blood sample and checking the DNA pattern of a gene (to look for an alteration in the gene; that is, "proofreading" the gene for a typo).

Results of genetic testing are most informative if a person who has been diagnosed with cancer is tested first. If an altered gene is identified in that person, the individual's blood relatives can be tested easily. Then, if the relative has the altered gene known to cause the cancer in the family, he or she would have an increased risk of developing cancer. If the relative does not inherit this altered gene, his or her risk of developing cancer will be the same as that of an individual in the general population. If the person with cancer does not have an identifiable alteration in a gene, genetic testing would not be helpful for the rest of the family.

IF I TEST POSITIVE FOR AN ALTERED CANCER SUSCEPTIBILITY GENE, HOW LIKELY IS IT THAT I WILL GET CANCER?

A person with an altered cancer susceptibility gene has a higher chance (or risk) of developing cancer than someone with two normally functioning cancer susceptibility genes. Risk is sometimes a difficult concept to grasp. One person with a 99 percent chance of getting cancer may not get it, while someone with a chance of 1 in a 1000 may. Risks apply to groups of people, and statistics don't dictate what will happen to an individual. A higher risk does mean that a particular event is more likely to happen, but it doesn't mean that the event will definitely happen.

The likelihood (or risk) that a person with an altered cancer susceptibility gene will develop cancer is described by a concept called *penetrance*. Penetrance is usually expressed as a percentage. An altered gene with a "100 percent penetrance" implies that a person with that altered gene is 100 percent likely to develop cancer (i.e., he or she will definitely get cancer). If an altered gene is 30 percent penetrant, then a person with the altered gene has a 30 percent (or roughly one in three) chance of developing cancer in his or her lifetime.

The vast majority of cancer susceptibility genes are not 100 percent penetrant and thus do *not* always cause a person to develop cancer. However, there are a few exceptions to this rule. For example, an alteration in a cancer susceptibility gene called *APC* is responsible for a disorder called familial adenomatous polyposis (FAP). People with FAP will always develop colon cancer at some point in their lives if the colon is not removed.

Most altered cancer susceptibility genes give a person an increased but not absolute risk of cancer. *BRCA1*, for example, is a gene that, if altered, predisposes a woman to breast and ovarian cancer. The likelihood that a woman with an altered *BRCA1* gene will develop breast cancer in her lifetime is about 55 to 85 percent. This is significantly increased over the risk of 11 percent that women in the general population have, but there are some women with altered *BRCA1* genes who never develop cancer.

It also is important to keep in mind that most cancer susceptibility genes give an increased risk of *specific* cancers—not *all* cancers. Take *BRCA1*, for example. We know that women with *BRCA1* alterations have increased risks of developing breast and ovarian cancer. As far as researchers can tell, however, women with an altered *BRCA1* gene do not have a higher risk of developing most other cancers, such as leukemias, lymphomas, or cervical cancers.

IF I TEST POSITIVE FOR AN ALTERED CANCER SUSCEPTIBILITY GENE, WHAT SHOULD I DO?

The first thing to do is to become informed. Talk with your genetic counselor and other health care providers about the cancer susceptibility gene and what it means. Next and most importantly, make sure you are screened appropriately for cancer. Most cancer susceptibility genes predispose individuals to specific types of cancers in specific organs of the body. Cancer monitoring should focus on those organs. Although using these screening strategies cannot prevent cancer, the overall goal of cancer surveillance is to identify a cancer at the earliest stage possible, when the chance of cure is the highest. Third, be healthy. The American Cancer Society has recommendations on maintaining a healthy lifestyle that are important for all people—especially those known to be at increased risk based on their genetic status (see Chap. 12 for more information about Internet sites related to your cancer or to cancer in general). Finally, some individuals might consider other specific interventions, such as prophylactic surgery (see below).

IF I TEST POSITIVE FOR AN ALTERED CANCER SUSCEPTIBILITY GENE, WHAT CAN I DO TO REDUCE MY RISK OF CANCER?

Unfortunately, there is nothing you can do to make sure that you absolutely won't ever develop cancer. What you can do, however, is to maintain a healthy lifestyle and hopefully *reduce your risk.* Following the American Cancer Society recommendations is a good idea for everyone, *including* those individuals known to have an altered cancer susceptibility gene. Some individuals with an inherited predisposition to cancer who want to reduce their risk even further might choose to undergo prophylactic surgery.

Prophylactic surgery is the removal of healthy (noncancerous) tissue before cancer can develop. This type of surgery is performed on the organs at increased risk, based on the specific altered gene. A person with an altered *APC* gene (and a 100 percent chance of developing colon cancer), for example, will often have his or her healthy colon removed so that cancer cannot develop in that organ.

Unfortunately, prophylactic surgeries will not eliminate the chance of developing cancer. For example, a woman with an altered *BRCA1* gene (and a high chance of developing breast cancer) may consider having her breasts removed (mastectomy) before a cancer develops. Prophylactic mastectomy, however, doesn't eliminate the possibility of developing breast cancer. It is virtually impossible to remove every single breast cell from a woman during a mastectomy. Although unlikely, it is feasible that one of these remaining breast cells could develop into a breast cancer. A mastectomy will reduce the risk of developing breast cancer substantially though, as was demonstrated in a recent study performed in the Netherlands. In this study, women who had either an altered *BRCA1* or *BRCA2* gene and who underwent a prophylactic bilateral (or "double") mastectomy had a lower incidence of breast cancer at 3 years of follow-up compared to women with one of the altered genes who did not undergo the surgery. Removal of the ovaries (oophorectomy) may reduce the risk of ovarian cancer by as much as 95 percent.

Prophylactic surgery has many emotional, psychological, and physical repercussions. For these reasons, it is important for a person considering this type of surgery to consult with many different health care professionals. These professionals may include a surgeon, plastic surgeon, oncologist, genetic counselor, and mental health professional.

CAN I RUN INTO PROBLEMS WITH MY HEALTH INSURANCE COMPANY IF THEY FIND OUT THAT I HAVE AN ALTERED CANCER SUSCEPTIBILITY GENE?

Many people are concerned about the threat of genetic discrimination. Genetic discrimination is the use of genetic information (such as results of testing for cancer susceptibility genes) by insurers or employers in a negative way (including increasing premiums and changing coverage to eliminate care for cancer). This is illegal in many states. The website (http://www.nhgri.nih.gov/) has a state-by-state listing of laws that protect against genetic discrimination. For the most part, though, these laws do *not* protect you in your ability to purchase life insurance. It is legal for a life insurance company to adjust your premiums and/or to choose not to insure you if they obtain this type of information. For this reason, some people choose to keep their test results confidential.

WHY DOESN'T EVERYONE GET GENETIC TESTING FOR INHERITED CANCER SUSCEPTIBILITY?

Altered cancer susceptibility genes are so rare that it just wouldn't make medical or economic sense to test everyone. For example, a 35-year-old woman with no relatives with cancer has a very small (1 in 500) chance of having an altered *BRCA* gene (Table 8-4). Genetic testing should be offered only to those members of families who have a reasonable chance (usually defined as greater than or equal to 10 percent) of having an altered cancer susceptibility gene (Fig. 8-4).

Even in families to whom genetic testing is offered, not everyone chooses to get tested. These people are usually willing to assume that they carry an altered cancer susceptibility gene and to undergo cancer surveillance accordingly.

TABLE 8-4 Risk of a 35-Year-Old Healthy (non-Ashkenazi) Woman
Having an Altered *BRCA* Gene

Family History	Chance of Having an Altered *BRCA* Gene*	
No relatives with cancer	0.2%	(1 in 500)
Mother with breast cancer at age 50	0.9%	(1 in 100)
Mother with breast cancer at age 38	1.8%	(1 in 50)
Mother with breast cancer at age 40 and a sister with breast cancer at age 40	13.3%	(1 in 8)
Mother with breast cancer at age 40, sister with breast cancer at age 40, and maternal aunt with ovarian cancer at age 50	38.3%	(1 in 2.5–3)

* Chance that the 35-year-old healthy woman has an altered gene. The chance that her relative with cancer (e.g., her mother) would have an altered gene would be twice this percentage.
Parmigiani G, Berry DA, Aquilar O: Determining carrier probabilities for breast cancer susceptibility genes *BRCA1* and *BRCA2*. Am J Hum Genet 62: 145–158, 1998. Or you could cite the website to get the program. www.isds.duke.edu/~gp/brcapro.html

IS IT ALL RIGHT FOR ME NOT TO FIND OUT IF I AM AT RISK FOR CANCER?

It is important that *all* individuals be screened appropriately for cancer. Members of families who have an inherited predisposition to cancer probably will be monitored more frequently. The goal is to keep an individual healthy and to detect a cancer (if it is to develop) at an early stage, when the cure rate is the highest. For this reason, members of high-risk families should understand their risk of cancer and learn how it translates into good medical care.

However, genetic testing for inherited cancer susceptibility is optional. Genetic testing is a personal decision, and an individual must make his or her own decision after weighing the risks and benefits of testing with the help of a genetic counselor. This is not to say that an individual should ignore his or her risk of developing cancer based on family history. If a member of a family with an inherited cancer susceptibility gene decides *not* to pursue genetic testing for whatever reason, that individual should be cared for as if he or she *had* the altered gene and thus is at an increased risk of cancer.

WON'T GENETIC TESTING JUST MAKE ME MORE WORRIED?

Undergoing genetic testing is stressful. Some people think that the psychological experience of being tested is just too much to handle. Even before getting their test results, many feel anxious and/or depressed. When people receive their results, they may experience many different emotions. Some people who are found to have an altered gene find that this is "empowering," and it helps them emotionally by allowing them to take charge of their lives. Others who find they have an altered gene have a difficult time dealing with this knowledge and feel "flawed." Still others feel guilty that they could have passed the altered gene on to their children. Discovering that one doesn't have an altered gene that runs in the family can be an emotional experience as well. Most people feel happy that they do not have an increased risk of developing cancer, but some feel guilty that they have "escaped" what others in their family have not. This is called "survivor guilt."

Finally, some people may not want to deal with the impact this information might have on their family members. If a person is found to have an altered gene, it may be difficult to share this information with other relatives. Some members of a family may absolutely not want to hear this type of information, and it may be difficult to *not* tell them when an altered gene has been identified. Additionally, some people may feel that knowing the test results will not change how they plan their health care, so it is not worthwhile to have the testing.

For all these reasons, you should weigh the risks and benefits *before* having genetic testing for inherited cancer susceptibility, and make sure that you have all your questions answered.

WHERE CAN I GET MORE INFORMATION ABOUT THE CONSEQUENCES OF BEING AT RISK FOR CANCER?

Most people with a family history of cancer, regardless of genetic testing plans, will benefit from genetic counseling and risk assessment. The NCI (*www.nci.nih.gov*) and the NSGC (*www.nsgc.org*) have state-by-state listings of programs that offer genetic counseling and risk assessment. Table 8-5 provides a listing of websites that some individuals may find helpful.

TABLE 8-5 Useful Websites

MGH Center for Cancer Risk Analysis	*www.cancer.mgh.harvard.edu/CancerCare/ genetics.htm*
The American Cancer Society	*www.cancer.org*
The National Society of Genetic Counselors	*www.nsgc.org*
Genetic Information and Health Insurance Enacted Legislation	*www.nhgri.nih.gov*
Facing Our Risk of Cancer Empowered (FORCE)	*www.facingourrisk.org*
The National Cancer Institute	*www.nci.nih.gov*
The Genetic Alliance	*www.geneticalliance.org*
The National Alliance of Breast Cancer Organizations	*www.nabco.org*
Hereditary Colon Cancer Association	*www.hereditarycc.org*

CHAPTER 9

The Meaning of Cancer to Children

ANNAH N. ABRAMS, M.D.

WHAT IS CHILDHOOD CANCER?

As discussed in previous chapters, whether it occurs in adults or in children, cancer involves the abnormal growth of cells. However, the types and rates of cancer in children and the meaning of cancer to children are different from those of cancer in adults.

HOW OFTEN DOES CANCER OCCUR IN CHILDREN?

Cancer in childhood is a rare disease. Only 2 percent of all cancers diagnosed each year occur in children below 15 years of age. Approximately 130 of every 1 million children are found to have cancer each year. Given this low frequency, when a child is diagnosed with cancer, often he or she is the only one in a community who has cancer. As a result, the child with cancer may become the cause célèbre of his or her town, or, alternatively, may feel like an outcast. No matter how rare cancer may be in children, once your child, sibling, granddaughter, nephew, neighbor, or friend is diagnosed with cancer, the statistics regarding the risks of cancer have little meaning to you.

WHAT TYPES OF CANCER OCCUR IN CHILDREN?

Leukemia and central nervous system tumors (brain tumors) are the two most common forms of childhood cancer. Some 55 percent of children with cancer have one of these types (leukemias account for 35 percent and brain tumors for 20 percent). Less common cancers in children include lymphomas (12 percent), neuroblastomas (tumors of nervous system tissue, 8 percent), Wilms' tumors (tumors of the kidney, 6 percent); rhabdomyosarcomas (soft tissue tumors, 3 percent), retinoblastomas (tumors of the eye, 3 percent), osteosarcomas (tumors of bone, 3 percent), Ewing's sarcomas (tumors of bone or soft tissues, 2 percent), and other tumors (8 percent).

The types of cancers that affect children vary according to age. Under the age of 6, the most common cancers are acute lymphoblastic leukemia (ALL), neuroblastoma, and Wilms' tumor. Hodgkin's lymphoma and bone tumors are seen most often in teenagers. Brain tumors and non-Hodgkin's lymphoma occur at the same rate across age groups.

IS CHILDHOOD CANCER AS BAD AS IT WAS 30 YEARS AGO?

Today, more than 70 percent of cases of childhood cancer can be cured. Although 30 years ago childhood cancer was often viewed as a terminal illness, significant advances in cancer diagnosis and treatment have been made. In slightly over two decades, the 5-year survival rate for children with ALL increased from 35 to 80 percent (1993 data). More recent statistics indicate that survival rates for children with this disease may be even higher. As a result, the approaches to children with cancer and to their care have changed.

WHAT DOES CANCER MEAN TO A CHILD?

A child's understanding of his or her diagnosis of cancer will depend on the child's age and the diagnosis. This chapter addresses the unique issues associated with the three age groups in childhood: preschool (2 to 6 years); grade school (7 to 12 years); and adolescence (13 years and above) (Table 9-1).

WHAT WILL MY PRESCHOOLER UNDERSTAND?

Children aged 2 to 6 engage in "magical thinking" (a mix of reality and fantasy) and have an egocentric point of view (seeing themselves as the center of everything) in interpreting the world around them. This combination of magical thinking and egocentricity leads a child to believe that his or her illness is a punishment for a bad thought or deed. The child's inability to differentiate fact from fantasy extends to the concept of illness. Children at this age are unable to understand the concept of chance. They tend to associate past acts with the development of their illness. For example, a 4-year-old boy may think he is sick because he took his sister's toy or ate too many cookies. As a result, these children need to be told that nothing they did or thought has caused them to be sick.

Cancer treatment often requires multiple hospital admissions and clinic visits. Therefore, frequent reminders are needed to ensure that your child does not think

TABLE 9-1 Age and Reaction to Cancer

Age	Reaction
2–6	Believes that his or her illness is a punishment for a bad thought or deed; may have body-image anxiety and a perception of whole-body vulnerability; fear of being left alone.
7–12	Better able to understand the concept of illness and to conceptualize how the illness or symptoms of the illness may occur; may temporarily lose some coping skills; may have concerns about looking different (e.g., losing hair) and the impact this will have on peer relationships.
13 and up	Particularly focused on independence, on physical appearance, and on acceptance by a peer group; noncompliance with medical regimens poses a significant obstacle to care within this age group, which uses the same coping styles as adults, including denial, anger, and eventual acceptance.

the treatment is a punishment for his or her behavior. This is particularly important because procedures and treatment side effects may often feel like punishment.
New medications and techniques can minimize the pain and suffering a child experiences during treatment. For example, EMLA cream, a local anesthetic, can be
applied to the blood draw site prior to the use of a needle; this decreases the child's
discomfort or pain. In addition, effective anti-nausea medications can be given to
children prior to the initiation of chemotherapy treatments.

Preschoolers are beginning to develop an awareness of their bodies and a pride
in their capabilities. This is accompanied by a heightened concern about their bodies, a concept referred to as body-image anxiety. Their perception is one of whole-
body vulnerability. A 4-year-old boy with a brain tumor may say, "my whole body
is sick," even though only one organ system is involved. He will think that not only
his head is sick but also his arms and stomach. The idea of illness in only one area
is difficult for a young child to grasp, especially as each of his body parts is involved
in his treatment. He may have intravenous lines (IVs) in his arms, lose hair from
his head, and have stomachaches from his medication. Frequently, the use of medical play dolls helps facilitate discussion with the child about the illness and its
treatment.

WHAT QUESTIONS WILL MY PRESCHOOLER PROBABLY ASK?

Preschoolers are completely dependent on adults. They rely on familiar family
members to protect them from unknown situations and to explain what is happening to them. Many parents try to anticipate their child's questions and worries.
Children ask many questions, but usually they are focused on the moment and not
on the severity of the diagnosis. It is important to follow the child's lead; try not
to assume that you know what his or her fears or concerns will be. For example,
in this age group, the fear of being left alone is paramount. When a procedure is
planned (e.g., a lumbar puncture or a computed tomography scan) or a hospital
visit is scheduled, preschool children will want to know who will be with them and
what will happen to them. Explain to the child in language he or she can understand where the procedure will take place, what the procedure will involve, and
who will be with him or her during and after the procedure. If the child asks if the
procedure will hurt, be honest. It will not help if you mislead your child and say
that a procedure is not going to hurt (as a way to get that child to agree to coop-
erate). If children cannot trust what you tell them, they will never know when to
believe you.

WHAT QUESTIONS DO PARENTS ASK REGARDING THE CARE
OF A PRESCHOOLER?

Parents often ask what their child will remember from their treatment, be it
chemotherapy, radiation therapy, or surgery. Most young children do not re-

member the details of their treatment. If pain is controlled, in future years a child likely will refer to the treatment as an important but not necessarily bad event that occurred in the past. One may hear, "I was sick 5 years ago and spent a lot of time in the hospital, but I am better now."

Parents frequently want to know which of their child's behaviors will change and how they can manage these changes. A child with cancer often regresses in some areas of behavior and development. Frequently, a previously toilet-trained child becomes a bed wetter; a child who loved to eat new foods refuses to eat; or a child who slept in his or her own room retreats to his or her parents' room nightly. Although these changes are common, they are not permanent. After a hospital admission, when the family is back at home, parents can address these issues individually and in a manner that feels comfortable for both the child and his or her parents. It is important to assess why some of these behaviors persist. A child sometimes sleeps with his or her parents because it is comforting for them all. After they have shared a hospital room with their child for weeks to months, some parents find it difficult not to be at their child's side. Encouraging one's child to regain milestones that were achieved in the past is healthy for both the child and for his or her parents.

Parents often wonder what expectations they should have of their child while that child is in treatment. Children typically respond to structure and to the setting of limits. If your daughter was previously responsible for picking up her toys, this expectation should continue when you are at home. It often is comforting for children to view their parents as omnipotent once again. Children do not want to be thought of as sick; the more they are treated in the same way as their healthy siblings or peers, the better they will feel.

WHAT WILL MY GRADE-SCHOOL (AGES 7 TO 12) CHILD UNDERSTAND?

Children aged 7 to 12 are in school and part of a peer group. Often, this period for a child is called the "mastery phase" of development. Children in this phase are learning to achieve goals and to accomplish tasks in school. They are better able to understand the concept of illness and to conceptualize how the illness or symptoms of the illness may occur. For example, a 9-year-old may say, "I have leg pain because of my bone tumor." School-age children also are able to appreciate the concept of "good" and "bad" cells. This allows them to understand better the idea and the need for chemotherapy and radiation therapy as a way to kill the "bad" cancer cells.

When children are confronted with the diagnosis and treatment of cancer, they may temporarily lose some of their coping (and cognitive) skills. They are at risk of developing a sense of inadequacy in the face of a serious illness. A 10-year-old who previously loved science and talked about how the body works may now have a distorted or magical notion about the etiology of his or her illness. It is important to elicit the child's current understanding and to correct any misconceptions.

Sharing with a child the names of medications or how an IV pump works can help facilitate his or her understanding and mastery of the disease and can enhance his or her ability to cope with these changes.

School-age children are developing peer groups and relationships outside of their nuclear family. Children want to "fit in" with their peers and to be perceived as the same as classmates and friends. They may have concerns about looking different (e.g., losing their hair) and the impact this will have on their peer relationships. To counteract a sense of alienation that may develop, it is important to encourage contact with classmates. If a child is medically able, attending school will decrease his or her sense of isolation. Often, parents arrange a part-time schedule for their child at school that allows for visits to the hospital and takes into account the child's energy level and medical condition. Children may be reluctant to return to school because they feel and/or look different than their peers. Most children will need support from family, staff, and their school to help with their reintegration into the classroom. Often, the oncology team offers assistance with back-to-school programs that facilitate the child's reentry into school and address the child's and the school's concerns. Teachers and school nurses may want to know what they should expect from the child and what information they should share with the child's classmates. The oncology team can help with this transition by speaking or visiting with the school. School reentry can be a positive and rewarding experience for the child as he or she gains a better sense of health and "normalcy."

WHAT QUESTIONS WILL MY GRADE-SCHOOL CHILD ASK?

Curiosity and inquisitiveness are prominent themes in this age group. School-age children often ask many questions. A child may want to know not only what kind of cancer he or she has but also what it means to have it. Parents and staff are sometimes confronted with questions they are not comfortable answering (e.g., "Will I die?"). Before responding, it is important to understand the source of the child's question. It may be that the only other person the child knew who had cancer (e.g., a grandfather) died, or that a child at school asked if he or she was going to die.

Identification of the underlying reason for a child's question helps in the formulation of a response. The best approach is to answer children as openly and honestly as possible. If you are uncomfortable answering a question or do not know the answer, it is reasonable to say to a child, "I don't know" and to promise to ask the doctor or nurse. This can give parents time to discuss how they want to answer a question as well as time to obtain more information.

WHAT IS THE IMPACT OF CANCER ON ADOLESCENTS?

Adolescence is a time of significant growth and development. Multiple developmental tasks are approached and pose challenges in this phase of life. Adolescents are particularly focused on their independence, on their physical appearance, and their acceptance by their peer group. Maintenance of their autonomy in the face of a diagnosis of cancer is difficult but possible. Although adolescents are cognitively able to understand the concepts of illness and death, they may be unable to apply this knowledge to their own situation.

At their stage of life, adolescents are struggling to establish independence from their parents; yet they may need and want to rely on their parents in new ways once they have been diagnosed with cancer. Finding a balance between these needs and desires is crucial during the treatment of an adolescent with cancer. Often, adolescents want to make their own decisions; this may be expressed as resentment of authority figures (including parents and physicians). Hence, noncompliance with medical regimens poses a significant obstacle to care within this age group. If a teenager knows that a particular treatment may cause unacceptable side effects (such as weight gain or baldness), he or she may decide to not take the required medication. It is important to encourage these youngsters to ask questions and discuss the actual and/or potential impact of the illness and its treatment on their appearance, ability, sexuality, and overall functioning. This will help increase compliance and facilitate a more open and honest relationship between the adolescent and his or her caregivers.

Peer-group acceptance and physical appearance are paramount to the adolescent. This is a time of significant physical change, including the development of secondary sexual characteristics (e.g., hair growth, breast development, or a deepening voice). Procedures and treatments that may alter an adolescent's appearance (e.g., amputation and baldness) or limit his or her participation in a defining activity (e.g., basketball, ballet, or band) may threaten his or her perception of acceptance in a peer group. Anticipating and appreciating the dilemmas and challenges a teenager with cancer faces will help facilitate compliance with treatment and an understanding of what is involved.

HOW WILL MY ADOLESCENT CHILD REACT AND FUNCTION?

Adolescents frequently use the same coping styles as adults, including denial, anger, and eventual acceptance. However, because these defenses are complicated by dependency issues, other factors also play a role in an adolescent's acceptance of his or her illness.

Frequently, parents will ask how their child will do during and after treatment. The best predictor of posttreatment function is pre-illness function. If a teenager was an honor student prior to a cancer diagnosis, it is likely that he or she will continue to do well in school after the diagnosis. Similarly, if a teenager was shy before the discovery of cancer, he or she will likely be shy during and after treatment.

Although adolescents try to establish themselves as independent, some regress as they become reliant on their parents in response to their diagnosis. Some teenagers may exhibit increased levels of anxiety and social withdrawal; others assert themselves through noncompliance with treatment and with risk-taking behaviors. When treatment ends, adolescents find themselves back in the middle of everyday adolescent issues with their peers; however, many feel more mature because of their experience. Some say they have gained a new perspective on life and on their future. Others say they feel like everyone else and they enjoy that feeling. Some express concerns that although their friends try to appreciate what they have been through, they really don't "get it."

HOW WILL SIBLINGS DEAL WITH THE CRISIS OF CANCER?

A child with cancer is part of a family system; each person in that system will be affected greatly by the diagnosis. The siblings of children diagnosed with cancer frequently feel left out. Parents spend a lot of time at the hospital and are often preoccupied when they are home with the needs of their ill child. Some children act up or act out (e.g., by doing poorly in school or by fighting at home) to obtain more attention from their parents or from other adults, even if it means getting negative attention. Others will take on more adult roles (e.g., by making their own school lunch or by not asking for help with homework) as a way to minimize their needs at home. Another way a sibling may cope is to spend more time away from home and from the ill sibling as a means of denying that anything is wrong.

It is important not to overlook the needs of the other children. A few important steps can help healthy siblings feel more a part of the family system during this difficult time. You should include siblings in discussions about the child's illness, maintain routines for them at home and school (as much as possible), and invite them to join you on a visit to the hospital or clinic. These steps will help demystify the child's illness and treatment and will allow siblings to feel more involved in their brother's or sister's care.

HOW WILL PARENTS REACT TO THEIR CHILD'S CANCER?

How do you even begin to understand and accept that your child has cancer? After hearing the diagnosis, parents frequently listen to the treatment plans, read and sign consent forms, and start treatments with their child without really digesting what they have been told. As time passes and as they obtain more information, they become better able to integrate the diagnosis and treatment plan for their child. Parents often ask if there is some activity in which they participated (e.g., taking a medicine during a pregnancy) that caused their child to develop cancer. Unlike many adult cancers, the types of cancer seen in children are not associated with lifestyle choices (such as smoking or drinking) and are much less likely to be associated with environmental exposures.

Many parents say they wish they could trade places with their child. Parents may feel that they are better able to face and to cope with the diagnosis and treatment of cancer. Bearing the physical pain of treatment may be less difficult than bearing the emotional pain of watching one's child go through treatment. Using these feelings to advocate for one's child can help ensure that he or she receives the best possible care.

Parents not only support their child through their treatment but also need the support of others. Seeking help from family, friends, and staff at the hospital is crucial in maintaining balance and caring most effectively for your child. It is difficult to recognize that your own needs are not being met when a child is ill. Many parents neither want to take time for themselves nor feel comfortable doing so when their child is ill. However, those who are able to care for themselves will often be better able to care for their child. For example, during a lengthy hospital admission, trading places with a spouse or relative for a couple of nights may give the primary caretaking parent a chance to get some sleep and restore energy while at home.

WHAT TYPES OF SUPPORTS ARE AVAILABLE?

Almost all children diagnosed with cancer are treated within a childhood cancer center. Cancer centers have a number of support systems in place for children and their parents (Table 9-2). Social workers are available to work with families and their children. Child psychologists and psychiatrists help address the individual concerns and needs of children in treatment. Child-life specialists use art projects and activities to help children cope with their hospitalizations. Support groups for parents of children with cancer are also available. Frequently, parents comment that these groups allow them to gain support from others in similar situations and to use their experience to assist other parents. Other important resources are religious institutions and community organizations.

Many organizations give children with cancer opportunities they otherwise might not be able to enjoy. Several summer camps for children with cancer are available at no cost to participants. These camps offer children nonmedical envi-

TABLE 9-2 **Supports Available for Those with Childhood Cancer**

Cancer center-based support groups
Social workers
Child psychologists
Child psychiatrists
Child-life specialists
Religious groups
Community organizations
Summer camps for children with cancer
Make-a-Wish foundations
Information found in libraries and on the Internet

ronments where they are able to enjoy themselves while talking freely about their illness; they need not be embarrassed by their baldness or their need to take multiple medications. Many establish lasting friendships with others they meet through these activities. Some camps include the whole family in the experience. Wish foundations also are widely used by children with cancer. Once designed for the child with a terminal illness, programs such as Make-A-Wish are now available for most children who are being treated for cancer. These organizations give children and their families the opportunity to enjoy dream vacations (e.g., meetings with movie stars) and to fulfill other wishes.

WHAT DOES TERMINAL CARE FOR THE CHILD WITH CANCER INVOLVE?

Although most children with cancer are cured, some do not survive. Taking care of these children at the end of life is an important and integral part of their treatment. Terminal care for the child at home has become more available and more accepted by families and medical teams alike. Quality of life is cited as one of the main reasons that parents and children choose this option. Use of hospice services is vital in facilitating families' wishes to provide terminal care for their children. Visiting nurses and access to medical care enable families to feel adequately prepared to care for their child at home. Pain relief and minimization of suffering are parents' and patients' main concerns; they are key factors in ensuring that a child's remaining time at home will be peaceful. Hospice care allows families to play a more active role in their child's last days.

On the other hand, some families feel more comfortable having their child in the hospital his or her last days. Being surrounded by the doctors and nurses who have cared for their child during the illness is comforting and reassuring for many. Respecting the wishes of the child and his or her parents as to where they would like to be taken care of is paramount.

HOW CAN I DEAL WITH THE DEATH OF A CHILD WITH CANCER?

The death of a child is an enormous tragedy. No one can be fully prepared for the impact of such a loss. After a child's death, the grieving process for a parent is life-long. Parents' grieving styles may differ. A mother may want to talk about her son and to maintain his room and keep his belongings where they were throughout the house, whereas a father may not want to hear his son's name mentioned or to see any of his possessions. Respecting each other's ways of grieving is important in the healing process. Support groups are available nationwide for those who have lost a child or family member to cancer (e.g., Compassionate Friends and Candlelighters). These groups are particularly important in helping people overcome their isolation after their loss (see Chap. 33 for more information).

SUMMARY

Childhood cancer is a rare occurrence. When cancer is diagnosed, it has a significant impact on the child, the family, and the community. Developments in diagnosis and treatment have changed the course of childhood cancer. New therapies are being developed and survival rates continue to rise. Addressing the needs of children in age-appropriate ways will improve the overall quality of their care.

CHAPTER 10

Helping Children Cope with a Parent's Cancer

Paula K. Rauch, M.D.
Stephen Durant, Ed.D.

OUTLINE

WILL MY CHILD BE OVERWHELMED AND MISERABLE BECAUSE OF MY CANCER?

Many parents feel overwhelmed about the diagnosis of cancer and feel guilty about the impact their illness may have on their children. Many imagine that this will be a magnified version of their own experiences. However, children are far more resilient than parents anticipate. Each child copes with a parent's illness according to his or her phase of development, temperament, and pre-illness coping style. Children take their coping cues from their parents. By understanding how a child at a given developmental stage views a parent's illness and by maximizing the key supports that help a child flourish, parents can ensure that their children will cope better than they ever could have imagined.

WHICH CHILDREN ARE LIKELY TO HAVE MORE TROUBLE COPING?

Children who have had difficulties (such as anxiety, depression, difficulty making or keeping friends, difficulty with schoolwork, or having conflicted relationships with close family members) before the onset of a parent's illness will be at greater risk for coping poorly with a parent's illness. Parents of such children will need to increase the supports that were helpful to their child before the onset of their illness and to anticipate that these difficult areas (which are already challenging for their child), will be further strained by the added stress of diagnosis and treatment.

Children of single-parent families or of families in which there is significant parental discord will also need additional support. During an ill parent's diagnosis and treatment, the child will be looking to the well parent for additional reassurances, security, love, and a shared concern for the ill parent. When the well parent is not viewed by the child as someone who holds the ill parent in high regard, he or she will need another loving adult or professional with whom these concerns can be shared.

DOES MY CHILD NEED TO KNOW ABOUT THE CANCER?

If your child is old enough to speak, you need to tell him or her about the cancer diagnosis. Children of all ages are perceptive and will sense a change in the emotional atmosphere of the family following such a diagnosis. Younger children are at risk of interpreting the shift in mood as evidence that their bad behavior is the cause of parental sadness, withdrawal, or tension. Older children are likely to learn of the diagnosis when they overhear discussions in the house, from a relative, or from another child.

Learning about a parent's cancer indirectly (by overhearing information about it) is problematic in many ways. It may suggest to your child that the news is too awful to speak about aloud. It may deliver the message that your child's feelings are not important enough to you to warrant direct attention, in contrast to others with whom you are engaged directly. News that is overheard is also most likely to be inaccurate, confused, and confusing. Perhaps most troubling, however, is that children who feel that key information is not being shared are left to ferret out information from "clues," which leads to a belief that the ill parent will not be honest or forthcoming.

CAN WE CALL THE CANCER BY ANOTHER NAME TO AVOID THE SCARY CONNOTATIONS OF THE WORD CANCER?

Using the words *cancer, brain tumor,* or *leukemia*, instead of using euphemisms such as *lump, bump, blood sickness,* or *boo-boo* is more protective of your children's feelings and gives you an opportunity to educate your children about your (the parent's) cancer. Euphemisms are confusing at any age and often leave a child feeling that serious illness and chemotherapy, hair loss, and radiation may follow their own lumps, bumps, or viral illnesses; this is scary. Furthermore, the naming of the cancer provides an important opportunity for you to talk with your child about how dissimilar different cancers are from one another and how even the same cancer can follow a different course in different people. This creates another opportunity for you to remind your child that he or she should not assume that what was heard about someone else's cancer is relevant to your condition. Rather, your child should share what he or she hears about cancer with you, so as not to worry unnecessarily or to be confused.

HOW WILL THE AGE OF MY CHILD AFFECT WHAT I TELL HIM OR HER ABOUT MY CANCER?

Simple explanations are best at any age, and the discussion you have with your child will be informed by his or her questions. Still, it is helpful to have a sense of how children of different ages may hear the explanation and how they are likely to understand the diagnosis of cancer.

Preschool Children

Preschool children (aged 3 to 6 years) engage in magical thinking; this means that they weave together fantasy and reality in their own idiosyncratic way and imagine themselves as the causal center of events that occur in their lives. For example, one 5-year-old might report that his mother's cancer grew inside her along with him, while another child might believe that her father got his cancer because she jumped on his chest on the day that he said she was hurting him. Feeling as though they were the cause of events (i.e., normal preschool egocentricity) leads to a sense of responsibility for the parent's illness (which can increase the child's anxiety or aggression). The anxious child feels frighteningly powerful and is fearful of causing additional harm to the people he or she loves. Such a child will become either clingy or withdrawn.

In contrast, aggressive children feel too overwhelmed to contain their feelings and frequently try to control other situations by overpowering peers or using force to get their own way. Preschoolers are often anxious or aggressive even without an ill parent, so it can be difficult to decide what part of this behavior can be ascribed fairly to the parent's cancer and what part is consistent with normal development. In general, you should remind your children that your cancer was not caused by something they did, thought, or said. Children will need to be reminded repeatedly that they are not responsible for the fatigue of chemotherapy or your irritability because of gaffes in scheduling. In addition to these reminders, they should be invited to talk about what they think is causing the cancer or the mood in the household in order to make sure that potential misconceptions are dispelled.

School-Age Children

School-age children (aged 7 to 12 years) are old enough to understand that a parent's cancer is not caused by a child's actions. Nevertheless, under the stress of changes in family life, they may regress at times and feel somehow responsible. They, too, need to be invited to voice thoughts about the cause of the cancer. Typically, school-age children understand that the world is ordered. They expect that illness should follow a set of rules and respond fairly to treatment, and that if the parent follows the doctor's rules for treatment, the cancer should be cured. Relapse and recurrence are especially hard for children of this age to accept. Most understand that germs are the means of illness transmission. In the setting of cancer treatment, the focus on protecting a parent with a compromised immune system from exposure to viral illnesses and emphasizing careful hand washing is often interpreted by children as evidence that it is possible to catch the cancer. Unless this misconception is corrected, the child may become anxious and withdraw from the ill parent. Finally, children of this age think that cancer is the result of cigarette smoking and therefore feel it is unfair if a nonsmoking parent gets cancer.

Adolescents

Adolescents can understand the full meaning of a cancer diagnosis, including the uncertainty about prognosis and the absence of guarantees despite adherence to a treatment regimen. A teen bearing this worrisome uncertainty may try to force his or her parents to make promises (such as the promise not to die) that cannot be kept. When parents make promises that cannot be kept, the adolescent becomes angrier and more mistrustful. Rather than promises, adolescents need parental empathy regarding the stress of uncertainty and hopeful strategies (e.g., "I cannot promise that the cancer will be cured, but I plan to live every day believing that is true until I learn otherwise" or "I have worries sometimes, but I also have lots of times when I forget that I am sick and I hope you will try to do the same").

Many adolescents will throw themselves into peer relationships and activities and thereby minimize the time with the ill parent or the family. Parents need to find a balance between facilitating this age-appropriate engagement, adopting a healthy coping strategy, and protecting some one-to-one time and family time. Two key reasons exist to protect some family and parent-child time. First, it is impossible to supervise teens or to be aware of their mood and functioning if they are never at home. Second, if the parent dies from the cancer, the teen may regret having spent so little time with the family, particularly with the ill parent.

Adolescents often have a better relationship with one parent and a more prickly relationship with the other. When the ill parent is the one with whom the child has the prickly relationship, it is helpful for the child to hear that people who love each other get irritated or mad at each other. This does not mean that the parent is unloved by the child or vice versa.

HOW CAN I GET MY CHILD TO TALK WITH ME ABOUT MY CANCER?

It is essential for you to give your child an age-appropriate explanation of your cancer and its treatment. This gives your child the necessary tools to talk with you. Next, you should create an atmosphere that welcomes discussion whenever it occurs. Some children are talkers and some tend to keep their thoughts to themselves. If your child was not a "big talker" before your diagnosis, he or she is unlikely to become one now. When new information is shared, your child should be invited to ask questions and then be invited to ask questions again several hours or a day later, after having some time to mull over the new information. Parents usually discover that there are settings that lend themselves to a particular child's opening up. Often, children choose to talk in the car, at bedtime, or while doing an activity, like cooking, with a parent.

When your child asks a question, you should encourage elaboration of the question. The goal is to be sure that you understand the real question on your child's mind. As adults, we may imagine that a question is more comprehensive than it is. For example, a child might ask, "Will you be all better by the summertime?" You might think your child is looking for a guaranteed cure. However, after asking, "What are you wondering about?" he or she might in turn reply, "If you're sick, how will I get to swim lessons?" Teasing out the real question helps you (the parent) address the real worry; many times, what is revealed is a concrete concern that has an easy solution.

The less talkative child may not come up with many of his or her own questions but may engage more readily in questions about the way your illness or treatment affects him or her. For example, asking, "How do you feel about my breast cancer?" may get a shrug or a grunt, while asking "How is it working out having Billy's mom do all the driving to soccer practice?" may get more of a response. You also can try specific questions about the effect of the cancer on you: "Has anyone commented on my bald head?" or, "Am I grumpier since I started on chemotherapy?" Following up on questions that get shrugs or one-word answers with a general explanation (to convey why you are asking) is helpful. For example, "I know there are changes in me and changes in our regular schedule because of my cancer, and I really care about how it is going for you."

Sometimes parents who feel that their children are not talking enough about the cancer actually need another adult to talk to about it. Remember, having a parent with cancer is a different experience from having a spouse with cancer or having cancer yourself. Children may want to have fewer and shorter conversations than an adult would. So be patient. If your child is continuing to engage in favorite activities with friends and family and doing okay at school, you should feel reassured.

WHAT IF MY CHILD ASKS ME A QUESTION I CAN'T ANSWER?

You can welcome questions warmly without having an immediate answer. Ask your child what got him or her wondering about this question, and tell your child that it is a good question. Good questions deserve thoughtful answers; you should determine whom else you might want to talk with (such as your spouse, doctor, or clergyperson) so that you can give a quality answer. It also is reasonable to reply that the question being asked is a hard one and that you want to think about your answer to be sure that it is what you really believe before actually responding. The key is to understand the question and to let your child know you will come back to him or her with an answer in the near future. Some questions are hard to answer because no one knows the right answer. Uncertainty is hard for anyone at any age, but it is especially hard for children (who rely on parents to have all the answers). It is acceptable to say that you too find "not knowing" difficult and that you cope with uncertainty by keeping busy, doing fun things, or trying to be optimistic.

ARE THERE THINGS I CAN DO AT HOME THAT WILL HELP MY CHILD DURING MY CANCER TREATMENT?

Protect your family time. Turn on the answering machine during meals and don't answer the phone. Encourage friends and family to call during times when your children are at school and to communicate by e-mail, so that the children are not listening (after school and in the evening) to endless talk about your illness. Ask a family member or a close friend to be the "point person" and direct any acts of kindness toward activities or gifts that will help the children. For example, let people know that if they want to cook a meal, your children will eat macaroni and cheese; the duck in orange sauce will go untouched.

It also is important to explain to your children that chemotherapy makes you feel queasy and that you take antinausea medicine that makes you sleepy on treatment days. The more they can differentiate the effect of the cancer from the effect of the treatment and how these factors affect life at home, the better. This helps explain new household routines and makes the home time feel more stable.

SHOULD I TELL MY CHILD'S SCHOOL ABOUT MY CANCER?

Yes. It is important that your child's teachers know what is going on at home. Teachers also need to know that school should be allowed to be, as much as possible, a haven from the cancer for the child. If your child chooses to talk about your illness with friends, that is his or her choice. Teachers should not introduce this information into the classroom discussion. If a child shares worries or concerns with a teacher about the parent's cancer, the teacher should let the parents know. Most teachers are relieved to hear that parents want them to continue to act as teachers, not as counselors. If a child is having academic difficulties, the teacher should let the parents know sooner rather than later. Some teachers may think they are protecting already stressed parents by withholding this information. To the contrary, knowing early allows you and your child to come up with an action plan that may include a reduced workload, tutoring, or special homework time.

Some teachers who have experienced cancer treatment or lost a family member to cancer may feel it helpful to share this with the child—that it will make the child feel less alone. A teacher may feel that your child's learning about such details will help your child. In fact, children younger than adolescents find this information burdensome and unsolicited. While with adolescents a teacher may try to connect around a shared experience, even a teen should not be flooded with the details of the teacher's experience.

SHOULD MY CHILD VISIT ME IN THE HOSPITAL?

A child of any age who wants to visit a parent should be allowed to do so if possible. The child does need to be prepared with a description of how the parent looks (including having intravenous medicine and a roommate or wearing an oxygen mask or a hospital gown) in the hospital. Some parents may even send home a Polaroid picture of themselves to show a child in advance of the visit; this should help decrease the discomfort of being surprised and overwhelmed.

If you have more than one child coming for a visit or if the family member bringing the child or children also wants to visit with you, it is important to bring another familiar adult. This person should be comfortable staying only as long as the child feels comfortable in the hospital room. This other adult can take one or more children down to the cafeteria or outside for a walk (if after a minute or two the child is ready to leave). For younger children, it is especially nice to bring some art materials—paper and markers—so that while in the room or in another location the child can draw or even make a picture for the parent's bedside.

Parents may worry that looking ill or hooked up to machinery is too frightening for a child. Experience suggests that for most children, particularly those who are asking to visit, imagination creates a more frightening scenario than the real setting. If a parent has just completed a surgical procedure and expects to feel much better in 24 to 48 hours, the parent may elect to postpone the visit for a short time so that he or she can be more interactive when the children do visit. This presupposes that no one believes the parent to be in any immediate medical danger and that the parent will see the children after this short recuperative period. If a parent is gravely ill, the children should have the option to see and to speak to the parent without delay.

WHAT SHOULD I DO AFTER THE CHILDREN VISIT?

After a visit, each child needs an opportunity to talk about how it felt to see the parent in the hospital. Often, this occurs on the trip home. The adult taking the child home should inquire whether the child was surprised by what he or she saw or felt; answer questions stirred up by the visit; and inquire whether the child is pleased or regretful at having visited. The child's range of positive and negative feelings should be validated. This dialogue will help both you and your child think about structuring, facilitating, or limiting future visits according to your child's responses. One healthy message to your child is that you want to help him or her find coping strategies that may be useful in dealing with challenging circumstances. Using the responses of your child is always better than assuming that you know what is best for your child.

IS IT DIFFERENT TO HAVE A CHILD VISIT IF THE PARENT IS DYING?

At the end of life, it is usually recommended that children have a chance to say goodbye. If your child wants to have this opportunity or even is neutral about it, he or she should be supported in having the chance to do so. If a child is adamant that he or she does not want to see you, that child may accompany others to the hospital and stay with a familiar adult in the waiting area outside the room but on the hospital floor. Here, the reluctant-to-enter child may speak or write a message to the parent, which can be conveyed by another loved family member or friend, or the child may be invited to go into the room for a few seconds to say or think some good-bye words.

When a parent is in a coma and unresponsive, telling the child that we do not know what someone in this state can hear (but we believe that he or she may sense loved ones in the room) seems helpful. Then, the child can be encouraged to say aloud or to think anything he or she wants the parent to know. Often, the child will simply say "I love you," "good-bye," or "I will miss you." This is an important time for other loving adults to remind the child that the parent knew that he or she was loved by the child and loved the child in return. If there was conflict in the relationship between the parent and the child, acknowledging this fact and re-iterating the shared love is helpful. For example, "Even though you and Dad got into lots of arguments, people who love each other often get really mad at each other, and Dad always loved you and knew you loved him."

IS THERE ANYTHING I CAN DO BEFORE THE END OF MY LIFE TO HELP MY CHILDREN?

It is important that you continue to live every day that you have (Table 10-1). Do not underestimate the value of your children being able to tell you about the daily activities of life (such as the grade on a spelling test, who scored at the soccer game, or the unfair thing a classmate said). Children flourish when they feel that the minutiae of their lives are important to a loved parent. Take advantage of opportunities to celebrate (e.g., birthdays, holidays, a first lost tooth, a great basketball season, or a prom). Take pictures or videos of the happy times so they will be recorded (and available) for the child. Some parents write letters to each child describing their early years together as well as their special memories and admirable traits. Sometimes, these letters also give the child some general advice (such as work hard and be true to yourself, or surround yourself with people who see the best in you).

Either in conversations with the child or in such a letter, it is useful to let the child know that you hope he or she will be close to other loving adults; in addition, you can give the child permission to attach to other adults without feeling disloyal to the dying parent. For example, telling the child, "I hope you will get closer and closer to Aunt Janet, and other quality women like Sarah's mom. Using those relationships to make good choices for yourself will make me proud."

Celebrate your own birthdays or special events. You can use one of these occasions as an opportunity to ask friends and family to collect old pictures of you and to write down funny stories about you as a child or in more recent years. Collecting these accounts provides the children with another vehicle for really knowing

TABLE 10-1 **Strategies to Help Your Children as You Near the End of Life**

Continue to live every day you have.

Do not underestimate the value of your child being able to tell you about the daily activities of life (such as the grade on a spelling test, who scored at the soccer game, or the unfair thing a classmate said).

Take advantage of opportunities to celebrate (e.g., birthdays, holidays, a great basketball season).

Take pictures or videos of the happy times so that they will be recorded for your child.

Write letters to your child describing your early years together.

Communicate to your child that you hope he or she will be close to other living adults.

Celebrate your own birthday.

Create a photo album for each child, annotated with stories about your family life.

you. It may be of interest now and can provide an opportunity for telling stories about your past; alternatively, these accounts may become interesting to a child later in childhood or in adulthood. Creating a photo album for each child, beginning with photos of you and your spouse together, pregnancy, baby pictures, and later ones can also serve as a memory book annotated by a parent or used as a stimulus for telling stories about different times in the life of the family.

CAN MEMORIAL SERVICES BE HELPFUL TO THE CHILDREN?

Memorial services can be meaningful to a child. They provide an opportunity for a child to see that the community cared for and valued the loved parent, and to share in the sadness of the loss. Memorial services are a special opportunity to ask friends and family to send photos and stories instead of flowers, which can enrich the children's knowledge of the parent who died. Children should be encouraged to participate in the services in ways that feel comfortable. Some children may want to speak, to play music, or to display something created for the parent. Some children may want to listen and to grieve privately. A child's emotional tolerance for being present at the memorial service, wake, shiva, or funeral needs to be respected. Older children need permission to go to a quiet place when they have had enough, and younger children need a familiar adult assigned to take them out of the service as needed.

WHEN SHOULD I THINK ABOUT HAVING MY CHILD SEE A MENTAL HEALTH PROFESSIONAL?

Any child who requests the opportunity to speak with someone outside the family should be assisted in doing so. Children who have had psychological difficulties that necessitated therapy prior to your cancer diagnosis may benefit from returning for support. Children who have a conflicted relationship with either the sick or the well parent may benefit from some counseling. If the child is in conflict with the well parent, he or she may feel particularly frightened by the vulnerability of the parent with whom he or she has a good relationship. If the parent with whom the child has the conflicted relationship is ill, the child may feel guilty about past behavior and haunted by angry, hurtful words exchanged in both directions. If there is significant discord between the parents, the child may benefit from having a counselor act as a neutral adult, one who can support the child's attachment to both parents as the parent's cancer is experienced.

Children who have symptoms of depression should be referred for help. These include a depressed mood for more than a couple of weeks, a change in sleep pattern, a change in appetite, a loss of interest in favorite activities, feelings of guilt, a loss of energy and concentration, and feelings that life is not worth living. Suicidal thoughts should be taken seriously and support should be sought quickly, even if the child is resistant to the idea.

Children who become anxious also need professional help. These children have anxiety that interferes with age-appropriate activities, including sleep, school, and friendships.

Some children may exhibit risk-taking behavior, including driving recklessly, taking dangerous dares, or abusing substances. These children need referral for professional help so that they do not hurt themselves or others.

ARE THERE SOME GUIDING PRINCIPLES FOR HELPING MY CHILD THROUGH MY CANCER DIAGNOSIS AND TREATMENT?

1. Try to maintain the child's usual daily routine. This includes sleeping, mealtimes, school, and leisure activities.
2. Demonstrate an active interest in the regular events of your child's day. Pay attention to the small stuff, because this makes home feel safe and makes the child feel important.
3. Give news bulletins so that your child does not learn new information by overhearing it. Overhearing difficult news leaves a child confused, undervalued, and silenced.
4. Be honest. Don't make promises you can't keep; once your child is uncertain about whether you can be trusted, he or she will always be looking for clues and won't believe your words.
5. Welcome all questions warmly and work to understand where and why the question originated. Don't feel you have to answer questions immediately. It is fine to take time to get helpful input and to think about your answer.
6. Remind children to share what they hear about your cancer from others. This allows you to correct misinformation and to encourage your child not to worry alone.

7. Prepare children for hospital visits by describing what they will see, especially how you will look. Bring along an adult who is happy to stay only as long as the child feels comfortable. Discuss the visit after leaving, including questions about what may have surprised the child, what was hard, what was fun, and how he or she feels about having made the visit.

8. Protect family time from intrusive, constant discussion of the cancer by limiting calls and visits during family time.

9. Let the school know about your cancer diagnosis and treatment. Encourage the teacher to take his or her lead from the child about how private this information should be kept. Ask to be informed about expressed worries concerning you, and to be informed early about any decline in school performance.

10. Seek professional counseling and support if your child asks to talk with someone outside of the family. Get assistance if he or she is anxious or depressed enough for it to interfere with favorite activities, with ongoing school performance, with friendships, or with sleep or appetite. Consultation is also beneficial when the picture is accompanied by risk-taking behavior, by substance use, or by expressions of life not being worth living.

CHAPTER 11

Diagnosis and Staging

WILLIAM KIM, M.D.

OUTLINE

WHAT TESTS ARE USED TO MAKE A CANCER DIAGNOSIS?

Numerous tests are used to make a diagnosis of cancer (Table 11-1). In some cases, there is a diagnostic test of choice (for example, a bone marrow biopsy is almost always used to make a diagnosis of leukemia), but often a battery of complementary tests is required to make a cancer diagnosis. The range of tests doctors order is highly dependent on the type of cancer suspected, but all of the tests share the common goal of either proving or disproving the diagnosis. In general, the types of tests used can be broadly grouped into (1) radiologic tests, (2) tissue biopsies (or obtaining pathology samples), and (3) blood tests. Each specific group of tests is described in more detail below.

Radiologic Testing

When the diagnosis of cancer is suspected, radiologic tests are frequently performed. These tests assist in the evaluation of a person's symptoms. They are also ordered purely for screening purposes. For example, a computed tomography (CT) scan of the chest might be obtained when a person complains of coughing up large amounts of blood, whereas a mammogram might be obtained for a woman beyond the age of 50 without complaints (i.e., for annual screening).

The types of radiologic tests vary. They include direct x-rays, such as mammograms and plain x-rays, both of which are classic radiographic imaging tools. A chest x-ray, for example, might show nodules (or masses) in the lungs, suggestive of cancer.

TABLE 11-1 Types of Tests Frequently Used to
Prove or Disprove a Cancer Diagnosis

Radiologic tests
    X-rays (e.g., chest x-ray, mammography)
    Computed tomography (CT) scans
    Magnetic resonance imaging (MRI) scans
    Ultrasound images
    Nuclear medicine scans
        Bone scans
        Gallium scans
        Positron emission tomography (PET) scans
Tissue biopsies
    Biopsies of tissues in specific organs or structures
        Lymph node biopsies
        Bone marrow biopsies
Blood tests
    Tumor markers
        Prostate-specific antigen (PSA)
        Carcinoembryonic antigen (CEA)

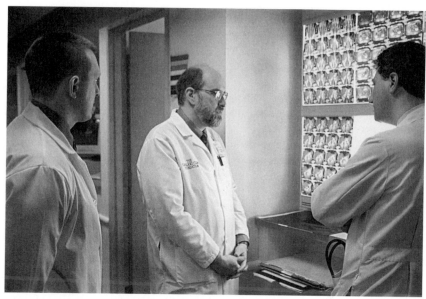

FIGURE 11-1 X-rays are one type of radiologic test.

More high-tech x-ray machines include CT and magnetic resonance imaging (MRI) scanners, which are able to take multiple sequential pictures of the body, much like looking at each slice of a loaf of bread. This allows doctors to visualize the internal organs with tremendous precision (Fig. 11-1). A CT scan of the abdomen might be performed in a patient with abdominal pain, and that scan could, for example, show a mass suggestive of cancer within the liver. Much like CT and MRI scans, ultrasounds also can be used to visualize internal organs and may be able to identify a mass within the liver.

Tests such as bone scans, gallium scans, and positron emission tomography (PET) scans, collectively called *nuclear medicine scans*, use a safe radioactive tracer that is injected into the bloodstream. These radioactive elements concentrate in areas of cell growth, such as tumors or infections. The tracer then can be seen when a picture of the body is taken. These studies are particularly good for imaging bone metastases (spread of cancer to bones) and lymphomas.

Finally, some words of caution are required regarding radiologic testing. First, high-tech tests such as MRI and PET scans are not always better than basic x-rays. Take, for example, the disease multiple myeloma, in which the bone lesions (tumors in the bone) tend to be lytic (i.e., they cause holes in the bone). In this setting, plain x-rays of the major bones detect the bone lesions much better than a sophisticated bone scan (which may overlook these lesions). More importantly, although x-rays, CT scans, mammograms, bone scans, gallium scans, PET scans, and MRIs can each be suggestive of cancer, it is impossible to make a diagnosis of cancer by radiologic tests alone. A presumptive diagnosis of cancer should almost always be verified by obtaining a pathologic specimen—a piece of tissue.

Tissue Biopsy and Pathology

Typically, the diagnosis of cancer is made by obtaining tissue from the organ thought to be involved with the cancer. This is called a *biopsy*. The tissue being biopsied may be the primary site (where the cancer originated) or a secondary site (where the cancer has spread to involve nearby lymph nodes or other organs). Often, a preliminary procedure—such as a CT or ultrasound-guided needle biopsy, colonoscopy, or bronchoscopy—will be done in an attempt to make the diagnosis of cancer. Sometimes this is sufficient and no further procedures are needed. However, in a fair percentage of cases, either the mass is not accessible by a minimally invasive procedure or an inconclusive biopsy (i.e., no diagnosis can be made from the tissue obtained) results and more invasive procedures, typically performed by a surgeon, are needed.

In some cancers—the "liquid tumors" (which include leukemia, myeloma, and lymphoma)—the cancerous cells may be readily accessible directly from the blood. Some types of leukemia can even be diagnosed by inspection of blood samples alone. However, most of the time (as is the case with solid tumors), the diagnosis rests on analysis of pathologic tissue samples. With lymphomas, samples are obtained from either a needle or surgical biopsy of a lymph node. In leukemia and myeloma, the pathologic sample is obtained directly from the bone marrow, using a procedure called a *bone marrow biopsy*.

After a piece of tissue is obtained, it is processed and examined under a microscope by a pathologist (Fig. 11-2). Depending on how the cells appear, either with or without special immunologic stains (dyes added to the tissue sample), the diagnosis of cancer is confirmed or disproved. A specialized tool in the detection of liquid tumors is *flow cytometry,* which involves use of a machine that sorts cells based on the "signature" of proteins that appear on the cell's surface as if the machine were reading bar codes on the cells to separate them. This test is often helpful in diagnosing and subclassifying leukemias.

Blood Tests and Tumor Markers

As mentioned above, the ultimate diagnosis of cancer depends on the analysis of a tissue sample. However, some blood tests, specifically tumor markers, can be helpful in making a cancer diagnosis. Tumor markers are proteins or chemicals found in the bloodstream that are produced by both cancerous and normal cells. Often, cancerous cells overproduce the tumor marker. Thus, when high levels of tumor markers are detected in the bloodstream, a diagnosis of cancer becomes more likely.

You might easily imagine that the use of tumor markers would be a quick and easy way to diagnose cancer. Unfortunately, the test is not foolproof. Because tumor markers are produced by both normal and cancerous cells, the presence of a

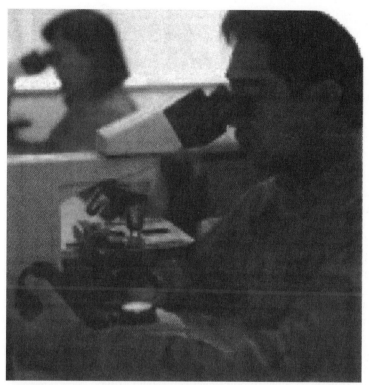

FIGURE 11-2 *After a piece of tissue is obtained from a biopsy, it is processed and examined under a microscope by a pathologist.*

marker does not always confirm a cancer diagnosis. For example, PSA (prostate-specific antigen) can be made by both normal prostate cells (and may be "elevated" in benign prostatic hypertrophy, or BPH) and cancerous cells of the prostate. Thus, detection of PSA proteins in the blood does not mean that a man has prostate cancer. Also, many other nonspecific disease processes can elevate tumor markers. For example, carcinoembryonic antigen (CEA), which is produced by many organs (including the colon, liver, and lungs), can be elevated either because cancer is present somewhere in the body or because of liver damage (which may occur with liver trauma or surgery on the liver).

Finally, with the exception of the PSA marker, which is used to detect prostate cancer, tumor markers are not tissue-specific. Thus, the detection of an elevated CEA does not point specifically toward colon cancer. It is produced by most gastrointestinal cancers and by cancers of the breast and lung. In summary, tumor markers do not reliably diagnose cancer. However, they can be useful to assess response to certain types of therapy or to detect a recurrence of a cancer.

WHAT INFORMATION SHOULD I BRING WITH ME TO MY FIRST APPOINTMENT WITH AN ONCOLOGIST?

The materials a person brings to the oncologist are important (Table 11-2). Information can expedite the evaluation process and lead to better medical care. Oncologists, like any other type of medical doctor, are interested in your general medical condition and in your medical and personal history.

In general, it is best to think ahead and to list the following:

1. Your medical history, including surgeries, along with the time of treatment. Pay particular attention to problems with your heart, lung, and kidneys and to medical conditions such as high blood pressure, diabetes, heart disease, and stroke.
2. Your allergies to medications and foods (and their specific effects upon you).
3. The medications you are currently taking. You should bring an updated list of each medication with doses and frequency of use.
4. Your family history of medical illnesses, paying particular attention to cancer.
5. Your pattern of smoking and drinking (e.g., how many packs per day you have smoked and how many alcoholic beverages do you drink in a week or month).

In addition, you should bring copies of your medical records from your doctor's office; these will be extremely helpful.

Specifically for an oncology appointment you should bring:

1. Office notes from the referring physician (even better is a summary of your recent medical history).
2. Results of radiology tests, including both the reports and the actual x-rays, MRI, and CT scans themselves.

TABLE 11-2 **Important Information to Bring with You to Your Oncologist's Office**

Your medical history
A list of your allergies to medications and foods
A list of your current medications
A list of the medical illnesses experienced by your family members
A description of your pattern of smoking and drinking
Copies of your medical records, including:
    Office notes from your physician
    Results of radiologic tests (and the actual x-rays or scans if available)
    Results of pathology reports (and the actual slides if available)
    A list of prior chemotherapy treatments (and the timing of them)
A list of questions for your doctor

3. Results of pathology reports and even the actual pathology slides; these reports are critical.

4. A list of previous chemotherapy treatments with their approximate dates.

By providing the above data, your first visit with the oncologist will run more smoothly. This will allow your oncology team to collect the needed information efficiently and to focus on important issues, such as explaining your disease and reviewing the pros and cons associated with your treatment options.

Last, it can be helpful to bring a friend or family member to your appointment. People who accompany you to appointments can be invaluable, not only for emotional support but also to help remember or to write down what you and your doctor discuss. Most people remember only a small fraction of what took place during a doctor's appointment. Prior to the appointment, you should think carefully about the questions you have for your doctor and write them down so you won't forget to ask them. If you have any unresolved questions following an initial consultation, you should address them with your oncology team, either by phone or during a subsequent appointment.

WHAT IS A CANCER STAGE?

Cancer staging is a system used to separate people with cancer into groups based on the characteristics of their cancer and the extent to which their cancer has spread. Each individual cancer can have a wide range of presentations—i.e., ways in which the cancer affects the individual when he or she first comes to a doctor's attention. For example, breast cancer can range from a small, pea-sized nodule in the breast (found on a screening mammography) to widespread disease involving multiple bones, the liver, or even the brain. Because both the treatment and prognosis of these different breast cancers differ so widely, knowledge of a person's stage allows an oncologist to form an idea of that person's overall prognosis and to determine what the treatment options might be. On a more mundane level, grouping cancer patients by stage enables health care providers and medical researchers to speak the same language when referring to a person with cancer.

When thinking about staging, keep three things in mind:

1. In general, cancers have only one commonly used staging system, although some have several types (for example, colon cancer can be staged by either the Duke's stages or the TNM staging system).
2. Staging is extremely helpful to physicians, but it is not necessarily definitive. Even within a particular stage there can be wide variations in the extent of the cancer, the prognosis, and the therapy.
3. Staging can be defined either clinically (based on the physical exam and radio-

logic studies) or pathologically (through surgical resection or biopsies). Thus, the "stage" of a tumor can change before and after a tissue biopsy.

WHAT TESTS ARE USED TO DEFINE CANCER STAGE?

Tests used to define a cancer stage are actually quite similar to those used to diagnose cancer. These tests include physical examination, radiographic studies (e.g., CT scans, MRI scans, and x-rays), blood tests, and surgical biopsies, along with pathologic evaluation. Depending on the type of cancer you have and the types of tests that were used to diagnose your cancer, additional testing may or may not be needed to define cancer stage.

WHAT IS THE "TNM" STAGING SYSTEM?

The majority of cancers are staged using the American Joint Committee on Cancer (AJCC) classification scheme (Table 11-3). This staging system is based on the tumor or T stage (typically based on the size of the primary tumor); nodal status or N stage (typically based on the number or location of lymph nodes involved with cancer); and metastases or M stage (typically defined by either the presence or absence of tumor spread to other organs, or metastases). These three important variables (T, N, and M) are then used to group cancer patients into an overall stage—usually classified as stages 1 to 4 (or I to IV), with the higher numbers indicating more advanced disease.

Certain cancers, in particular the liquid tumors (leukemias, myelomas, and lymphomas) are staged a bit differently. These tumors' staging systems take into account variables such as the number of lymph node areas involved, the level of the blood counts (how high or low the red blood cells, white blood cells, and platelets appear in the bloodstream), the results of pathologic testing, and whether a person has symptoms from the cancer.

TABLE 11-3 **The TNM Staging System of Tumors**[a]

T stage
    Typically based on the size of the primary tumor
N stage (nodal status)
    Typically based on the number or location of lymph nodes involved with cancer
M stage (metastases stage)
    Typically defined by either the presence or absence of tumor spread to other organs

[a]Typically classified as stages 1 to 4 or I to IV, with the higher numbers indicating more advanced disease.

WHY IS STAGING IMPORTANT?

Staging has become an important component of the evaluation of people with cancer for several reasons. It enables physicians to group cancer patients into broad categories, which aids communication between physicians and facilitates research. It thus allows physicians to speak the same language in discussing cancer. A woman with stage 2 breast cancer in Iowa will have a similar prognosis and treatment options as a woman with stage 2 breast cancer in Maine or elsewhere in the world. In the end, this benefits patients, as physicians can inform their patients more accurately about their disease and can then present pertinent facts, such as the likelihood of cure, average length of survival, and, most importantly, treatment options. However, as mentioned above, prognosis and treatment may vary widely even within a specific stage. Always remember that every person with cancer is an individual.

HOW SOON AFTER DIAGNOSIS SHOULD I START THERAPY?

The answer to this question varies depending on what type of cancer you have, what types of tests were performed to make the diagnosis, and what your symptoms are.

After a cancer diagnosis has been made, the appropriate staging workup needs to be completed. This is extremely important, as many rational treatment decisions are based on the stage of the cancer. For example, many isolated tumors without evidence of involvement of nearby lymph nodes or spread to other organs are amenable to surgical resection (and thus possibly to cure). However, for the majority of cancers that have spread to other organs (and thus are in a more advanced stage), surgical resection is not the treatment of choice, as taking out one site of tumor will have no effect on the other metastatic sites and will not prolong survival. In this setting, the surgery may actually incur side effects and delay possible therapy (such as chemotherapy). Exceptions to this rule include cases in which not resecting the primary tumor leads to complications. An example of this would be a colon cancer that grows large enough to cause an obstruction of the colon.

After proper staging has been completed, the next question to ask is whether or not further therapy (e.g., surgery, radiation, or chemotherapy) is needed. Again, this decision is based upon multiple factors, but it is heavily influenced by the stage of the tumor and whether the tumor is causing symptoms. For example, after the complete surgical removal of a breast lump and lymph nodes, further therapy may not be required if the tumor has been properly and fully resected.

Another reason for forgoing further therapy lies at the opposite end of the staging spectrum. In certain cases there is no known cure for a cancer. Because most therapy (either chemotherapy or radiation therapy) is toxic and has side effects, the decision to treat a person is often based on whether the therapy being considered has been shown to change the natural history of the disease (i.e., by prolonging survival) or is thought somehow to allay specific symptoms (for example, the use of radiation therapy for pain caused by bone metastases). This decision also will depend on a person's age, other medical problems, and in general his or her ability to tolerate the rigors of therapy. Most importantly, it will depend on the individual's personal preferences.

If the decision is made to undergo further therapy, in most cases it should be done sooner rather than later. In the majority of cases the therapy is not an emergency; thus, if you have special plans (such as upcoming holidays, anniversaries, or a planned vacation), you can delay therapy or schedule it around these dates. In some cases, as with acute leukemia, chemotherapy should not be delayed more than a few hours or a day or two. Again, the cancer stage and the purpose of the therapy should be kept in mind in making these decisions.

In cases where the intent of therapy is a cure, as in the surgical resection of colon cancer or therapy for localized lymphoma, the treatment should be started within a reasonable time frame, such as 2 to 3 weeks from the time of diagnosis and the completion of staging. On the other hand, in cases of metastatic lung cancer without symptoms (a treatable but incurable disease), chemotherapy or radiation can be delayed a bit longer.

CHAPTER 12

Information Resources

Robert Dean, M.D.

OUTLINE

HOW CAN I BECOME MY OWN EXPERT?

Now that you've learned some basic facts about cancer, you may be thinking about digging deeper to gather specific information about your particular illness. This chapter will help you find the information you need to make informed choices. Some people want to learn just enough to understand what their doctor is saying. Others would rather know just enough to get through their treatment. And some people dedicate themselves to finding out everything they can about their disease and the different ways it can be treated.

There is no right or wrong way to go about this; everyone deals with cancer in his or her own way. However, there are some advantages to "becoming your own cancer expert:"

- It is natural for most people to have some anxiety following a cancer diagnosis. Understanding your diagnosis (including the manifestations of your type of cancer, the course the disease may run, and your prognosis), as well as the available treatments, usually helps to ease that anxiety and many unspoken fears.
- By becoming more informed, you also can help your family and friends understand your diagnosis; this may help those close to you feel less nervous about the changes that are happening in your life, making it easier for them to give you the support you need as you face cancer.
- Learning more about your illness usually makes it easier to choose the treatment that is best for you.
- Becoming more informed enables you to choose the most appropriate treatment setting, including your own home, a nearby doctor's office, or a major academic center.

WHERE CAN I TURN FOR RELIABLE INFORMATION?

You'll be surprised by how much information you can find about cancer, once you start looking. For example, a search for books about cancer in the Library of Congress produced 6387 entries! Now, not everybody is able to go to the Library of Congress, but even my local library branch lists approximately 100 books on cancer. On the Internet, a search of Amazon.com revealed over 8000 books and almost 40 videos dealing with cancer. Using the search engine on Yahoo! identified almost 1800 Internet sites that dealt with cancer, while a search using Google.com revealed almost 9 million sites!

It's only natural to feel a little overwhelmed by all of this information. Most people with cancer don't want to read everything that's ever been written on the subject. Instead, you need reliable information about *your* cancer to help you understand your specific diagnosis and to make informed choices about your treatment. In this section, we'll describe some excellent resources to use as starting points on the road to becoming your own cancer expert.

Your first stop for information about cancer should be a visit to your oncologist, who can give you answers that are tailored to the specifics of your condition. Talking with your doctor also gives him or her an opportunity to address your concerns and to understand your point of view; this almost always helps people feel more comfortable with the treatment they have chosen (if any) and with the doctor who is prescribing it. You also may find it useful to talk with a nurse or social worker at your doctor's office; these members of your health care team often have years of experience and plenty of knowledge to share.

Besides discussing your questions one-on-one, your oncologist may have printed literature that explains various aspects of your cancer and its treatment. For some, this information may be enough; others may still want to pursue other avenues of inquiry (discussed below). Many oncology centers keep a broad collection of printed and multimedia educational materials in a "patient resource room" that you can explore (Fig. 12-1). Beyond your doctor's office, there are vast resources at your command. The following list is by no means intended to be all-inclusive; however, it should give you a starting point for some of the most dependable resources available.

WHERE CAN I FIND INFORMATION ABOUT CANCER-RELATED ORGANIZATIONS?

American Cancer Society

For information about cancer in general as well as for specific details about many types of cancer (most likely including yours), the American Cancer Society (ACS) is one of the oldest and most respected resources. Founded in 1913 (as the American Society for Cancer Control), the ACS today raises funds for cancer research, conducts public awareness campaigns about cancer prevention, diagnosis, and treatment, and provides a variety of services to people with cancer and their families. It is a community-based organization with over 3400 local chapters nationwide. The ACS has developed an outstanding Internet website with a wealth of information, including links to local ACS chapters and to other resources.

To reach the website, go to http://www.cancer.org/. To reach the ACS 24-hour information service, call 800-ACS-2345.

From the home page of the ACS website, you can follow links to pages with information for practically anybody who wants to learn more about cancer. For patients, their families, and friends, the website provides specific information about different types of cancer. Interactive tools can help you understand treatment options and make treatment decisions. There are guides to clinical trials, tips on coping with cancer and its side effects, and suggestions about getting support from

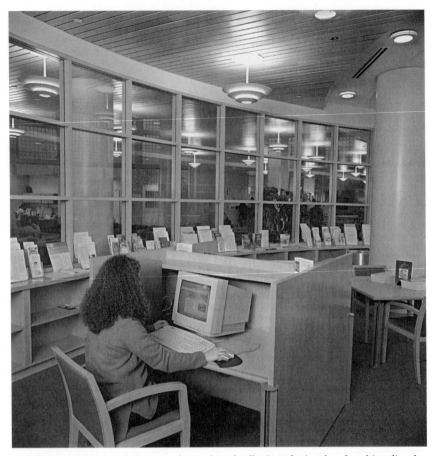

FIGURE 12-1 Many oncology centers keep a broad collection of printed and multimedia educational materials in a "patient resource room" that you can explore.

both local resources and national organizations. Cancer survivors can learn about staying healthy after their treatment is finished, and learn of ways they can help other people who are facing cancer, in their community or online. The website provides cancer statistics, a discussion of risk factors for developing cancer, tips on cancer prevention and early detection, and news reports on recent research studies in cancer. You can search online, by city or ZIP code, to learn what cancer organizations have chapters in your community, what kind of activities they are conducting, and how people can get involved through donations or volunteering.

National Cancer Institute

Another great source of both general and disease-specific cancer information is the National Cancer Institute (NCI). Based in Bethesda, Maryland, and formed by the federal government in 1937, the NCI is the largest of the National Institutes of Health. It offers the following resources:

The Cancer Information Service, in operation for 25 years as a free service, interprets cancer research findings in a clear and understandable manner. Cancer information specialists are available to provide personalized answers to your questions Monday through Friday from 9:00 a.m. to 4:30 p.m. (EST). You can also listen to recorded information about cancer at any time or use CancerFax to obtain printed summaries, fact sheets, and literature searches.

800-4-CANCER (1-800-422-6237)
TTY: 800-332-8615
800-624-2511 or 301-402-5874 (CancerFax)

The NCI's website, Cancer.gov, is a centralized source for trustworthy information about cancer. Cancer.gov provides credible, current, and comprehensive knowledge for people with cancer and their physicians, including up-to-date cancer information summaries on more than 80 types of adult and childhood cancers. Visitors to Cancer.gov can obtain assistance from a cancer information specialist through an online instant messaging service called Live-Help. This service is available Monday through Friday from 9:00 a.m. to 10:00 p.m. (EST) and is accessible from the Cancer.gov home page.

http://www.nci.nih.gov/ or http://cancer.gov/ (main NCI web page)

The Cancer.gov website is organized so that you can find information by general topics or by specific cancer types, with sections on cancer information, clinical trials, statistics, research programs, and research funding by the NCI. For most types of cancer you will find integrated information on treatment, prevention, genetics, causes, and screening, with versions prepared for both patients and health professionals. Physician Data Query (PDQ), the NCI's comprehensive cancer database, contains reviewed summaries of published cancer research, a registry of cancer clinical trials from around the world, physician directories, and organizations that provide cancer care. A section on treatment information even includes the role of complementary and alternative medicines and provides general facts as well as reviews of specific topics. To help people cope with cancer, there is information about cancer complications, treatment side effects, nutritional recommendations, emotional problems, and end-of-life issues. Cancer.gov also includes information for cancer patients and their families about support organizations, finances, insurance, hospice care, and home care. For more information, visitors can search CANCERLIT, a database of published research articles, or browse collections of NCI publications.

If you are interested in clinical trials, you can use Cancer.gov to search for them by cancer type, geographic location, and kind of treatment. The website also explains some general concepts about clinical trials and summarizes the results of noteworthy studies that have been completed. Cancer statistics are presented by type of cancer. You can also use an interactive system to display information from the NCI's national statistical database.

Other Organizations

The American Society of Clinical Oncology (ASCO) and the American Association for Cancer Research (AACR) are organizations that seek to advance the care of cancer patients through training, research, advocacy, and communication. ASCO's and AACR's main audiences are oncology professionals and scientists, but both societies provide some patient-oriented information. ASCO's website emphasizes clinical trials and recent advances as reported in the *Journal of Clinical Oncology* and at the ASCO Annual Meeting, while AACR's Internet site contains fact sheets on several common forms of cancer, with links for patients to participate in advocacy efforts.

http://www.asco.org/   http://www.aacr.org/
703-299-1044   215-440-9300

Another organization, the National Comprehensive Cancer Network (NCCN), publishes treatment guidelines for physicians on specific types of cancer. In partnership with the American Cancer Society, NCCN is producing patient-friendly versions of these documents; it currently offers summaries for cancer pain, nausea and vomiting, and cancers of the breast, colon, and prostate.

http://www.nccn.org/
800-909-NCCN (800-909-6226)

In addition to the wide range of information available from the sources identified above, there are specific organizations dedicated to education and advocacy for most common forms of cancer. The list in Table 12-1 will help get you started.

WHAT OTHER INTERNET SITES CAN I USE TO LEARN MORE ABOUT MY CANCER?

Through the World Wide Web, electronic mail lists, news groups, and chat rooms, the Internet can bring a world of information about cancer to your home, office, or library. In a matter of hours, a person with average computer skills can obtain information online that used to take days to gather through telephone calls and trips to the library.

Most organizations that serve people with a specific type of cancer maintain their own websites (see Table 12-1). Along with the many Internet sites listed elsewhere in this chapter, three others deserve special mention here.

TABLE 12-1 Useful Websites for Information about Specific Cancers

Bladder cancer	American Foundation for Urologic Disease http://www.afud.org/ 800-242-2383 410-468-1800
Brain tumors	American Brain Tumor Association (ABTA) http://www.abta.org/ 800-886-ABTA (800-886-2282) The Brain Tumor Society http://www.tbts.org/ 800-770-TBTS (800-770-8287) National Brain Tumor Foundation http://www.braintumor.org/ 800-934-CURE (800-934-2873) 510-839-9777
Breast cancer	The Susan G. Komen Breast Cancer Foundation http://www.breastcancerinfo.com/ 800-462-9273 Y-ME National Breast Cancer Organization http://www.y-me.org/ 24-Hour Hotline: 800-221-2141
Cervical cancer	National Cervical Cancer Coalition http://www.nccc-online.org/ 800-685-5531 818-909-3849
Colon cancer	Colorectal Cancer Network http://www.colorectal-cancer.net/ 301-879-1500 Colon Cancer Alliance http://www.ccalliance.org/ 877-422-2030
Head and neck cancer	Support for People with Oral and Head and Neck Cancer http://www.spohnc.org/ 800-377-0928
Kidney cancer	Kidney Cancer Association http://www.kidneycancerassociation.org/ 800-850-9132 847-332-1051 American Foundation for Urologic Disease http://www.afud.org/ 800-242-2383 410-468-1800
Leukemias and lymphomas	Cure for Lymphoma Foundation http://www.cfl.org/ 800-CFL-6848 (800-235-6848) 212-213-9595 Leukemia and Lymphoma Society http://www.leukemia-lymphoma.org/ 800-955-4572

(*continued*)

TABLE 12-1 (*continued*)

Leukemias and lymphomas (*continued*)	Leukemia Research Foundation http://www.leukemia-research.org/ 847-424-0600 Lymphoma Research Foundation of America http://www.lymphoma.org/ 800-500-9976 310-204-7040
Lung cancer	Alliance for Lung Cancer Advocacy, Support, and Education (ALCASE) http://www.alcase.org/ 800-298-2436 360-696-2436
Melanoma	The Skin Cancer Foundation http://www.skincancer.org/ 800-SKIN-490 (800-754-6490) 212-725-5176
Multiple myeloma	International Myeloma Foundation http://www.myeloma.org/ 800-452-CURE (800-452-2873) 818-487-7455 The Multiple Myeloma Research Foundation http://www.multiplemyeloma.org/ 203-972-1250
Ovarian cancer	National Ovarian Cancer Coalition http://www.ovarian.org/ 888-OVARIAN (888-682-7426) 561-393-0005 Ovarian Cancer National Alliance http://www.ovariancancer.org/ 202-331-1332
Pancreatic cancer	Pancreatic Cancer Action Network (PanCAN) http://www.pancan.org/ 877-2-PANCAN (877-272-6226)
Prostate cancer	CaP CURE http://www.capcure.org/ 800-757-CURE American Foundation for Urologic Disease http://www.afud.org/ 800-242-2383 410-468-1800
Sarcomas	Amschwand Sarcoma Cancer Foundation http://www.sarcomacancer.org/ 713-838-1615
Testicular cancer	The Lance Armstrong Foundation http://www.laf.org/ 512-236-8820

OncoLink

OncoLink, founded in 1994, is a project of the University of Pennsylvania Cancer Center. It was the first multimedia oncology information resource on the Internet, and it remains one of the most comprehensive.

Its address is http://oncolink.upenn.edu/.

Association of Cancer Online Resources

The Association of Cancer Online Resources contains a large collection of cancer-related Internet resources, including mailing lists that serve as online support groups for people with various kinds of cancer.

Its address is http://www.acor.org/

People Living with Cancer

ASCO has developed an excellent website specifically for patients, called People Living with Cancer. Its purpose is to provide accurate and comprehensive information for people with cancer. The site features a general introduction to cancer, with sections devoted to coping with cancer, managing side effects, learning about clinical trials and genetic testing, and describing the kinds of oncologists who make up a cancer treatment team. You can find information organized by types of cancer, including the most recent research updates from ASCO's annual meeting. Another section offers live online chats with cancer experts, recorded presentations from the ASCO annual meeting, and tools to help you find an oncologist or support resources in your community. You can search in a medical dictionary or a drug database to learn more about terms you have encountered or medications you have been prescribed. There are also links to additional resources, such as scientific abstracts from ASCO's annual meeting, the PubMed database of biomedical research articles, and consumer magazines that discuss detecting, treating, and coping with cancer. Another section provides news updates on recent developments in cancer research.

http://www.peoplelivingwithcancer.org/
or http://www.plwc.org/

HOW CAN I JUDGE THE ACCURACY OF INTERNET SITES?

In using the Internet, the challenge is to find information that is reliable and relevant to your situation. Remember that much of the content on the Internet is *unmoderated*; this means that individuals can create websites or post messages with nearly total freedom to say what they want. In this section, we'll give you a few simple rules of thumb to help you decide which Internet sources to trust for cancer information (Table 12-2). We'll also highlight some sites that most people with cancer will find useful.

Rule #1: Consider the Source

This is probably the most important rule about cancer information on the Internet. If your source is a respected cancer organization, research facility, medical center, or educational institution, then the information will generally be reliable—meaning that most cancer experts would agree with what you're reading and would give you similar information. Also, a trustworthy site should support its statements with clear references to other reliable sources. In contrast, sites that do not offer professional credentials or do not identify sources for their information should be regarded with skepticism until their claims can be verified.

Rule #2: If It Seems Too Good to Be True, It Probably Is

It takes tremendous resources to develop effective treatments for cancer. By comparison, it costs little to design an Internet site that is polished and persuasive. Unfortunately, the Internet has become an effective tool for promoting treatments that are either unproven or, worse, proven useless. Such treatments still attract attention, though, through skillful presentations and misleading advertisements that capitalize on people's fears and on their hopes for a cure. As the saying goes, *caveat emptor*—let the buyer beware! Look for sales pitches, which you can often identify by asking, "What will this author gain if I believe what I'm reading?" If there is an obvious benefit for the people providing the information, don't accept it without verifying the claims through an independent source.

Rule #3: Know the Facts (and the Opinions) and Make Comparisons

Standard practices in oncology are based on the best medical evidence available, and reliable sources of cancer information should draw from the same evidence. However, when the available data are limited or conflicting, authorities study the

TABLE 12-2 **Rules to Remember When Using the Internet**

Consider the source.
If it seems too good to be true, it probably is.
Learn the facts (and the opinions) and make comparisons.

information to give the best advice possible. In these cases, there is usually more than one valid interpretation, and most dependable sources (on the Internet and elsewhere) will be honest about the basis for—and limitations of—their conclusions. Obtain information from more than one source; a trustworthy Internet site will usually confirm what you've learned elsewhere. With this in mind, be skeptical of sites that contain radically different information—especially if references aren't provided to support their claims.

National Cancer Institute's "Ten Things to Know"

For more tips on judging the quality of online information about cancer, see the National Cancer Institute's website, "10 Things to Know about Evaluating Medical Resources on the Web." The guidelines on this excellent page apply to medical information from any source, not just the Internet:

http://www.cancer.gov/cancerinfo/ten-things-to-know

HON Code

Another great tool to help you identify trustworthy Internet sites is to look for the HONcode seal on the website's home page. The Health On the Net Foundation (HON) is a not-for-profit organization whose mission is to guide laypersons or non-medical users and medical practitioners to useful and reliable online medical and health information. HON sets ethical standards by promoting eight "HONcode principles" designed to help websites practice responsible self-regulation and to make sure a reader always knows the source and the purpose of the information he or she is reading. Websites that adhere to these principles are certified by HON and permitted to display the HONcode seal. Clicking on the HONcode seal from any website that bears it should take you to the Health On the Net Foundation's website, where you can verify the certification status of the original website and learn more about the HONcode principles.

http://www.hon.ch/HONcode/Conduct.html (HONcode principles)
http://www.hon.ch/home.html (Health On the Net Foundation homepage)

Briefly, the HONcode principles encourage websites to do the following:

- Provide medical advice from qualified professionals;
- Offer information to support, not replace, the relationship between a site visitor and his/her physician;
- Respect the confidentiality of information about patients or site visitors;
- Give references and revision dates for the site's information;
- Provide scientific evidence to support claims on behalf of a specific treatment or product;

- Present information clearly, including contact information for website authors;
- Identify clearly who sponsors the website (including commercial and non-commercial contributors); and
- Indicate clearly if the website obtains any funding from advertisements, with a description of the site's advertising policy.

CHAPTER 13

Lifestyle Modifications

David R. Spigel, M.D.

OUTLINE

IN GENERAL, HOW CAN A CANCER DIAGNOSIS HAVE A MINIMAL EFFECT ON MY LIFESTYLE?

Facing a new diagnosis of cancer can be difficult. For many, this is a sudden and unexpected event. One important and often underestimated challenge for people with cancer is the change in lifestyle that this new diagnosis brings. Any treatment—be it chemotherapy, radiation, surgery, or a combination of treatments—can have an important impact on your lifestyle. Fortunately, advances in cancer care have helped to lessen this impact. Today, most treatments can be given in the outpatient setting and do not require a hospital stay. Many new medications, including those that help with nausea and sleep, have reduced the side effects of these therapies dramatically. Health care teams have expanded to include nutritionists, social workers, and pharmacists routinely. In short, many resources and services are designed to help with the lifestyle changes a new diagnosis can bring.

SHOULD I STOP DRINKING ALCOHOL, SMOKING CIGARETTES, OR DRINKING COFFEE?

Many people in the United States either drink alcohol, smoke cigarettes, drink coffee, or partake in more than one of these activities. Whether you do so for pleasure or because one of these activities has become a habit, you may find it difficult to stop when given a cancer diagnosis. Does a person newly diagnosed with cancer need to stop drinking alcohol, smoking, or drinking coffee?

Smoking is the easiest of these to address. Most doctors would agree that quitting is an important first step toward improving your health. While smoking cessation is easier said than done, it cannot be overemphasized how important this is to your care. Smoking can promote the growth of some cancers, and it has the potential of interfering with the beneficial effects of chemotherapy and radiation therapy; moreover, it may slow wound healing following surgery. As worrisome as its ill effects are on your heart, lungs, and overall fitness, the therapies for cancer can be more difficult to withstand when you are exposed to the stress of smoking (Table 13-1).

For example, people who smoke and receive the drug bleomycin and/or receive radiation therapy for Hodgkin's disease (see Chap. 14 for more information about this drug) are more likely to have lung damage, a limited exercise capacity, and possibly to develop lung cancer following treatment than those who do not smoke.

TABLE 13-1 **Some Adverse Effects of Smoking**

Smoking can promote the growth of some cancers.
Smoking may interfere with the beneficial effects of chemotherapy and radiation therapy.
Smoking slows wound healing following surgery.
Smoking can combine with radiation therapy to cause subsequent cancer.

The side effects of quitting, while at times difficult to tolerate, tend to be short-lived. In the long run, your body will be healthier once you have quit smoking, and you will be better able to meet the challenges of therapy.

With alcohol use, quitting is ideal in most circumstances; at the very least, moderation is important. As with smoking, alcohol has the potential of interfering with your therapy. Some cancers (such as cancers of the head and neck, esophagus, liver, and breast) are directly linked to alcohol use. It makes sense that people with these cancers attempt to abstain if possible. In addition, certain chemotherapies, such as methotrexate, can put extra stress on the liver. Alcohol, which is processed (metabolized) by the liver, can add to this.

Alcohol also interferes with the cells in the bone marrow that produce the red blood cells (which provide oxygen to your tissues), white blood cells (which fight infections), and platelets (which help stop bleeding). Many types of chemotherapy and radiation therapy similarly interfere with the function of these cells, and the combined effect of these treatments and alcohol could lower blood counts even more dramatically. With these therapies, your doctor might ask that you abstain from using alcohol throughout your treatment course.

In addition, both radiation therapy and some chemotherapies can irritate the lining of the gastrointestinal tract, including the esophagus, stomach, and duodenum (a condition called *mucositis*). Alcohol can cause a similar irritation and may worsen the effects of these therapies. Finally, the sedative effects of alcohol can be dangerously additive to the sedative effects of some of your medications used to treat pain and nausea. For that reason alone, limiting intake as much as possible makes sense (Table 13-2).

In summary, for many therapies, alcohol intake should be eliminated. If you drink alcohol regularly (more than one or two drinks every night), your intake of alcohol should be tapered gradually, with assistance from your physician, and not stopped suddenly, as sudden cessation can cause serious side effects. If you cannot or are unwilling to stop drinking alcohol, you should drink it in moderation, never in excess. Moderation is usually defined as one to two drinks a day

---

TABLE 13-2 **Some Adverse Effects of Alcohol**

Alcohol interferes with the cells in the bone marrow that produce red blood cells (which provide oxygen to your tissues).

Alcohol interferes with the cells in the bone marrow that produce white blood cells (which fight infections).

Alcohol interferes with the cells in the bone marrow that produce platelets (which help stop bleeding).

Alcohol has the potential to interfere with your therapy.

Alcohol can irritate the lining of the gastrointestinal tract.

The sedative effects of alcohol can add to the sedative effects of some of your medications used to treat pain and nausea.

Alcohol can adversely affect the function of your liver.

(one drink = 5 ounces of red/white wine, 12 ounces of beer, or 1 ounce of hard liquor).

Coffee is becoming an increasingly common part of our lives; many fear giving this up more than they fear giving up cigarettes or alcohol. There is no evidence that coffee has any ill effects on your health or that it is a risk factor for any type of cancer. It is a stimulant (similar to the nicotine in cigarettes, but the opposite of alcohol) and can contribute to anxiety and, rarely, to heart rhythm disturbances. Coffee is also a diuretic (like a water pill) and might contribute to dehydration; finally, it is a stomach irritant (like alcohol). The best advice is to drink in moderation and to be aware of its adverse effects (including its impact on your sleep cycle).

IS IT SAFE TO EXERCISE WHILE RECEIVING TREATMENT FOR CANCER?

Exercise is another important aspect of your lifestyle that is often overlooked as cancer therapy gets under way. Clearly, there are instances when exercising may be dangerous while you are receiving treatment. In general, these are isolated periods when you might be too weak from dehydration, loss of appetite, or lowered blood counts, particularly low red blood cells. For the majority of people with cancer and for most treatments, however, exercise is strongly encouraged, though again in moderation. Exercising to excess or in extreme conditions (such as days when the heat index or humidity is too high) can be dangerous for anybody, regardless of whether that person has cancer. In addition, treatments can cause fatigue and make what used to be an easy workout seem a bit more challenging.

Exercising in moderation for 30 minutes or more on most days, particularly aerobic exercise (such as walking, running, or swimming), can have significant benefits for your heart, lungs, and overall stamina. Simply walking most days for 30 minutes can have important health benefits. There is even a protective effect of exercise on the development of colorectal cancer. Being as active as you can be goes a long way toward helping you get through your therapy. Remember, discuss this with your doctor before starting any new exercise regimen, and be careful not to "push yourself" to exercise too much while on therapy. People with other medical illnesses (such as heart or lung disease) should exercise in a monitored setting, such as a cardiac rehabilitation program.

SHOULD I ALTER MY DIET IN ANY WAY TO DECREASE MY RISK OF CANCER?

This is a common question for many, and unfortunately not always an easy one to answer. Tremendous advances have been made over the last decade in the areas of nutrition and health. Prevention has been at the center of these advances. Learning which foods lead to cancer is difficult; such knowledge requires well-designed studies. Unfortunately, many recommendations about the impact of nutrition on health are reported in the media, though these recommendations may not be based on well-designed studies. For example, while obesity is related to breast, colorectal, and endometrial cancers, the reduction of dietary fat has not been shown to prevent these cancers. Similarly, recent evidence has raised doubts about the beneficial effects of fiber in preventing colorectal cancer. Dietary fat and red meat may contribute to prostate cancer, though this has not been proven fully. Vitamin E and selenium have shown promise in preventing prostate cancer and possibly other cancers, but again are unproven. Folic acid (folate) may also have a benefit in preventing colorectal cancer, though this relationship has not yet been established definitively. So what's the best advice?

The best advice is to consume a diet low in saturated fat and red meat and rich in whole grains, fruits, and vegetables. This diet has known benefits for people with cardiovascular disease and diabetes and may have benefits for people with cancer. As mentioned above, obesity is associated with a number of cancers. Addressing this through diet and exercise may have preventive benefits.

SHOULD I ALTER MY DIET TO HELP TREAT MY CANCER?

Many people with cancer are concerned about how diet can affect their treatment. Chemotherapy, radiation therapy, and surgery can place increased nutritional demands on the body, creating a need for more calories. In addition, treatment often takes away your appetite, and meeting these increased requirements can be difficult. Fortunately, we are better able to control nausea today, and appetite can be improved with activity and even with some medications.

Medications to help treat nausea include odansetron (Zofran), granisetron (Kytril), dolasetron (Anzemet), prochlorperazine (Compazine), promethazine (Phenergan), trimethobenzamide (Tigan), dronabinol (Marinol), and droperidol (Inapsine); relaxation techniques, acupuncture, and other complementary or alternative therapies can also be of help (see Chap. 21). Appetite stimulants include megestrol (Megace) and dronabinol (Marinol).

Occasionally, your usual pattern of eating may be altered, either because of a lack of desire to eat (anorexia), nausea, or because you have to time eating around a medication schedule. Smaller and more frequent meals/snacks may temporarily suit you better than the more traditional "three meals a day." In advanced cancer, avoiding foods high in fat is actually discouraged. Supplements in the form of shakes (e.g., Ensure, Boost, or Sustecal), snacks, or vitamins are helpful in meeting your body's increased needs during therapy. For more detailed recommendations, a nutritionist should be consulted. Often, a detailed assessment of your needs and what you are currently achieving can be made. Ask your doctor to set up a meeting with a nutritionist early in your therapy. This is a valuable step toward being in control of your body and treatment.

CAN MY DIET INFLUENCE THE EFFECT OF THE MEDICATIONS I AM TAKING?

This is an important question, as you likely will be taking many new medications as part of your treatment. Several of these medications accompany your primary chemotherapy, radiation therapy, or surgery and include medicines for nausea, insomnia, or constipation. As previously mentioned, these medications and treatments may affect your diet and place increased metabolic demands on your body. Similarly, your diet can affect your medications.

For example, diets deficient in calories cause your body to "burn" fat and muscle for energy. This breakdown in tissues can have important consequences on how your medications are absorbed and distributed throughout your body. These medications then can become more concentrated in the bloodstream and may be more likely to cause unwanted side effects, as if you took higher doses of the medicine.

In addition, some medications require food to aid in their absorption in the stomach and small intestine. An inadequate diet, then, may result in underdosing of these medications. Some foods also may cause nausea and thus make it difficult for you to take all of your necessary medications. Finally, some foods may interfere with the absorption or have an effect on the metabolism (breakdown) of important medications, as is the case with grapefruit juice and the drug tacrolimus (or FK506), used in people who have received a bone marrow transplant. A pharmacist works hand-in-hand with your doctor and nutritionist and is readily available to help ensure that all of your medications are well tolerated, safe, and effective.

WHICH MEDICATIONS EITHER DECREASE OR INCREASE MY APPETITE?

Therapies for cancer are strong and, unfortunately, some therapies can have potentially significant effects on your appetite. Chemotherapies and radiation therapies can cause nausea. While this is somewhat predictable, depending on the medication or radiation dose and on the chemotherapy agent, individual responses can vary. Nausea is often temporary and tends to occur at the time of treatment or in the few days following it. In some, nausea can occur several days or even weeks later. Fortunately, medications that combat nausea are effective and well tolerated.

Loss of appetite also can be due to narcotic pain medication. Again, this is usually related to nausea. As new pain medications are started or doses increased, nausea can be a troublesome side effect. For many, this toxicity diminishes with time without compromising the pain-relieving effect. Constipation—whether from narcotics, antinausea medications, or other medicines—also can decrease your appetite. It is important to communicate changes in bowel habits regularly with your team as this can be prevented readily or treated if caught early.

Some therapies decrease appetite. These tend to be the more intensive chemotherapy and radiation regimens. Nausea and constipation may be only small components of this decrease in appetite, which can be long-lasting and difficult to overcome at times. Addressing appetite problems early with the help of medications (listed above) and your nutritionist can be helpful.

While cancer treatments historically have been associated with the loss of appetite, the opposite can be true. That is to say, sometimes therapy can increase appetite. It's a common phenomenon for some people to actually gain weight during therapy. Theoretically, the reasons for this relate to the treatment's effect on the cancer itself. Many tumors release chemicals that contribute to diminished appetite. In fact, one such chemical, now called *tumor necrosis factor*, used to be named *cachexin* because it caused anorexia and weight loss (cachexia) in people who had tumors that produced the chemical. With treatment, tumor growth—and thus chemical production—is disrupted, allowing some people to eat more and to gain weight.

Some drugs, such as steroids (commonly used in the treatment of lymphomas and multiple myeloma and as an antinausea medication in many other cancers), are well known to stimulate appetite and weight gain. Steroids are even used to treat people who have had poor appetites for prolonged periods of time. Table 13-3 offers a list of drugs commonly used in cancer treatment that can have effects on appetite.

TABLE 13-3 **Selected Drugs That Affect Appetite**

Drugs that *decrease* appetite
    dotorubicin (Adriamycin), diphenhydramine (Benadryl), bicalutamide (Casodex), irinotecan (Camptosar), cyclophosphamide (Cytoxan), dacarbazine (DTIC), fentanyl (Duragesic), amitriptyline (Elavil), etoposide (VePesid), flutamide (Eulexin), fludarabine (Fludara), gemcitabine (Gemzar), trastuzumab (Herceptin), hydroxyurea (Hydreu), interferon (Intron), leucovorin, diphenoxylate and atropine (Lomotil), dronabinol (Marinol), morphine, vinorelbine (Navelbine), granulocyte colony stimulating factor (G-CSF, Neupogen), rituximab (Rituxan), thalidomide (Thalid), vincristine (Oncovin), fluorourucil (5-FU, Xeloda).

Drugs that *increase* appetite
    bicalutamide (Casodex), prochlorperazine (Compazine), dexamethasone (Decadron), leuprolide (Lupron), dronabinol (Marinol), Megestrol (Megace), prednisone, docetaxel (Taxotere)

WHAT IS "PERFORMANCE STATUS" AND WHY IS IT IMPORTANT?

Simply put, performance status (PS) is a measure of how functional you are while living with cancer. Specifically, this is a measure of how independent you are in performing everyday activities and personal care—and, more importantly, how much cancer interferes with this. Commonly used systems for assessing PS include the Karnofsky Performance Status (KPS) scale, the Eastern Cooperative Oncology Group (ECOG) PS scale, and the Lansky PS scale for children. Each scale provides a single numerical "score" (for the KPS, a score of 0 to 100; for the ECOG, a score of 0 to 5; and for the Lansky scale, a score of 0 to 100) that correlates with your ability to perform activities. These scales are shown in Tables 13-4, 13-5, and 13-6.

Your doctor will assign a PS score to you. In doing so, he or she will consider several aspects of your daily life, such as whether you are having symptoms (ranging from mild to severe), whether you are in bed most of the day, or whether you

TABLE 13-4 **Karnofsky Scale of Performance Status**

	Condition	%	Complaints
A.	Able to carry on normal activity and to work. No special care needed.	100	Normal. No complaints. No evidence of disease.
		90	Able to carry on normal activity. Minor signs or symptoms of disease.
		80	Normal activity with effort. Some signs or symptoms of disease.
B.	Unable to work. Able to live at home, and care for most personal needs. Some degree of assistance is needed.	70	Cares for self. Unable to carry on normal activity or to do active work. Some degree of assistance is needed.
		60	Requires occasional assistance but is able to care for most needs.
		50	Requires considerable assistance and frequent medical care.
C.	Unable to care for self. Requires equivalent of institutional or hospital care. Disease may be progressing rapidly.	40	Disabled. Requires special care and assistance.
		30	Severely disabled. Hospitalization is indicated although death is not imminent.
		20	Hospitalization necessary. Very sick, active supportive treatment necessary.
		0	Dead.

Source: Karnofsky DA, Ableman WH, Craver LF, et al: The use of nitrogen mustards in the palliative treatment of carcinoma. *Cancer* 1:634–656, 1948.

TABLE 13-5 Eastern Cooperative Oncology Group (ECOG) Scale of Performance Status

Value	Description
0	Normal activity
1	Symptoms, but nearly fully ambulatory
2	Some bed time, but needs to be in bed < 50% of time
3	Bedridden > 50% of daytime
4	Totally bedridden

SOURCE: Zubrod CG, Scheiderman M, Frei E III, et al: Cancer—Appraisal of methods for the study of chemotherapy of cancer in man: Thiophosphoramide. *J Chronic Dis* 11:7–33, 1960.

TABLE 13-6 Play-Performance (Lansky) Scale for Children—Parent Form

Child's name:
Date of birth:
Your name:
  Relationship:
    Mother
    Father
    Other
Today's date:
Directions for parents: On this form are a series of descriptions. Each description has a number beside it. Think about your child's play and activity over the past week. Think about both good days and bad days. Average out this period. Now read the descriptions and pick the one that best describes your child's play during the past week. Circle the number besides that one description.
100: Fully active, normal
 90: Minor restrictions in physically strenuous activity
 80: Active, but tires more quickly
 70: Both greater restriction of, and less time spent in, active play
 60: Up and around, but minimal active play; keeps busy with quieter activities
 50: Gets dressed, but lies around much of the day; no active play; able to participate in all quiet play and activities
 40: Mostly in bed; participates in quiet activities
 30: In bed; needs assistance even for quiet play
 20: Often sleeping; play entirely limited to very passive activities
 10: No play; does not get out of bed
  0: Unresponsive

SOURCE: Lansky SB, Lis MA, Lansky LL, et al: The measurement of performance in childhood cancer patients. *Cancer* 60:1651–1656, 1987.

can walk without difficulty. This number is useful because the PS can be remeasured at each visit as well as at the start, middle, and end of therapy. The number can change or stay the same, and it gives you and your health care team an idea of whether you will be able to tolerate treatment. The PS number also can determine eligibility for certain clinical trials (see Chap. 18 for more information about these). Many studies have shown that being able to care for yourself independently

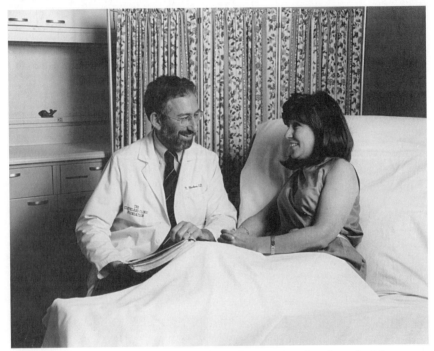

FIGURE 13-1 Treatment is sometimes challenging, but every member of your health care team should do everything possible to help make it easier and more effective for you.

and being able to perform daily activities, while having few disabling symptoms, can be an indicator that you are more likely to do well with treatment. A change in your PS can be an important signal that perhaps treatment should be delayed or altered or, alternatively, that your cancer is shrinking in response to the treatment. It is one of several ways your medical team can make sure that your care is optimal and safe.

In conclusion, there are several ways in which your life changes when you learn you have cancer. Sometimes, these changes are obvious to you and to your health care team. However, sometimes they can be subtle though just as meaningful. The key to helping to modify your lifestyle as you begin treatment is to communicate with your medical team. Communicating your concerns, questions, fears, and hopes is a critical aspect in your care. Treatment is sometimes challenging, but every member of your health care team should do everything possible to help make it easier and more effective for you (Fig. 13-1).

Chemotherapy

Vincent T. Ho, M.D.

WHAT IS CHEMOTHERAPY, AND WHAT IS THE HISTORY OF CHEMOTHERAPY?

The term *chemotherapy* was coined originally by Paul Ehrlich, a renowned nineteenth-century physician/scientist who used animals to screen chemical compounds for activity against various infections. It was not until the twentieth century, however, that similar programs were used to develop drugs against cancer. *Chemotherapy* literally means the use of chemical agents in the treatment or control of disease. While this definition can be applied both to antibiotics used to treat or control infection and to drugs used to treat and control cancer, it is more commonly used in reference to cancer therapy.

The first chemotherapy agents used to treat cancer were discovered by accident during World War II, when it was observed that soldiers exposed to mustard gas subsequently developed low blood cell counts. This led scientists to investigate nitrogen mustard compounds as a treatment for patients with leukemia and lymphoma, which are cancers of the blood cells.

Dr. Sidney Farber, a physician in Boston who was caring for children with cancer, was responsible for the next major advance in chemotherapy. Dr. Farber made the important observation that a vitamin, folic acid (folate), accelerated the growth of cancer cells in some of his patients with acute lymphoblastic leukemia (ALL), the most common leukemia in children. Convinced that folic acid was vital to the survival and continued growth of these malignant cells, he proceeded to treat these children with compounds that blocked the actions of folate and was able to demonstrate arrested growth of the leukemic cells—that is, the cancer cells stopped growing. The important work of Dr. Farber led to the development of an antifolate drug called methotrexate, which to this day remains an important chemotherapy agent in the treatment of leukemia, lymphoma, and other cancers. In fact, going back to the definition of the word *chemotherapy*, methotrexate can be thought of as an extremely potent form of the antibiotic combination drug trimethoprim and sulfamethoxazole (Bactrim), which kills bacteria by a similar mechanism.

By the 1960s, the first cures of leukemia and lymphoma in humans using a combination of chemotherapy drugs were recorded, and efforts to use chemotherapy to treat solid tumors (e.g., cancers of the lung, breast, and colon) began. The impact of chemotherapy is best exemplified by the greater than 90 percent cure rates now attainable in cancers such as Hodgkin's lymphoma and testicular cancer. Although chemotherapy has not been curative in some other conditions, such as advanced cancer of the lung or colon, it has had significant benefits in terms of prolonging survival, decreasing pain, and improving the quality of life for people living with these cancers.

HOW DOES CHEMOTHERAPY WORK?

Chemotherapy drugs use many different mechanisms to kill cancer cells. In general, they prevent the growth of tumor cells by interfering with some process that is required for cell division. As described in Chap. 1, cancer is the abnormal growth of cells, the basic building blocks of body structures. The genetic blueprints for a cell's function, development, reproduction, and eventual death are contained in structures called DNA, short for *deoxyribonucleic acid*. When a cell is ready to divide, long strands of DNA reproduce, or *replicate,* and coil together to form chromosomes; these chromosomes migrate to the center of a cell and are then pulled apart when a cell undergoes division into two cells. This process ensures that each resulting *daughter cell* receives an equal number of chromosomes, and thus DNA.

A number of chemotherapy agents work by blocking DNA replication, either by damaging the DNA directly or by interfering with the enzymes (proteins) necessary to make DNA or its building blocks. Other agents interrupt the growth of cancer cells by interfering with the migration of chromosomes. Drugs with different mechanisms are commonly used in combination to maximize the cancer cell kill rate and minimize side effects and the development of *resistance*, the word used to describe the cancer cell's survival mechanism to avoid being killed by chemotherapy.

WHAT TYPES OF CHEMOTHERAPY ARE AVAILABLE?

Many types of chemotherapy drugs have been developed since nitrogen mustard was first tested in the 1940s on patients with cancers of the blood. These drugs vary greatly in their mechanisms of action (i.e., how they work) as well as in their side-effect profiles, details of which are beyond the scope of this chapter. However, as an introduction, chemotherapy drugs can be grouped into several classes based roughly on which stage of the cancer cell's life cycle they inhibit. For example, nitrogen mustard and other compounds that kill dividing cancer cells by preventing the cell's DNA from functioning properly can be grouped into one class, while chemotherapy drugs that interrupt the microtubules, or "scaffolding" for the migration of chromosomes during cell division, belong in a separate class. The general classes of chemotherapy agents currently available are outlined in Table 14-1.

Because chemotherapy agents in different classes use different mechanisms to kill cancer cells, and because they frequently cause different side effects, they are often used in combination to maximize cancer cell kill rates without compounding toxicities. For this reason, many chemotherapy treatments have eponyms that stand for the combination of agents involved. Some common examples include: CAF [**c**ytoxan, **A**driamycin (doxorubicin), 5-**f**luorouracil (5-FU)], ICE (**i**fosfamide, **c**arboplatin, **e**toposide), or MAID (**m**esna, **A**driamycin, **i**fosfamide, **d**acarbazine).

TABLE 14-1 Classes of Common Chemotherapy Agents

1. Alkylating agents: Cyclophosphamide (Cytoxan); ifosfamide; melphalan; chlorambucil; mechlorethamine (Mustargen); thiotepa; mitomycin C, busulfan, BCNU (carmustine), CCNU (lomustine), procarbazine, dacarbazine (DTIC), temozolomide (Temazol).

Mechanism of action: Alkylating agents represent the oldest class of chemotherapy drugs; they include nitrogen mustard, which was first used to treat patients in the 1940s. As a class, these drugs react with, or *alkylate*, the DNA inside cells and cause DNA strands to be inappropriately cross-linked to each other. Because DNA is the genetic blueprint of every cell, it must be "copied," or replicated, before the cell can divide. DNA that has been cross-linked by alkylating drugs cannot be replicated, and this damage renders the cell unable to reproduce, which leads to eventual cell death.

Applications: Alkylating agents have been used extensively in combination with other chemotherapy agents in the treatment of cancers of the blood (including leukemia, lymphoma, and multiple myeloma) as well as in the treatment of many solid tumors (including sarcoma, melanoma, and carcinomas). These agents are used commonly in high doses in patients undergoing bone marrow transplantation.

Side effects: As a class, alkylating agents are considered toxic, causing significant suppression, or lowering, of blood counts. They also are associated with a high incidence of hair loss, nausea, mouth sores, and infertility. Exposure to alkylating agents increases the risk of developing acute leukemia years later. Cyclophosphamide and ifosfamide, two of the more commonly used drugs in this class, can damage and cause bleeding in the urinary bladder. These drugs are sometimes given together with a bladder protectant called Mesna. BCNU (carmustine) at high doses may cause damage and scarring of the lungs.

2. Platinum analogs: Cisplatin, carboplatin, oxaliplatin.

Mechanism of action: Agents in this class are compounds of the precious metal platinum. They react with DNA, resulting in the formation of platinum-DNA cross links, which interfere with cellular division and promote cell death.

Applications: Platinum agents are an important class of drugs used in the treatment of solid cancers. Cisplatin is a major component of chemotherapy regimens used for testicular cancer, ovarian cancer, head and neck cancer, bladder cancer, and lung cancer. Carboplatin has similar applications in most of these cancers. In contrast, oxaliplatin is a newly-developed agent that appears to be active in colon cancer, particularly colon cancer that has spread to other organs (i.e., metastatic cancer).

Side effects: The side effects most often associated with platinum agents are related to the gastrointestinal tract. Cisplatin is extremely nausea-provoking and can cause severe damage to the kidneys. As a result, cisplatin must be administered with intravenous fluids—i.e., fluids given by vein. Carboplatin is a relative of cisplatin that is better tolerated by most people. Carboplatin and oxaliplatin cause less nausea and are more forgiving on the kidneys. However, carboplatin can lead to a significant drop in blood counts. Along with the other platinum agents, oxaliplatin can damage nerves, and result in numbness and a sensitivity to cold temperatures.

3. Antimetabolites: Methotrexate, 5-fluorouracil (5-FU), capecitabine (Xeloda), cytarabine (Ara-C), gemcitabine (Gemzar), 6-mercaptopurine (6-MP), fludarabine, cladribine (2-CdA), and 2-deoxycoformycin (Pentostatin).

Mechanism of action: Agents in this class interfere with the production of folate, or other building blocks of DNA. Without DNA, cancer cells cannot replicate.

(continued)

TABLE 14-1 *(continued)*

Applications: Antimetabolite agents are used extensively in the treatment of hematologic (blood) and solid cancers. Methotrexate is active against a wide range of cancers, including leukemia, lymphoma, breast cancer, sarcoma, head and neck cancers, and bladder cancer. 5-Fluorouracil (5-FU), capecitabine, and gemcitabine are common agents used against gastrointestinal (GI) malignancies, including cancer of the colon, stomach, and pancreas. Cytarabine is an important agent in the treatment of acute leukemias and aggressive lymphomas. Fludarabine, cladribine, and 2-deoxyforcomycin are commonly used against indolent (slow-growing) lymphomas and leukemias.

Side effects: The toxicity associated with agents in this class are quite variable. Methotrexate and 5-FU can cause significant GI side effects, including mouth sores and diarrhea. At high doses, methotrexate can also cause a significant drop in blood cell counts, including the white and red blood cells and platelets, and kidney damage. These effects may be lessened by administration of a protective drug called leucovorin. A major toxicity of fludarabine, cladribine, and 2-deoxyforcomycin is suppression of the immune system. Patients receiving these drugs often require antibiotics to prevent the development of certain infections.

4. **Inhibitors of Topoisomerases:** Doxorubicin (Adriamycin), daunorubicin, idarubicin, epirubicin, etoposide (VP-16), temiposide, mitoxantrone, irinotecan (CPT-11, Camptosar), and topotecan (Hycamtin).

Mechanism of action: As a class, these agents work by blocking enzymes (proteins called topoisomerases) that unwind and untwist DNA. DNA that cannot be unwound or untwisted cannot be duplicated. This inhibition leads to breakage of the DNA strands and to subsequent cell death.

Applications: Doxorubicin, daunorubicin, idarubicin, and epirubicin have been used extensively in combination regimens in the treatment of lymphoma and acute leukemia. Doxorubicin and epirubicin also have activity against a number of solid tumors, including sarcomas, breast cancer, stomach cancer, and bladder cancer. Etoposide is an important agent in many chemotherapy regimens for the treatment of lymphoma and leukemia. It also is used in the treatment of testicular cancer and the small cell subtype of lung cancer. Camptothecin is a recently developed agent that has activity in colon cancer and small cell lung cancer.

Side effects: An important side effect of doxorubicin, daunorubicin, idarubicin, epirubicin, and mitoxantrone is the potential for heart muscle damage that results in heart failure. Prior to treatment with some of these agents, a cardiac evaluation is often performed to ensure adequate cardiac function. Etoposide is not associated with heart injury but can cause significant bone marrow suppression (with a drop in blood cell counts including the white and red blood cells and platelets) and allergic reactions in some patients. Etoposide exposure has been associated with the development of acute leukemia years later. Camptothecin is associated with significant diarrhea in many patients.

5. **Antimicrotubule agents:** Paclitaxel (Taxol), docetaxel (Taxotere), vincristine (Oncovin), vinblastine (Velban), vindesine, and vinorelbine (Navelbine).

Mechanisms of action: Drugs in this class block the assembly or disassembly of microtubules, the scaffolding required for chromosome migration (and subsequent DNA and cell replication) during cell division.

(continued)

TABLE 14-1 (*continued*)

Applications: This is an important class of agents in the treatment of many cancers. The taxanes (Taxol, Taxotere) have activity in a number of solid tumors, including ovarian cancer, lung cancer, breast cancer, head and neck cancers, and some sarcomas. Vincristine is a staple in chemotherapy regimens used against lymphoma and lymphoblastic leukemia. Vinblastine, vindesine, and vinorelbine have been used in solid tumors (including bladder cancer and lung cancer), and vinblastine is used in some Hodgkin's disease regimens.

Side effects: The single most important side effect associated with agents in this class is injury to nerve endings. With increasing cumulative doses, most patients will develop sensory numbness (losing the sense of touch) in their fingers and toes. On rare occasions, weakness may result. With the taxanes (Taxol and Taxotere), allergic reactions are common during the infusion and can be prevented by the administration of steroids and other medications beforehand.

Using multiple drugs in combination also decreases the chance that any given cancer cell will develop resistance to chemotherapy. To illustrate this point, envision a tumor (made up of millions of cells) that is exposed to a single chemotherapy drug, such as cyclophosphamide. Cyclophosphamide works by damaging DNA directly. Most of the cells in this tumor are killed by cyclophosphamide; over time, however, a few cells may survive because they have evolved a mechanism to repair the DNA damage or because they have developed a protein that pumps the cyclophosphamide out of the cell before it has had a chance to damage the cell's DNA. When this happens, that cell is no longer susceptible to the effects of cyclophosphamide; it will continue to grow throughout treatment and eventually will reconstitute a tumor resistant to cyclophosphamide. Now envision the same tumor being treated with the three-drug regimen CAF, mentioned above. In this case, the chance of the same cell's developing resistance would be much lower because that cell would now have to evolve not only escape mechanisms from cyclophosphamide but also from the Adriamycin and 5-FU, all at the same time!

HOW IS CHEMOTHERAPY GIVEN?

Although most chemotherapy is administered intravenously (IV, through the vein) (Fig. 14-1), some agents are taken by mouth. Whether a drug can be given by mouth depends on whether the stomach's digestive enzymes inactivate the drug, rendering it useless, and whether the drug can be absorbed into the bloodstream in adequate amounts. Some chemotherapy agents cause irritation of small veins and are administered through *central* IV lines. These are large catheters placed in the chest wall or neck that tunnel into large veins at the base of the neck or under the collarbone. Central lines have an additional advantage in that they can be used for drawing blood, thus sparing a person repeated needle sticks.

In terms of timing, most chemotherapy is given periodically, or in *cycles*. A common cycle length for many combination chemotherapy regimens is 21 days. Us-

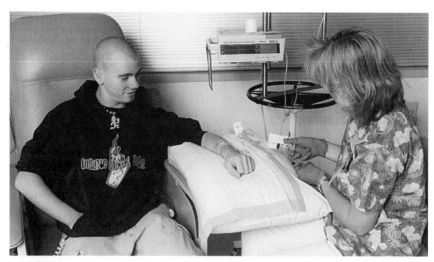

FIGURE 14-1 Most chemotherapy is administered intravenously (by vein).

ing this cycle length as an example, the chemotherapy is given by vein or by mouth on day 1 (referred to as cycle 1), and then again on day 22 (actually, day 1 of cycle 2). Chemotherapy dosed at intervals, such as 21 days, allows a person a long-enough period of time to recover both strength and blood counts but not so much time that the cancer can start growing again. For certain chemotherapy drugs, such as 5-FU, paclitaxel, gemcitabine, and vinorelbine, which have fewer side effects and are less suppressive of blood counts, a weekly dosing schedule can be used effectively.

WHAT ARE THE COMMON SIDE EFFECTS OF CHEMOTHERAPY, AND WHAT CAN BE DONE TO MINIMIZE THEM?

For many, the mere mention of *chemotherapy* conjures up the poignant but distressing image of a pallid cancer patient with no hair who is emaciated, constantly vomiting, and miserable. While loss of hair (*alopecia*) and nausea are significant side effects of many chemotherapy drugs (Table 14-2), they are by no means universal. In fact, with many of the newer chemotherapy agents, most people keep their full head of hair and have few or no gastrointestinal side effects (e.g., nausea, vomiting, and diarrhea).

For those who do have significant nausea, there are now a number of extremely effective medications that can ameliorate or eliminate the nausea altogether. It is important to remember that the nausea is temporary; it usually improves within a few days to a week after administration of chemotherapy.

TABLE 14-2 Effects Commonly Associated with Chemotherapy

Bone marrow suppression
    A decreased *white blood cell* count which increases the risk of infection
    A decreased *red blood cell* count which produces anemia (with fatigue) and reduces
        the oxygen-carrying capacity of the blood (leading to shortness of breath, chest pain,
        and a rapid heart rate)
    A decreased *platelet* count which increases the risk of bleeding and bruising
Infertility
Hair loss
Nausea
Vomiting
Fatigue
Diarrhea
Loss of appetite

Alopecia can be a traumatizing side effect for many. The timing of alopecia is variable, with most people noticing some hair loss 2 to 3 weeks after chemotherapy and complete baldness after a few cycles. Fortunately, hair growth almost always returns after the completion of treatment. For those who feel uncomfortable without hair during chemotherapy, most cancer centers have a service that will provide a wig (or *hair prosthesis*) for the individual with hair loss. There are also new medications in development that will prevent hair loss.

Fatigue and loss of appetite probably are the most common adverse effects after chemotherapy administration. These symptoms tend to worsen with cumulative doses of treatment—the more chemotherapy a person receives, the more likely he or she will become fatigued or experience loss of appetite. An element of fatigue may be related to the anemia caused by chemotherapies that decrease production of red blood cells in the bone marrow. In most cases, however, people receiving chemotherapy complain of fatigue even though they are not anemic. Adequate rest, a healthy diet, and even stimulant medications may be helpful in alleviating this fatigue. Appetite stimulants, including megestrol (Megace) and dronabinol (Marinol), may be added to encourage fluid and food intake.

The dose-limiting side effect of most types of chemotherapy drugs is bone marrow suppression. The bone marrow is a highly active organ, constantly producing the white blood cells that fight infection, the red blood cells that provide oxygen to body tissues, and the platelets that assist in blood clotting. These three types of cells circulate in our blood. The bone marrow contains cells that divide constantly to produce these three types of cells; it is therefore susceptible to the effects of chemotherapy, because these drugs target mainly dividing cells. By affecting dividing cells in the bone marrow, chemotherapy treatments often lead to decreased counts in white cells, red cells, and platelets. The consequences of this marrow suppression are described below.

Leukopenia, Neutropenia

The condition with a low white blood cell count (a low number of total white blood cells) is referred to as *leukopenia*, and, in more severe cases, *neutropenia*, or a low number of bacteria fighting white blood cells. People with neutropenia are at risk for severe, potentially life-threatening infections. Hospitalization for intravenous antibiotics is necessary if fever develops while a person is neutropenic. Daily injections of growth-factor drugs such as [granulocyte colony stimulating factor (G-CSF) or filgrastim (Neupogen), or granulocyte-macrophage colony stimulating factor (GM-CSF) or Sargramostim (Leukine)] that stimulate white blood cell production may shorten the duration of neutropenia after chemotherapy, though growth factors may not decrease the incidence of infections.

Thrombocytopenia

The condition defined by a low platelet count is known medically as *thrombocytopenia*. Platelets can be thought of as little "Band-Aids" in our blood. They help form blood clots and minimize bleeding after injury. Low platelet counts (the total number of platelets) following chemotherapy place a person at increased risk for bleeding and bruising. These bleeding complications are often minor and include tiny bleeds just under the skin surface that resemble pinpricks (called *petechiae*), nosebleeds, or cuts after shaving that ooze for a long time. However, on rare occasions, life-threatening hemorrhages, such as bleeding in the brain, can occur. To prevent major bleeding episodes, it is important for people with thrombocytopenia to avoid contact sports or heavy/dangerous activities when their platelet counts are low. When platelet counts fall below certain critical levels, platelet transfusions are indicated.

Anemia

Anemia refers to a low red blood cell count (the total number of red blood cells) in the blood. Red blood cells carry oxygen from our lungs to our tissues and vital organs, and they return carbon dioxide to the lungs, where it is exhaled. Anemia can develop from bleeding (e.g., someone who has just been in a car accident may lose blood through a wound and thus become anemic), or from decreased production of red cells in the bone marrow, which occurs with nutritional (iron, folate, vitamin B_{12}) deficiency or chemotherapy. Common symptoms of anemia include fatigue, pallor (an overall pale appearance), shortness of breath, chest pain, and rapid heart rate. Red blood cell transfusions often are given when the hematocrit, which measures the percent of red cells in the blood volume, drops below a certain level. Injections of a medication (e.g., erythropoietin, also known as Epogen or Procrit) to stimulate red blood cell production may improve the anemia and decrease the need for blood transfusions.

Infertility after chemotherapy is a major issue for male and female patients of reproductive age. This subject is covered in more detail in Chap. 24. It is important to remember, though, that not all chemotherapies are sterilizing and that the risk for infertility varies with both the type and the dose intensity of the chemotherapy drugs as well as with the recipient's age. In addition, newer chemotherapy regimens are less likely to cause infertility.

For example, Hodgkin's disease, a lymphoma that affects predominantly young adults, is one of the more curable forms of cancer. The classic chemotherapy combination for Hodgkin's disease, called MOPP (**m**echlorethamine, vincistine (**On**covin), **p**rocarbazine, and **p**rednisone), carries with it a high incidence of infertility because it contains two potent alkylating agents (mechlorethamine and procarbazine). In contrast, another Hodgkin's disease chemotherapy regimen, called ABVD [doxorubicin (**A**driamycin), **b**leomycin, **v**inblastine, and **d**acarbazine], has been found to be equally effective to MOPP yet is associated with significantly less infertility. This major advantage has resulted in ABVD becoming the regimen of choice for young people with Hodgkin's disease. For chemotherapy regimens that are not as forgiving as ABVD, all male and female patients of reproductive age should consider sperm or ovum banking if they desire children in the future. Women in this age group may be encouraged to take oral contraceptives that suppress ovarian function while chemotherapy is administered.

Related to fertility issues, it is important to mention that many chemotherapy agents are highly *teratogenic*—i.e., they cause birth defects. It is therefore imperative that sexually active patients, male or female, adopt strict birth control measures while taking chemotherapy and that they inform their physician promptly if there is any chance that a pregnancy could have occurred.

Last, before starting any chemotherapy, it is important to discuss with the oncologist the side effects expected from the regimen that is planned for you and to understand the risks involved. Work with your doctor to minimize side effects, such as nausea, and, most importantly, always call if you have a fever, no matter what time of day.

IF I DO NOT GET SICK FROM CHEMOTHERAPY, IS IT STILL WORKING?

The short answer is yes. The theoretical concern here is that if your body is tolerating the chemotherapy so well, the cancer may be doing so as well and the treatment won't be effective. While there have been anecdotal reports that Hodgkin's disease patients whose hair did not fall out after ABVD chemotherapy did less well than those who experienced alopecia, these reports have not been substantiated. There also have been many instances in which excellent cancer responses were observed in patients who tolerated chemotherapy without difficulty.

CHAPTER 15

Cognitive Impairment Associated with Cancer and Its Treatment

JASON HERSHBERGER, M.D.
THEODORE A. STERN, M.D.

OUTLINE

WHAT IS THINKING?

WHAT IS THE ANATOMY OF THINKING?

HOW DOES CANCER AFFECT THINKING?

WHAT ARE THE PSYCHOLOGICAL CAUSES OF DISORDERED THINKING?

WHAT ARE THE MEDICAL CAUSES OF DISORDERED THINKING?

WHAT ARE WARNING SIGNS OF TROUBLE?

WHEN SHOULD I TELL MY DOCTOR ABOUT THE DIFFICULTIES I AM HAVING WITH THINKING?

WHAT WILL MY DOCTOR LOOK FOR IN DIAGNOSING ALTERATIONS IN THINKING?

WHAT CAN BE DONE TO HELP WITH DISORDERED THINKING?

WHAT ARE SOME OF THE WAYS IN WHICH THINKING CAN BE DISORDERED?

WHAT IS THINKING?

Many people notice changes in aspects of their thinking when they have a medical illness or receive treatment for an illness. What is loosely described as "thinking" is a complicated process involving many mental faculties, including perception, attention, concentration, memory, decision making, and actions.

Facing cancer is a challenge to the body and to the mind. The ability to solve problems, make decisions, and understand this process is crucial to the well-being of every person with cancer. Furthermore, the diagnosis of cancer doesn't keep the rest of life's problems at bay; a clear head remains necessary.

WHAT IS THE ANATOMY OF THINKING?

There are 10 billion neurons (nerve cells) in the human brain. Each neuron connects with 1000 to 10,000 other neurons. All of these cells and connections work together to allow us to perceive, process, contemplate, and act on the world around us. Different areas of the brain are involved in different steps in this process.

During information processing, the *thalamus* is the first structure in the brain to take in information. The thalamus is the "gateway of the senses." All information from the body (i.e., what the senses perceive) travels from nerve cells outside of the brain to the thalamus. The thalamus is located in the middle of the brain and serves as the central relay point for incoming information. In the thalamus, the information is refined and then sent to the outermost layers of the brain.

This outermost section of the brain is called the *cerebral cortex*. The thalamus divides the incoming information by type and sends it to areas of the brain that specialize in sorting through that kind of information. For example, visual information might start with light reflected off a jumping rabbit. This light strikes the back of the eye and stimulates light-sensitive cells, which then send messages to the thalamus. The thalamus receives this information and recognizes that this is visual information. It, in turn, sends this information to the back of the brain, to a territory called the *occipital lobe* (which houses the visual cortex), where the information is processed. Different subsystems identify characteristics (e.g., How bright was the light? Was the object moving? What color was it? How big was it?) of the information. After these basic questions are answered, the different subsystems pool their information into a complicated visual image of a hopping rabbit. But without information from the other senses, this image is solely a silent movie of the rabbit.

At the same time, the ears receive the sound of the rabbit's feet on the ground. This noise vibrates the eardrum and stimulates nerves cells in the inner ear. As with vision, the information is carried along nerves to the thalamus. It is recognized as auditory information and is sent to the hearing center of the cortex (in the temporal lobe). There, basic questions of volume, pitch, and location are answered by different subsystems of the brain. Once a complicated sound is interpreted, the brain is ready to complete the experience.

Both the visual cortex and the auditory cortex send their work to another area of the cortex, called the medial temporal lobe. *Medial* means in the middle, and the temporal lobe is the part of the brain nearest to the ears. The purpose of the medial temporal lobe is complicated. First, it integrates the information from multiple senses (mixing the sound and the visual image) to allow that information to be stored in a person's memory. Next, it attaches an emotional value to the experience. Does the experience of seeing and hearing a rabbit create fear, sadness, anger, amusement, or joy? Is it emotionally noteworthy at all? Threats to one's safety take a higher priority in information processing: the fears attached to the sight of a ferocious bear assume a higher priority than the image of a rabbit. Then, the experience is recorded in the person's memory, so that it can be recalled immediately, in a minute, and possibly even years later. Thus, the medial temporal lobe organizes experiences and places an emotional importance on the elements of those experiences. Finally, it stores the experiences so that you can act on them and learn from them.

An experience can be recorded in several kinds of memory according to the emotional importance of the experience and according to how it relates to previously recorded memories. For example, the phone number you read on a piece of paper is placed in working memory long enough for you to dial it and then is forgotten. The schedule for the day's events may be placed in a short-term memory that allows you to remember a lunch date. If the experience is important enough that it becomes encoded in the long-term memory, it can be remembered years later. The medial temporal lobe is critical in recording all levels of these experiences.

Other parts of the brain also participate in classifying experiences. The frontal lobe (the part of the brain closest to the forehead) plays a crucial role in maintaining attention to ongoing experiences and in formulating a response. The frontal lobe controls *executive functions*. Like the executive of a company, the frontal lobe must make decisions based on the information at its disposal. The frontal lobe is in constant communication with the temporal lobe as it compares the current situation with those that were previously recorded.

Creatively, it attempts to imagine responses to a situation, pick a plan, and suppress the other options. It asks, for example, "Should I run? Stop? Take a picture?" Clearly a good action plan depends on the information available to the frontal lobe. If a rabbit is hopping away quickly, the brain may have only a fraction of a second to evaluate its experience and organize the response of taking a snapshot. If a surly bear approaches, the importance of a speedy and rational decision is even greater.

Once a plan is chosen, it is communicated to the *motor cortex*. The motor cortex, in combination with structures in the base of the brain called the *basal ganglia*, sends impulses to the body; this allows you to move, speak, stay quiet, or take a picture.

Although simplistic, this is a basic model of how the brain works. Now that we have discussed how the brain functions, we can move on to how those functions can be disrupted during illness.

HOW DOES CANCER AFFECT THINKING?

Cancer can affect thinking in a multitude of ways. Thinking is an activity of the brain, and any disturbance of brain function can disrupt the normal flow of thought.

The brain is necessary for the performance of basic life functions, such as controlling the heart rate and breathing. It regulates basic needs (such as hunger, thirst, and body temperature) as well as the higher functions of intellectual life, discussed above.

The brain is also fragile. Brain tissue has a high demand for basic nutrients: sugar and oxygen. Without a steady supply of these nutrients, brain cells quickly lose their ability to function, become exhausted, and ultimately die. The body has a number of mechanisms designed to guarantee that the fragile brain will remain viable.

For example, the hard, protective skull encases the brain. This protects against injury and ensures that a large proportion of the blood flowing from the heart reaches brain tissue to support its metabolic needs. A filter known as the *blood-brain barrier* further purifies the blood that does reach the brain. This barrier prevents many potentially toxic chemicals from reaching the brain.

Unfortunately, in the course of any illness, the defenses of the brain can be overwhelmed. Causes of dysfunctional (poor or disordered) thinking include psychological factors, the effects of medical illness, and the unwanted effects of medical treatments.

WHAT ARE THE PSYCHOLOGICAL CAUSES OF DISORDERED THINKING?

Receiving a diagnosis of cancer and treatment for the disease can be profoundly disturbing. Although we all realize that most people get sick at some point during their lifetimes and that all people, whether or not they have cancer, eventually die, developing a serious illness is traumatic. It attacks our fundamental wish to feel well and it can affect our expectations for the future.

Thus, it is not surprising that many people faced with a serious illness find that they suffer from a depressed mood. It is difficult to think clearly when you are flooded with profound sadness and negative thoughts (Table 15-1). Often, taking some time to regroup with loved ones provides enough of a cushion to return a

TABLE 15-1 Possible Causes of Disordered Thinking in a
Person with Cancer

Psychological factors
    Anxiety
    Depression
    Fear
The effects of medical illness on the brain and other organs
The unwanted effects of medical treatments

---

sense of control and well-being. Occasionally, depression takes on a life of its own, and there seems little that the sufferer or those who care about him or her can do to relieve the sadness. When this occurs, physicians consider the diagnosis of major depression (see Chap. 25).

Major depression is a syndrome of mood and behavioral changes that typically can be relieved with treatment (see Chap. 17). Besides having a depressed mood, people with depression can suffer from a variety of cognitive problems; some of these, like negative thinking, seem related to the depressed mood. Other individuals experience problems with their ability to focus and concentrate. People with depression, for example, often complain of an inability to complete cognitive tasks (such as reading a newspaper or watching a movie). This can occur because of a loss of pleasure and interest in things or a constant distraction by negative thoughts or feelings.

Another common psychological cause of cognitive problems is anxiety. Facing a serious illness and dealing with the decisions involved in its treatment can provoke overwhelming fear. The course of the illness and the choice of treatments may be uncertain; because of this uncertainty, a person may feel that any decision is likely to be wrong. Sometimes, the anxiety about these choices and about the future becomes an obstacle to hearing, remembering, and acting on important information. In general, this is a normal experience when a person is faced with a health crisis. When high anxiety begins to affect most of your decisions over an extended period, however, you and your doctors should consider whether an anxiety disorder is impairing your ability to function.

WHAT ARE THE MEDICAL CAUSES OF DISORDERED THINKING?

Medical causes of disordered thinking include the cancer itself, cancer therapy, and other illnesses to which a person with cancer is susceptible.

Cancer itself may affect a person's ability to think clearly. Some types of cancers originate in the brain and cause damage to this fragile organ. Other cancers begin in distant organs of the body, such as the lung or the breast, and can spread via the bloodstream (or metastasize) to the brain. The brain then becomes a site of new cancerous growth. If indicated, a doctor will perform a neurologic exam and obtain a picture of the brain [e.g., a computed tomography (CT) or magnetic resonance imaging (MRI) scan] to assess this possibility.

Cancers that have not spread to the brain may release chemicals that affect the brain, thus altering thinking. For example, some lymphomas or leukemias cause flu-like symptoms of fevers, chills, and sweats. Any person who has had the flu understands how difficult it is to think and function normally with these symptoms. Alternatively, some cancers cause anemia (a low red blood cell count), which can compromise the brain's oxygen supply. Rarely, a cancer causes elevation of one of the blood's components (the white blood cells or platelets), which, in turn, can compromise blood flow to the brain.

Cancer therapy or other illnesses may also compromise a person's ability to think clearly. Cancer is an abnormal growth of cells in the body, and most treatments attempt to slow and eradicate this growth (see Chap. 1). Unfortunately, many of the treatments (including surgery, radiation therapy, and chemotherapy) also affect healthy cells. Doctors refer to these phenomena as *side effects.*

All treatments for cancer carry the risk that the person receiving the treatment may experience side effects. Occasionally, side effects of treatment cause disturbances in thought. For example, medicines that cause fatigue, malaise, or sedation as unwanted effects can interfere with attention and concentration. Similarly, medicines that prevent some of the side effects of chemotherapy (e.g., antinausea medicines) also have the side effects of sedation and forgetfulness. Without the functions that engage the world around us, our memory of events suffers.

Side effects of treatments have the potential to adversely affect normal brain cell function, thereby impairing the flow of normal perceptions, thoughts, and feelings. The best way to detect such side effects is by obtaining a careful history of the timing of thinking problems and by relating them to any change in the individual's treatment. People receiving cancer therapy often are the best judges of how a treatment has affected them. A doctor's job is to listen with a trained ear for side effects. See Chaps. 14 and 16 for more details about these treatments and their potential side effects.

A third source of thinking problems results from other illnesses that can affect a person with cancer. Infections that an otherwise healthy person could fight off can have more dramatic consequences in a person with cancer. Both cancer itself and the many treatments for cancer weaken the body's immune response to viruses, bacteria, and even yeasts and fungi. Cancer, radiation therapy, and surgery can disrupt the anatomic barriers, such as the skin, that keep infectious organisms from invading the body. Infection in the body can elevate body temperature (fever), cause malabsorption of essential foods and fluids, and release toxins into the bloodstream. This may result in impaired brain function and cognitive disturbances.

WHAT ARE WARNING SIGNS OF TROUBLE?

Often, the signs of cognitive problems are subtle. People with cancer, their families, and their doctors often notice slight changes in memory, mood, or concentration before a stranger or casual acquaintance does. You may be aware of losing small objects, such as keys, or feel unable to follow the drift of a television show or newspaper article. One common complaint is losing a healthy sleep cycle (and either sleeping all day or lying awake all night).

Thinking is an incredibly complex and flexible process; many people with impaired thinking have difficulty describing what is wrong or what has changed. Occasionally, it takes a meeting among the person with cancer, his or her caregivers and family, and the medical staff to begin to put words to any difficulties.

WHEN SHOULD I TELL MY DOCTOR ABOUT THE DIFFICULTIES I AM HAVING WITH THINKING?

The sooner you can detect trouble, the sooner an appropriate diagnosis and treatment plan can be created. Too often, cognitive problems associated with cancer go undetected or unreported until they have reached dangerous proportions. Thus, as with any change in your body, your doctor wants to learn about alterations in your thinking when they change your ability to function or to enjoy life. Often, people are too embarrassed to discuss abnormal mood, perceptions, or memory problems with their physicians. In addition, because cognitive problems can rob a person of the insight that there is a problem, thinking disorders may escape detection until family members or caregivers notice the shift in mood, or a loss of memory.

WHAT WILL MY DOCTOR LOOK FOR IN DIAGNOSING ALTERATIONS IN THINKING?

First, your doctors should listen closely to your concerns about your ability to perceive, organize, feel, remember, plan, and act. Try to be as specific as possible about what activities are troublesome. Ask yourself the following questions: "Do I feel as if my senses aren't as sharp as they were? Am I having difficulty maintaining a focus on tasks that I used to perform without difficulty? Am I feeling more anxious or sad than seems normal? Am I forgetting things easily? What am I forgetting? Am I forgetting things from the distant past? Do I feel unable to make simple decisions? Am I having trouble performing everyday tasks, such as putting gas in the car, tying a tie, or navigating the neighborhood?" Try to recall when you first noticed such a problem and how it has changed since you first noticed it.

After hearing about your concerns, your doctor will examine you in a way that will best check for possible causes of your problems. Most doctors will do a physical examination with emphasis on the neurologic system. Testing your reflexes, strength, and gait can often give valuable information about how your body is receiving and processing basic sensory and motor information.

Once the basic physiology of your body is better understood, your doctor will likely ask you a series of questions that test attention, memory, calculation, mood, and perception. This is referred to as the *mental status examination*. Many of these questions may appear simple and even unrelated to your problem, but a thorough exam helps everyone better understand both the nature of what is impaired and also what is not.

Once your doctor has heard your story and performed an examination, he or she may ask for special tests to better understand your problem or to look for specific causes of cognitive dysfunction. Commonly, doctors order basic blood and urine tests to check for infections, and they will check your thyroid, liver, and kidney functions as well as the levels of your medications. Sometimes, physicians will ask for more elaborate testing of your thinking. This is called *neuropsychiatric testing* and is performed by a specially trained psychologist, who can look for and describe the specific problem that is troubling you. Occasionally, a doctor will look for an abnormality in the anatomy of your brain. Brain imaging usually comes in two forms: CT or MRI scans of the brain, which provide more detailed information about the soft tissue structures of the brain. Overall strategies for evaluating impaired or disordered thinking are specified in Tables 15-2 through 15-4.

WHAT CAN BE DONE TO HELP WITH DISORDERED THINKING?

Sometimes just identifying the problem and its cause can be comforting and will enable a person to begin to address the problem he or she is having. If the cause of the problem is understood, treatments can be tailored to that specific cause. For example, when attention is impaired by the addition of a new medicine, perhaps trying an equally effective alternative medicine will eliminate that side effect. Or, if the cancer has spread to the brain, surgery or radiation therapy may be able to reduce the tumor's pressure on brain tissue, thus ameliorating the symptoms. If another illness, such as anemia, has reduced the brain's supply of oxygen, a blood transfusion and supplemental oxygen can restore the oxygen supply and a person's ability to think clearly. Finally, if a mood or an anxiety disorder is affecting a person's ability to think clearly, a psychiatrist can be consulted and psychotherapy and/or medicine can be prescribed.

If the cause of the cognitive disturbance cannot be found or cannot be fully reversed by treatment, specific rehabilitation services can assist a person in using

TABLE 15-2 **Strategies for the Evaluation of Disordered Thinking**

Review the history of the symptoms
    Timing
    Severity
    Duration
    Quality
    Context
    Modifying factors
    Associated signs and symptoms

Determine the baseline mental function

Obtain a medical and psychiatric history
    Procedures
    Medical illnesses
    Head trauma
    Medication use
    Medical symptoms

Obtain a family history

Conduct an appropriate physical examination
    General appearance
    Vital signs (heart rate, respiratory rate, temperature, and blood pressure)
    Skin
    Head, eyes, ears, nose, and throat
    Neck
    Lymph nodes
    Thyroid gland
    Chest
    Heart
    Abdomen
    Genitalia
    Extremities
    Nervous system

Conduct an appropriate mental status examination
    Level of consciousness
    Appearance and description of motor activity (movement)
    Speech
    Affect
    Mood
    Thought
    Perception
    Cognition
    Abstracting abilities
    Insight and judgment

Order appropriate laboratory tests

TABLE 15-3 Laboratory Tests Often Used to Assess Disordered Thinking

Tests of brain function
   Electroencephalography (EEG)
   Functional MRI (magnetic resonance imaging)
   PET (positron emission tomography) scans
   SPECT (single photon emission computed tomography) scans
Radiologic tests
   CT or MRI scans
   Chest x-ray
   Noninvasive studies of the carotid artery
Tests of the cerebrospinal fluid
   Lumbar puncture and cerebrospinal fluid (CSF) analysis
Neuropsychological tests
   Attention and concentration
      Trail-making tests, part A and B
      Mental control subtests of the Wechsler Memory Scale III
      The WAIS (Wechsler Adult Intelligence Scale)-II Digit Span, Digit Symbol, and
      Arithmetic subtests
Receptive and expressive language
   Simple word recognition
   Reading comprehension
   Verbal fluency
   Naming ability
   Writing
      WAIS-III Verbal IQ subtests
      Boston Naming Test
      Verbal Fluency Test
Memory
   Visual memory
   Auditory memory
   Immediate and delayed recall
   Pattern and rate of new learning
   Recognition memory
   Unaided recall
Visual-spatial constructional ability
   Rey-Osterreith Complex Figure
   Hooper Visual Integration Tests
   Draw-a-clock face test
   Performance IQ subtests of the WAIS-III
Executive functions and abstract thinking
   Judgment
   Planning
   Logical reasoning
   Modification of behavior based on external feedback
      Wisconsin Card Sorting Test
      Stroop Color Word test
      Similarities and Comprehension test of the WAIS
Motor and sensory functioning
   Finger tapping test
   Grip strength

(*continued*)

*TABLE 15-3 (**continued**)*

Finger localization test
Two-point discrimination and simultaneous extinction test

General intelligence
  WAIS
  Verbal intelligence
    Vocabulary
    Similarities
    Arithmetic
    Digit span
    Information
    Comprehension
  Nonverbal visual spatial intelligence
    Picture completion
    Digit symbol
    Block design
    Matrix reasoning
    Picture arrangement

Emotional function
  MMPI-2 (Minnesota Multiphasic Personality Inventory)

Tests of the blood and urine

TABLE 15-4 Tests of the Blood and Urine Often Helpful in Identifying the Source of Neuropsychiatric Dysfunction

Tests of the urine
  Urinalysis

Tests of the blood
  HIV testing
  Rheumatoid factor
  Antinuclear antibody
  Drugs levels
  Heavy metal screening
  Complete blood count
  Vitamin B_{12} level
  Folate level
  Sedimentation rate
  Glucose
  Calcium
  Magnesium
  Phosphorus
  Electrolytes
  Liver function tests
  Thyroid function tests
  Tests of renal (kidney) function (creatinine and blood urea nitrogen)
  Cholesterol
  Triglycerides
  Syphilis serology

TABLE 15-5 Types of Neuropsychiatric Symptoms Associated with Disordered Thinking

Diagnosis	Description
Abulia	A lack of will or motivation
Agnosia	A lack of sensory ability to recognize familiar objects despite intact sensory function
Apathy	Absence of emotion; indifference
Aphasia	A difficulty with the transmission of language (e.g., speaking, reading, writing, or repeating)
Aprosodia	A lack of pitch, rhythm, and modulation of speech
Confabulation	The making up of tales and a readiness to give a fluent answer, with no regard to the facts
Delusions	Fixed, false beliefs
Dyslexia	A difficulty in reading
Dysarthria	A disturbance in articulation due to paralysis, incoordination, or spasticity of the muscles of speaking
Dysgraphia	A difficulty in writing
Dyscalculia	A difficulty in computing or calculating
Echopraxia	An involuntary imitation of movements made by another person
Hallucinations	Subjective perceptions of what does not exist, in any of the five sensory modalities
Illusions	Sensory misperceptions
Logorrhea	Garrulousness
Prosopagnosia	A difficulty in recognizing faces
Reduplicative paramnesia	A delusion that an impostor has replaced a person

other intact cognitive abilities to maintain function and quality of life. In this case, a thorough neurocognitive assessment can assist with identification of the strengths, as well as the impairments, in cognition. This assessment can guide and refine rehabilitative treatment.

WHAT ARE SOME OF THE WAYS IN WHICH THINKING CAN BE DISORDERED?

The brain can malfunction in a variety of ways; in part this reflects the portion of the brain that is affected and the degree to which that portion is affected. The definitions of several terms used to describe abnormalities in brain function (e.g., abulia, agnosia, apathy, aphasia, aprosodia, attentional deficits, confabulation, delusions, dyslexia, dysarthria, dysgraphia, dyscalculia, echopraxia, hallucinations, illusions, logorrhea, poor planning, prosopagnosia, and reduplicative paramnesia) are listed in Table 15-5.

Radiation Therapy

BRIAN CHON, M.D.

WHAT IS RADIATION THERAPY?

In 1895, a German physicist named Wilhelm Conrad Roentgen was the first to use radiation for medical purposes. He discovered that a new kind of ray, which he dubbed an *x-ray*, could blacken photographic film. He produced the first radiograph by placing his associate's hand between an x-ray tube and the film, which resulted in a picture of a white image of the hand against a dark background. Thus, the field of diagnostic radiology (the science of interpreting images taken of internal structures) was born.

By 1897, the first therapeutic use of radiation occurred when radiation therapy was used to eradicate a hairy mole from the skin of a German patient. This, in essence, was the beginning of radiation oncology—the treatment of cancer with radiation. The genesis of both diagnostic radiology and radiation therapy (the science of eradicating tumor cells with radiation) are clearly linked to the discovery of the x-ray, though the goals of each discipline and the tools employed to achieve their respective aims are very different. While diagnostic radiology [e.g., the use of x-rays, computed tomography (CT) and magnetic resonance imaging (MRI) scans, positron emission tomography (PET) scans, and ultrasounds] is applied to the population as a whole to determine whether disease is present, radiation therapy actually treats disease in a limited population—namely, people with cancer.

HOW DOES RADIATION WORK?

Basically, radiation given in high doses kills cells. Cells are the basic building blocks of body structures. Millions of cells attach to, and interact with, each other to form, say, the liver, the lungs, or the bones. Each cell, in turn, functions as its own mini-factory, contributes to the general function of the organ to which it belongs (for example, enabling the stomach to digest food) and ensures its own self-preservation. The blueprints for a cell's ability to function, grow, divide, and eventually die are housed in structures called deoxyribonucleic acid (DNA). Radiation therapy works by damaging the tumor cell's DNA, thus preventing cancerous cells from growing and dividing. Radiation therapy preferentially kills cells that are growing and dividing rapidly. Because cancer cells tend to grow more quickly than do normal cells and have a limited capacity to repair damaged DNA (no matter what type of cancer), they are more susceptible to the effects of radiation therapy than are normal cells in the body.

Unfortunately, normal cells in the body are affected to some extent by radiation. For example, a person with lung cancer may receive radiation therapy to the chest. While the radiation will be aimed at the portions of the lung affected by tumor, some radiation may hit the esophagus (the tube through which food passes when you swallow), which also sits in the chest. Because the esophagus is lined with normal mucosal cells that divide fairly frequently, some of those cells may be killed by radiation, causing the person receiving radiation therapy to experience pain with swallowing, possibly some bleeding, or even chest pain.

Consequently, the ultimate goal in giving radiation therapy is to target tumor cells and limit the radiation exposure of normal cells. Unlike cancer cells, when normal cells are exposed to radiation, most recover from the exposure by repairing themselves. Still, a person receiving radiation therapy experiences side effects (such as pain with swallowing) until those normal cells recover their function. To protect normal cells and hopefully to prevent many side effects, radiation oncologists (doctors who treat cancers with radiation) carefully limit the overall doses of radiation a person receives and may give only a small dose of radiation at any given time. In addition, most of the normal tissues are shielded from the path of the radiation through the use of "blocking" materials—objects impermeable to radiation that are placed over areas of the body not affected by cancer.

IS RADIATION THERAPY AS GOOD AS CHEMOTHERAPY FOR MY CANCER?

Tumors are as different as people. Some tumors that do not shrink when exposed to chemotherapy are killed by radiation. The converse is also true. Consequently, the selection of treatment, whether chemotherapy or radiation, depends on the specific type of tumor. Interestingly, many cancers are treated with both chemotherapy and radiation at the same time. Studies have shown that when these two treatment modalities are given simultaneously, many tumors are more likely to be eradicated. This strategy has become the standard of care for many lung cancers, anal cancers, and head and neck cancers.

HOW IS RADIATION THERAPY GIVEN?

Radiation therapy can be delivered in one of two ways: externally (from outside the body) or internally (from inside the body, through the use of radiation implants) (Table 16-1). Depending on the clinical situation, a combination of both therapies also may be necessary.

External Beam Radiation

Most people undergoing radiation receive it externally. With external beam radiation therapy, a machine directs high-energy rays at the cancer and at a small margin of normal tissue surrounding it. It is assumed that tiny, microscopic cancer

TABLE 16-1 **Ways in Which Radiation Therapy Is Delivered**

Externally
    X-rays
    Electron beams
    Cobalt-60 gamma rays
    Proton beams
    Neutron beams

Internally (brachytherapy)
    Intracavitary
    Interstitial (temporary and permanent)
    Surface molds

cells have invaded normal tissue in the area immediately surrounding the tumor and that this apparently normal tissue (which probably contains microscopic cancer cells) should be treated with radiation therapy to prevent a cancer recurrence. Depending on the location of the cancer, appropriate energy x-ray beams of known penetrating ability are chosen. Thus, superficial tumors (e.g., skin cancers) are treated with x-ray beams that penetrate the skin only slightly (so as not to affect deeper body structures unnecessarily), while deep tumors (e.g., cancer of the prostate) are treated with x-ray beams that penetrate deeply.

Five types of high-energy external radiation beams are used to treat cancer. These types include x-rays, electron beams, cobalt-60 gamma rays, proton beams, and neutron beams. *X-rays* are the most common. X-rays vary in the amount of photon energy (a measure of the intensity of the x-ray beam, described as the number of "packets" of energy released into cells) they deliver to a tumor. Machines called *linear accelerators* create these x-rays.

Electron beams and *cobalt-60 gamma rays* are also used clinically. Historically, both of these beams have been used to treat relatively superficial (i.e., close to the skin surface) tumors, including skin tumors, head and neck tumors, and brain tumors.

The two final types of radiation beams, comprised of *protons* and *neutrons*, are considerably heavier in mass than the other beams and require special machines to create them. Only two centers in the United States, one at the Massachusetts General Hospital and the other at Loma Linda Medical Center in California, currently have the capacity to create protons to treat tumor cells. Although proton beams are as effective as other beams in killing tumor cells, the advantage of using proton beams lies in their ability to deliver a full dose of radiation therapy to the tumor cells while minimizing the radiation to normal tissue.

It is important to note that the external types of radiation described above do not render the recipient "radioactive" or transmit radioactivity to others around him or her. The radiation is deposited immediately within the tumor as energy, much like heat. No residual radiation lingers within the body, and none is emitted to the environment or to other people.

Internal Radiation (Brachytherapy)

When high doses of radiation must be delivered to a small area, internal radiation therapy, or *brachytherapy,* can accomplish this goal in a shorter time than can external radiation. Internal radiation therapy places radiation sources as close as possible to the cancer cells. Instead of using large machines that emit radiation, radioactive materials are placed directly into the affected tissue or organ. This method of treatment concentrates the radiation on the cancer cells and lessens the radiation dose to surrounding (normal) tissue. A variety of radioactive sources—including iodine, palladium, cesium, and iridium—are used as brachytherapy implants.

Three techniques (intracavitary, interstitial, and surface molds) exist for the internal implantation of radiation. In *intracavitary* radiation, the radioactive sources are placed "within a cavity" or body orifice. Cesium sources, or implants, are examples of intracavitary implants commonly placed within the vaginal "cavity" for the treatment of cervical cancer.

In *interstitial* brachytherapy, radioactive implants in the form of needles, wires, or seeds are inserted directly into the tumor, called the *target tissue.* There are two types of interstitial implants: temporary and permanent. The selection of implants is largely based on the tumor type. For instance, prostate cancer is treated with permanent implants, while cervical cancer requires temporary implants. Cervical cancer implants usually require a total of 40 hours of radiation. Some head and neck tumors may be implanted for only 6 to 9 hours. With a temporary implant, the radioactive sources are removed after the desired dose has been delivered. The duration of radiation "implanted" in the tumor is largely dependent on the total amount of radiation delivered. The treatment schedule will also depend on the type of cancer, the tumor location, and the general health of a person with cancer. For instance, if a person cannot physically tolerate lying flat in bed for 40 hours, three 30-minute sessions with a different radiation source (iridium instead of cesium) can be used.

With a permanent implant, the sources are left indefinitely in the implanted tissue, as with seed implants for prostate cancer. When permanent implants are left in the tumor, the radioactive substance administered (the source) will lose radiation quickly and become nonradioactive in a short time. The half-life of the radioactive source specifies the rate at which the source becomes inactive (i.e., the time it takes for half of a substance's radioactivity to disappear is called its *half-life*). For all radioactive sources, five half-lives are required for the radiation to become essentially undetectable. This could take as little as 11 days for gold seed implants and as long as 300 days for iodine seeds. However, implants are designed to give off all of their dose to the implanted tumor with almost no radiation going to surrounding tissues. Consequently, the time required for implants to become entirely inactive is not a clinically important issue.

Last, *surface molds* are specially prepared to conform to the external contour of the specific cancer to be treated. The radioactive sources are securely positioned on the outer surface of the mold. A typical clinical example is a scalp mold used to treat superficial skin tumors of the head. A mold is designed to fit the shape of a person's head closely, with radioactive sources positioned along the outer surface.

Because the placement of most types of radioactive implants may be painful, general or local anesthesia is given to alleviate or eliminate pain. To ensure proper implantation with minimal discomfort, most internal radiation placement is done in the operating room, where anesthetics or analgesics (pain medicines) can be administered easily.

There are two types of temporary implants: low-dose-rate (LDR) and high-dose-rate (HDR). LDR implants are left in place for several days and require hospitalization in a special radiation-protected room, as these implants can emit radiation to other people and to the surrounding environment. HDR implants are left in place for several minutes in a special procedure room, which is also radiation-protected; HDR implants generally do not require hospitalization overnight.

HOW DOES THE DOSE OF RADIATION I AM RECEIVING COMPARE WITH THE RADIATION ASSOCIATED WITH A CHEST X-RAY?

The total dose of radiation used to eradicate a tumor is significantly higher than the dose used to image the chest for a chest x-ray. However, unlike a chest x-ray, which emits radiation to the entire upper body (including the lungs, heart, esophagus, ribs, and spinal cord), radiation therapy is targeted to specific tumor locations. For instance, a person with lung cancer will not receive treatment to both lungs, the heart, and the ribs. Radiation will be delivered only to the portion of the lung that contains the tumor. The strategy of radiation oncologists is to deliver a "bomb" of radiation to the tumor while keeping the otherwise healthy tissues from receiving any radiation.

HOW ARE OTHERS PROTECTED FROM IMPLANTED RADIATION?

The radiation sources implanted in tumors deposit nearly all of their radiation into the cancerous tissue. In fact, as the distance from the source increases, the dose drops exponentially: tissue 1 inch from the radiation source will be exposed to 10 times the amount of radiation as tissue 2 inches away and 100 times the amount of radiation as tissue 3 inches away. Consequently, the radiation dose affecting

TABLE 16-2 **Precautions for People with Temporary Implants**

Time limits are placed on visitor exposure to a person with a temporary implant and visits can vary from 30 minutes to several hours a day.
Children under the age of 18 should not visit a person with an internal implant.
Pregnant women should not visit a person with an internal implant.
Visitors should remain at least 6 feet from the person with the implant.
A rolling lead shield may be placed beside the bed and kept between the person with an implant and his or her visitors and staff members.

other people is extremely low and almost undetectable. However, to ensure the protection of others, including visitors and other health care professionals, time limits are placed on exposure to the implanted patient. Nurses typically will work quickly and often will speak from the doorway of a room, rather than at the bedside, to limit their exposure. This precaution is only germane to temporary implants because of the high energy of the radioactive sources. Permanent implants do not require such precautions because they emit only low energy—typically 200 times less energy than temporary implants. Nevertheless, health care professionals are able to give all necessary care by using radiation shields and other radioprotective devices. With the possible exception of prostate implants, urine and stool will be free of radioactivity.

Limits are set on visitors. Children under the age of 18 and pregnant women should not visit a person with an internal implant. Visitors should remain at least 6 feet from the person with the implant. The time of the visit can vary from 30 minutes to several hours a day. In most hospitals, a rolling lead shield is placed beside the bed and kept between the person with an implant, his or her visitors, and staff members (Table 16-2).

DOES THE DISTANCE FROM A RADIATION SOURCE MAKE A DIFFERENCE IN HOW MUCH RADIATION IS RECEIVED BY SOMEONE ELSE?

This is the precise principle behind brachytherapy, which involves both temporary and permanent seed implants. Implants deliver lethal radiation doses to the tumor while minimizing the radiation exposure of healthy tissues farther away from the implant. In fact, the radiation dose is exponentially lost as the distance from the radiation source is increased. Particularly for permanent implants, this effect is pivotal in keeping radiation doses at almost zero for normal tissues. For example, people who receive permanent prostate seed implants do not need to worry about being "radioactive" to their partners. Within a few millimeters of the prostate gland, radiation is hardly detectable. Consequently, people with permanent implants can carry on with their normal activities without worry.

WITH EXTERNAL RADIATION, HOW LONG DOES THE TREATMENT TAKE?

For most types of cancer, radiation therapy is usually given 5 days a week for 6 to 7 weeks. When radiation is used for palliative care (in other words, the treatment of side effects, such as pain, associated with a tumor but not for cure of the cancer), the course of treatment is shorter, usually 2 to 3 weeks. The total dose of radiation and the number of treatments required will depend on the size, location, and type of the cancer. The rationale for using fractions (i.e., small doses of daily radiation) rather than a few large doses is that small doses of radiation help protect normal body tissues by allowing them time to recover from the damage of radiation between treatments. Weekend rest breaks also allow normal cells to recover.

WHAT IS A RADIATION PLANNING SESSION (SIMULATION)?

A planning session (also called a *simulation*) is the first step of starting radiation therapy. This is an opportunity for the radiation oncologist to determine how best to deliver radiation to you. It is called a simulation because actual treatment positions and radiation fields that will be used for therapy are filmed and recorded (they are *simulated*), though no radiation is actually administered. It is like a dress rehearsal before the actual performance.

At a simulation, you will undergo the same rituals as in a typical treatment day. You will be asked to change into a gown and to lie down on a treatment table. Depending on the situation, you will either be asked to lie flat on your back or on your stomach. Once the radiation fields are determined, a few small "tattoos" no larger than freckles will be made on the skin. This ensures that the fields being simulated can easily be reproduced day after day. The simulation usually lasts 1 hour. This is much longer than a typical treatment session, which often lasts only 15 minutes. After the session, you are given an appointment to begin radiation therapy. The entire process is painless and as easy as having an x-ray.

WHAT HAPPENS DURING THE TREATMENT VISIT?

Before each external beam radiation treatment (Table 16-3), you may have to change into a hospital gown. In the treatment room, the radiation therapist uses marks on the skin to locate the treatment area (the area of skin that lies over the cancer) and to position you. Typically, you lie on your back, resting comfortably. To protect the normal tissue around the tumor, the radiation therapist may place special radiation blocking shields over these areas (Fig. 16-1).

TABLE 16-3 **What Happens during a Typical Radiation Therapy Visit**

You may need to change into a hospital gown.

The radiation therapist makes marks on the skin to locate the treatment area.

Typically, you lie on your back, resting comfortably.

To protect the normal tissue around the tumor, the radiation therapist may place special radiation blocking shields over these areas.

You may be repositioned with the assistance of "immobilization devices," such as foam or plaster.

The radiation therapist will leave the treatment room before the treatment begins.

The radiation beam is turned on for 1 to 2 minutes.

Though sometimes difficult, it is imperative to remain still during treatments to deliver radiation.

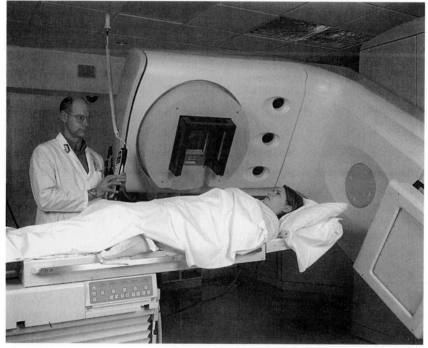

FIGURE 16-1 During an external beam radiation treatment, you will typically lie on your back, resting comfortably.

For each external radiation therapy session, you will remain in the treatment room for approximately 15 minutes. Much of that time is spent repositioning you with the assistance of "immobilization devices," such as foam or plaster. Once again, your position will depend on the simulation (treatment planning) session. Most commonly, people are asked to lie flat on their backs. Placing a person in different positions allows the radiation to penetrate the tumor at different angles, thus treating different areas of the tumor. The radiation beam is actually turned on for only 1 to 2 minutes. Though this is sometimes difficult, it is imperative for you to remain still during treatments to deliver radiation to the tumor precisely and consistently. External radiation treatments are painless, and you will not be able to see, hear, or smell the radiation.

The radiation therapist will leave the treatment room before the treatment begins. Immediately outside the treatment area, the therapist controls the radiation machine and is able to watch and to listen to you at all times. Although you may feel alone, the therapist can communicate with you by using the intercom in the treatment room. The machine can be stopped immediately at any time. These machines are large and produce a lot of noise as they move around the body. Once again, these machines are being moved and controlled by a radiation therapist, and the person receiving the therapy is constantly supervised.

WILL SOMEONE NEED TO ACCOMPANY ME TO AND FROM RADIATION TREATMENTS?

The answer to this question rests with your condition prior to beginning radiation treatments. If you were able to drive and come to the hospital alone before, then certainly you will be able to maintain this level of independence while on treatment. However, if you needed some assistance before beginning radiation therapy, then the same level of assistance will be required during radiation treatments.

WHAT ARE THE SIDE EFFECTS OF RADIATION TREATMENT?

Radiation therapy does not make the body radioactive. There is, in general, no need to avoid contact with others when receiving radiation therapy. Even hugging, kissing, or having sexual relations with others poses no risk of exposing them to radiation. The only exception to this rule occurs with permanent radiation implants for prostate cancer. People with these implants are advised against having children sit on their laps and against having sexual relations for several weeks after the initial date of the implant.

Most side effects of radiation therapy occur directly in the area that is being treated, and many people experience no side effects at all. Side effects are usually not serious and can be controlled with medication or diet. Typically, they disappear completely within a few weeks after treatment ends. The radiation oncologist should address the specifics of potential side effects with you prior to the first radiation delivery session.

People undergoing radiation treatments most frequently complain of fatigue and a lack of energy. Possible causes may relate to the disease process itself or to the treatment. Lowered blood counts, lack of sleep, pain, or poor appetite also contribute to these symptoms. Most people begin to feel tired after a few weeks of radiation therapy. This fatigue occurs because the body expends energy to heal. The added stress of coping with cancer, daily trips for treatment, and the effect of radiation on normal cells also contribute to fatigue. The fatigue gradually will disappear after the radiation treatments are completed.

Radiation therapy, like surgery, is local therapy—therapy that affects only one part of the body. The side effects generally will be limited to the tissue being irradiated. For instance, people with esophageal cancer may develop esophagitis (irritation of the esophagus) and may experience difficulty swallowing large, dry pieces of food. People with rectal cancer may have looser stools. People with breast cancer may develop skin reddening and irritation. These are all examples of radiation-induced side effects.

Throughout the course of radiation therapy, doctors will check regularly on the effects of the treatment. Although the changes in cancer size may not occur during treatment, symptoms like pain, bleeding, or discomfort should improve. Radiation continues to work over the next several months even after the completion of therapy, so tumor regression and improvement of symptoms will also continue.

WILL I LOSE MY HAIR FROM RADIATION TREATMENT?

Unlike chemotherapy, radiation remains in the irradiated tissue and does not travel to other parts of the body. Therefore, unless the brain or the scalp is being treated with radiation, hair loss will not occur.

IS THERE A LIMIT TO HOW MUCH RADIATION I CAN RECEIVE?

Every part of the body has a different radiation "tolerance." In other words, different parts of the body can tolerate different doses. For instance, bone can withstand 10 times more radiation than the lens of the eye. In treating cancer, physicians will not exceed this tolerance dose. The primary goal of radiation therapy is to kill tumor cells while letting the healthy, normal cells recover. This end will not be achieved if the tolerance dose is exceeded.

WHAT SHOULD I DO TO PREPARE MYSELF FOR RADIATION?

Reactions to radiation tend to be mild but may differ in magnitude depending on the site of your disease and your overall health. Not "overdoing it" is important during radiation therapy. If fatigue sets in, activities should be limited and leisure time spent in restful ways. People undergoing radiation treatments should not count on continuing a hectic work schedule, though some may be able to maintain full-time jobs. Short naps during the day and more sleep at night will help you cope with excess fatigue, as may light exercise, such as walking. It is important to try different approaches to the side effects of radiation therapy, as coping mechanisms vary from person to person. Cancer support groups can be a great source of ideas and recommendations for optimizing daily regimens.

WHAT CAN I EXPECT AFTER RADIATION THERAPY?

People who have had radiation therapy need to continue with some of the special care they received during treatment, at least for a short period of time. For instance, skin irritation from radiation treatments can continue for several weeks after the treatment ends. Proper skin care needs to be followed for a short time after completing therapy.

Extra rest may be required after the completion of radiation therapy to allow for normal tissue recovery. Normal work schedules should be resumed gradually, being mindful of the sometimes subtle effects of radiation. A follow-up appointment, typically 3 to 4 weeks after completion of radiation therapy, is recommended.

WILL RADIATION THERAPY BE COVERED BY MY INSURANCE?

Absolutely! Radiation, along with chemotherapy and surgery, are considered standards of care.

SUMMARY

Radiation therapy is an important therapy used to eradicate cancer. It is used either alone or in conjunction with surgery and chemotherapy. Use of radiation is a painless, noninvasive way to preferentially kill tumor cells. It works primarily by damaging the DNA of tumor cells, which then cannot be repaired effectively. With either external or internal radiation, the principles of treatment and the mechanism of action are the same, though the precautions a person must take differ, as does the treatment time. For the most part, side effects of radiation therapy are limited to the treated area of the body, are usually minimal, and resolve after a short while. Most people can continue to work normally throughout their course of radiation treatment. Fatigue, however, is a common side effect of radiation therapy and typically persists for several weeks after the completion of treatment. Overall, radiation therapy is well tolerated and remains an important therapeutic tool in the fight against cancer.

CHAPTER 17

The Use of Medications to Alter Mood and Behavior Associated with Cancer

David Mischoulon, M.D., Ph.D.

WHAT TYPES OF DRUGS ALTER MOOD AND BEHAVIOR AS A SIDE EFFECT?

A variety of medications have been associated with the development of altered mood and/or behavior (Table 17-1). Among the more common offenders are the following:

Beta blockers [e.g., propranolol (Inderal)] and other medications for high blood pressure. These have been shown to cause depression, though evidence suggests that they may be less likely to do so when used in lower doses.

Steroids (e.g., prednisone), typically prescribed for respiratory and autoimmune illnesses as well as for cancer treatment, can dramatically affect mood and behavior. Depression and/or mood swings may result from taking these medications. In some cases, agitation, sleeplessness, anger attacks, bizarre thinking, confusion, or episodes of full-blown mania may result from steroid use, particularly at higher doses. If you notice any of these symptoms, you should notify your doctor immediately; it may be necessary to go to an emergency department for assistance.

Cimetidine (Tagamet), an antiulcer medication, may cause depression and bizarre thinking (e.g., paranoia), particularly in older individuals. Extreme cases may require administration of antipsychotic medications (also referred to as *major tranquilizers* or *neuroleptics*) to hasten the resolution of the thought disorder.

Oral contraceptive pills may cause depressed mood and/or irritability in some women. Often, this can be remedied by changing to another formulation of contraceptive medication with a different ratio of the hormones estrogen and progesterone.

Sedatives, sleeping pills, and antianxiety drugs, as their names indicate, can make you feel tired and sometimes "unmotivated." These symptoms may mimic depression, although they may not signify the presence of a depressive disorder per se. Also, stronger sedatives [such as diazepam (Valium) or lorazepam (Ativan)]

TABLE 17-1
**Medications Associated
with the Development
of Altered Mood
and/or Behavior**

Antianxiety medicines
Antinausea medicines
Beta blockers
Chemotherapy
Oral contraceptive pills
Sedatives
Sleeping pills
Steroids
Ulcer medicines

may result in temporary memory difficulties. These problems may be alleviated by decreasing the dose or switching to a milder sedative [such as buspirone (Buspar) or zolpidem (Ambien)].

Cancer chemotherapeutic agents may cause depression, either as a direct effect of the medication or possibly as a side effect of the medication (e.g., nausea and other physical symptoms that may limit one's lifestyle).

The chemotherapeutics most closely associated with depression are the *interferons,* which are used for the treatment of melanoma, cancer of the kidney, leukemia, and lymphoma. *Vinblastine* (Velban), *mitotane* (Lysodren), and *levamisole* (Ergamisole) have also been associated with depression in a few individuals.

Procarbazine (Matulane) has been reported to cause "depression." However, as this medication has a chemical structure similar to that of the monoamine oxidase inhibitor (MAOI) antidepressants, its apparent depressive effect may involve an overall depression of the central nervous system due to its sedating effect. In fact, it may cause an improvement in mood and even euphoria or mania.

Hormonal therapies for cancer, such as *flutamide* (Eulexin), *tamoxifen* (Nolvadex), and *megesterol acetate* (Megace), may be associated with depression, but the research in this area is limited.

By and large, there are no formal studies investigating the psychiatric side effects of cancer chemotherapies, and there is no solid evidence yet to determine conclusively whether these chemotherapies place people at risk for depression. It may be wise to discuss this issue with your doctor prior to initiating chemotherapy. In some instances, your doctor may want to consider adding an antidepressant before beginning treatment to prevent the onset of depressive symptoms.

Keep in mind that these warnings do not suggest that it is necessarily unsafe to take any of the above medications. However, it is important that you be aware of the risk of developing depression or other mood-related side effects. Most people, in fact, are able to tolerate these medications quite well. Remember that depression caused by a medication usually resolves quickly upon discontinuation of the medication.

Antinausea medications (antiemetics), like all medications, may have adverse effects, and some may cause mood changes, such as depression. The ones most commonly associated with depression include *trimethobenzamide* (Tigan) and *dolasetron* (Anzemet); *dronabinol* (Marinol) may exacerbate an already existing depression or manic state; *metoclopramide* (Reglan) may cause depression and, in some cases, suicidal thoughts. The actual mechanism for how depression develops in these cases is not well understood. Depression may be brought about by biochemical imbalances, similar to those seen in major depression not caused by medications, or it may be associated with sedation, which is a common side effect of antinausea medications. If you are taking medications for nausea and notice feelings of depression, you should discuss this with your doctor as soon as possible. Often, the mood changes resolve quickly upon switching to another medication.

HOW EFFECTIVE ARE ANTIDEPRESSANT DRUGS?

Approximately 60 to 70 percent of individuals who take antidepressant medications experience an improvement in their symptoms. However, despite the increasing number of marketed antidepressants, between 19 and 34 percent of depressed patients who take antidepressants will not respond to treatment. In addition, between 15 and 50 percent of patients who respond initially to an antidepressant will experience a recurrence of their depression, even if they are still taking an antidepressant. Individuals with coexisting medical or psychiatric illness may, in some instances, be less likely to respond to antidepressants or may respond only partially.

In cases in which an antidepressant helps only partially, higher doses and/or the addition of a second antidepressant (combination treatment) may be required to attain a more robust effect. Also, the addition of certain types of talking therapies is usually effective as an adjunct to medication treatment for depressed individuals.

WHEN SHOULD ANTIDEPRESSANTS BE PRESCRIBED?

Antidepressants are recommended when your doctor suspects that you are developing major depression, as manifest by a series of symptoms including the following:

Depressed mood; loss of pleasure or interest in ordinary activities

Feelings of guilt, worthlessness, or hopelessness

Decreased energy, fatigue, and unexplained aches and pains

Difficulty concentrating or making decisions

Restlessness or irritability, or feeling "slowed down" (psychomotor changes)

Inability to sleep well or oversleeping

Changes in appetite or weight

Thoughts of death or suicide

In these instances, antidepressant medications may be recommended, as they can relieve these symptoms within a few weeks. Some antidepressants, particularly those from the family of selective serotonin reuptake inhibitors (SSRIs), such as fluoxetine (Prozac) or paroxetine (Paxil), also have been shown to be helpful for some types of anxiety states, such as panic disorder or social phobia. Obsessive-compulsive disorder (OCD) also responds well to SSRIs and to some tricyclic antidepressants [e.g., clomipramine (Anafranil)]. Eating disorders, such as anorexia nervosa or bulimia nervosa, may respond to SSRIs. Some pain syndromes may be treated effectively with tricyclic antidepressants, SSRIs, or antiseizure medications, such as valproic acid (Depakote) or carbamazepine (Tegretol).

FOR HOW LONG SHOULD ANTIDEPRESSANTS BE PRESCRIBED?

Antidepressants typically require between 3 and 6 weeks to work. The response to these medications may come earlier, but in some instances, it can come later. Thus, it is important that you continue taking such a medication even if at first you do not feel better. It may take several weeks before you begin to see an improvement.

Once you have responded to an antidepressant, how long you will need to continue taking it will depend on several factors. If you have a history of a long-standing depression (depression lasting for many years) or of multiple depressive episodes throughout your life, you will have a higher risk of relapse when you stop taking antidepressants. In such cases, your doctor may recommend that you continue taking prescribed antidepressants indefinitely. If you are suffering your first episode of depression, you may be less likely to relapse when you stop taking the antidepressant. When your first depressive episode has been treated successfully, you may safely stop taking antidepressants about 6 to 12 months later. Even if you have to take antidepressants indefinitely, remember that these medications are, by and large, safe over the long term.

It is important that you do not discontinue your antidepressant without first consulting with your doctor, even if you are feeling well. Likewise, antidepressants must be taken daily, regardless of how you happen to be feeling on a particular day. Missing doses too frequently can decrease the overall effectiveness of antidepressants and may result in an unsatisfactory response.

WHAT ARE THE TYPICAL SIDE EFFECTS OF ANTIDEPRESSANTS?

Side effects depend on the specific type of antidepressant taken. People taking antidepressants may experience nausea, insomnia, fatigue, headache, dizziness, tremor, dry mouth, vomiting, weight gain (or loss), restlessness, pain, decreased sexual desire, delayed ejaculation and/or impotence (in men), increased urination, visual or taste abnormalities, coughing, yawning, and rapid heartbeat (Table 17-2). Given this extensive list, it might seem strange that these medications are prescribed so frequently. Fortunately, these side effects occur in a minority of those taking antidepressants. Some antidepressants, depending on their chemical structure, are more likely than others to cause certain side effects; in general, it is difficult to predict whether you will have a particular side effect from an antidepressant.

TABLE 17-2 **Infrequent Side Effects of Antidepressants**

Cardiopulmonary
  Coughing
  Yawning
  Rapid heartbeat
Constitutional
  Insomnia
  Fatigue
  Weight gain (or loss)
  Restlessness
Gastrointestinal
  Nausea
  Vomiting
  Dry mouth
Neurologic
  Headache
  Dizziness
  Tremor
  Pain
  Visual or taste abnormalities
Reproductive/urologic
  Decreased sexual desire
  Delayed ejaculation and/or impotence (in men)
  Increased urination

Some antidepressants have unusual, or idiosyncratic, adverse effects. For example, bupropion (Wellbutrin) may cause seizures if taken in doses higher than those recommended or by individuals with preexisting seizure disorders or eating disorders. Monoamine oxidase inhibitors (MAOIs)—e.g., phenelzine (Nardil) or tranylcypromine (Parnate)—require that you follow a special diet, as certain foods may result in your developing extremely high blood pressure, thus increasing the risk of stroke. Rarely, trazodone (Desyrel) may cause a prolonged erection (*priapism*) in men, which is considered a medical emergency requiring immediate medical intervention.

If you experience side effects while taking antidepressants, it may help to decrease the dose or to have your doctor switch you to another antidepressant. Sometimes adding another medication may help. For example, excessive sweating may be controlled by adding the antihistamine cyproheptadine (Periactin), sexual dysfunction may respond to sildenafil (Viagra), restlessness (akathisia) may be alleviated by adding a beta blocker (e.g., propranolol), insomnia may be treated by adding a mild sedative at bedtime.

It is important that you report all side effects to your doctor. In most instances, these adverse effects can be alleviated. You should not feel discouraged if you have side effects upon initiation of an antidepressant; there is a good chance that they will go away in a few days.

HOW EFFECTIVE ARE ANTIANXIETY DRUGS?

Antianxiety drugs are generally effective, with most people reporting at least some alleviation of anxiety (Table 17-3). They may be used for well-defined anxiety disorders (e.g., generalized anxiety or panic disorder) or for occasional episodes of anxiety brought about by stress or other demanding life situations. One attractive benefit of most sedatives is that they tend to work relatively quickly (sometimes within a few minutes), and therefore they can provide rapid relief of anxiety.

Some antianxiety drugs, such as those from the benzodiazepine family [e.g., diazepam (Valium)] are quite powerful and may, in some instances, be habit-forming. These should be prescribed with care, and it is important that you discuss with your doctor any concerns that you may have about your dependency on medications. People who have—or have had—problems with alcoholism or drug addiction may be better off avoiding these types of sedatives except in cases of severe anxiety that may not respond to milder sedatives. It is important that you never mix alcohol or "recreational" drugs with sedatives, as the combination may prove excessively sedating; in some extreme cases, it has been known to be fatal.

There are gentler sedative medications available as well. For example, buspirone (Buspar), which is effective for generalized anxiety, has a mild side-effect profile and is not habit-forming. However, it often takes up to 2 weeks to achieve its full effect. For people with mild insomnia, medications such as zolpidem (Ambien) or

TABLE 17-3 **Types of
Antianxiety Medications
(with Examples)**

Benzodiazepines
   Diazepam (Valium)
   Lorazepam (Ativan)
Gentler sedatives
   Buspirone (Buspar)
Sleeping pills
   Zolpidem (Ambien)
   Zaleplon (Sonata)
Blood pressure medicines
   Beta blockers
   Clonidine (Catapres)
Antidepressants
   Trazodone (Desyrel)
   Mirtazapine (Remeron)
   Tricyclics (Amitriptyline or Elavil)
Anticonvulsants
   Valproic acid (Depakote)
Antipsychotics
   Haloperidol (Haldol)

zaleplon (Sonata) may be helpful in promoting restful sleep without the risk of dependency or addiction.

Beta blockers and clonidine (Catapres), which are generally used to treat high blood pressure, also are useful for decreasing some of the physical symptoms associated with anxiety (e.g., rapid heartbeat). Certain antidepressants—such as trazodone (Desyrel), mirtazapine (Remeron), and some tricyclic antidepressants (e.g., amitriptyline)—may be useful in promoting sleep as well and are sometimes used in place of more conventional sedatives. Anticonvulsant agents, such as valproic acid (Depakote), may also alleviate anxiety. In some cases, the antipsychotic medications (*neuroleptics*) may be effective for extreme anxiety states that fail to respond to benzodiazepines or other sedatives.

FOR HOW LONG SHOULD ANTIANXIETY DRUGS BE PRESCRIBED?

This depends on the type of anxiety disorder being treated. Certain anxiety conditions, such as panic disorder, tend to be chronic and may require an indefinite course of antianxiety medication taken on a daily basis. Episodic anxiety, which occurs only in certain stressful situations, may be managed by "as needed" (or "p.r.n.") medication, to be taken only at the time that an anxiety episode develops. Chronic anxiety disorders tend to benefit from long-acting sedatives, such as clonazepam (Klonopin). Episodic anxiety may be treated with shorter-acting agents, such as alprazolam (Xanax) or lorazepam (Ativan).

Sometimes, if anxiety is brought upon by a specific stressor (such as visiting the doctor's office), certain types of psychotherapy (particularly cognitive-behavioral therapy) can be effective at reducing situationally driven anxiety and helping you to develop coping mechanisms for dealing with anxiety when it arises. These "talking therapies" can work along with medications and sometimes even function as an alternative to them. In some instances, avoidance (or decreasing the frequency) of the anxiety-provoking situation is an option.

WHAT ARE THE TYPICAL SIDE EFFECTS OF ANTIANXIETY DRUGS?

The main complaint people have about antianxiety medications is excessive daytime tiredness and/or light-headedness. Some people report reduced sexual energy and a depressed mood. In some cases, particularly with long-term use of benzodiazepines, memory difficulties may arise. People may even suffer brief episodes of amnesia, forgetting details of the day they received chemotherapy or portions of a hospitalization—not altogether bad side effects! Often these side effects may

TABLE 17-4 Common Side
Effects of Antianxiety
Medications

Excessive daytime tiredness
Light-headedness
Reduced sexual energy
Depressed mood
Memory difficulties
Brief episodes of amnesia

be reduced or eliminated completely by decreasing the dose of the antianxiety medication or by switching to a milder type of sedative (Table 17-4).

WHAT DRUGS CAN IMPROVE CONCENTRATION AND DECREASE IRRITABILITY?

Individuals with difficulties in concentration may benefit from the use of psychostimulants, such as methylphenidate (Ritalin) or dextroamphetamine (Dexedrine). These medications, used more commonly to treat attention deficit disorder (ADD), are quite effective, and most people report at least some improvement in focus and concentration. However, as with some sedatives, these medications must be prescribed with care, as they are potentially habit-forming. Also, they must be taken in the morning, as they may interfere with sleep if taken too late in the day. Individuals with certain types of heart problems or high blood pressure should not take stimulants. Side effects from stimulants include agitation, headaches, and mild loss of appetite (when used in moderately high doses). Modafinil (Provigil) is a nonstimulant medication that often improves daytime alertness and may be useful for people who feel too tired during the day.

Irritability may be treated with mood-stabilizing medications, such as lithium, valproic acid (Depakote), gabapentin (Neurontin), and others. Some mood-stabilizing medications can have serious side effects, including liver or kidney damage, and therefore require periodic monitoring of blood levels. Liver enzymes and kidney function also must be monitored in individuals who take these medications. Antidepressants (particularly SSRIs, such as fluoxetine) and some sedatives may also be effective in controlling irritability.

WHAT INTERACTIONS WITH OTHER MEDICATIONS SHOULD I BE CAREFUL OF WHEN USING THESE DRUGS?

Just as a car uses gasoline for fuel, breaks it down into smaller parts, and disposes of it as exhaust, so too does your body break down, or metabolize, medications so that they can be excreted in stool or urine. Antidepressants and antianxiety medications are, by and large, metabolized in the liver. There, they are usually broken down by a series of different enzymes, many of which break down several different types of drugs. Sometimes, different drugs may compete for the same enzymes, and sometimes a particular drug may inhibit (or stimulate) the function of a particular enzyme. This can affect the levels of other medications that you may also be taking. Most of the time, these interactions are benign and have little if any clinical significance. However, as medication regimens require at least a minimal dose to be effective, taking an assortment of medications puts you at greater risk of interactions that may decrease the effectiveness of some medications (if the medication level becomes too low). Conversely, the risk of toxicity (if a medication level becomes too high) also can increase with multiple medications.

When different doctors prescribe you medications, it is important that you discuss this with each of them, so that they will be aware of what you are taking. It is a good idea to always keep handy an up-to-date list of all your medications and their doses. This will prevent your doctors from prescribing a medication that could result in an adverse interaction with your other medications. It also is important to inform your doctors of any over-the-counter medications that you are taking, as these can also interact with your prescription medications.

Some drug combinations which may be troublesome include the following:

SSRIs plus warfarin (Coumadin): SSRIs can cause warfarin levels in the blood to get too high, and this can increase the risk of internal bleeding.

MAOIs [e.g., phenelzine (Nardil)] plus other antidepressants or opium-derived medications [e.g., meperidine (Demerol)]: these combinations may result in *serotonin syndrome,* a physiologic crisis which may include a rapid heartbeat, fever, sweating, and shaking and that may (in rare cases) be fatal.

SSRIs plus tricyclic antidepressants [e.g., amitriptyline (Elavil)]: although a common combination prescribed by psychiatrists, the tricyclic antidepressant blood levels may become too high in some individuals, and cause side effects or toxic reactions.

Lithium plus ibuprofen (Motrin, Advil) or other nonsteroidal anti-inflammatories: this combination may cause lithium levels in the blood to get too high, and thus result in toxicity and even kidney damage.

Again, these warnings do not suggest that these combinations may never be used but rather they must be used with extreme care and always under a doctor's supervision. The combinations listed do not represent a complete list of troublesome drug interactions.

SHOULD I TRY TO USE SOME OF THOSE NATURAL, OVER-THE-COUNTER REMEDIES TO TREAT MY DEPRESSION OR ANXIETY?

Natural or "alternative" remedies have been increasing in popularity in the United States and abroad over the past few years. Large numbers of people are self-medicating with them, either alone or in combination with conventional remedies. The evidence for the effectiveness of these treatments, however, is not clear. By and large, relatively few well-designed research studies have been performed to assess their effectiveness and safety; even fewer studies have compared them to more conventional treatments. The current state of knowledge suggests that natural remedies appear better suited for individuals with milder forms of depression and anxiety. More severe forms of these disorders do not seem to respond as well to natural treatments.

One advantage of natural remedies is that they generally have milder side-effect profiles than synthetic medications and often are more tolerable, particularly for those who are sensitive to side effects. However, certain natural remedies can have serious side effects. For example, the antidepressant *St. John's wort* may cause mania in individuals with bipolar disorder. The antianxiety medication *kava* may cause a toxic skin reaction or liver damage when taken for long periods or in very high doses. Therefore you should not assume that all natural treatments are automatically safe.

Finally, there has been increasing evidence demonstrating potentially adverse interactions between natural remedies and conventional remedies. For example, St. John's wort may decrease the blood levels of certain drugs (e.g., protease inhibitors) used to combat AIDS; individuals who are taking these should not use St. John's wort. People who have received organ transplants must also be careful, as St. John's wort may reduce blood levels of cyclosporine, which is used to prevent transplant rejection. Cyclosporine may also be used in the setting of bone marrow transplantation.

To conclude, while natural psychiatric medications may have a niche in the treatment of mood and anxiety disorders, they should be used with care and preferably under the supervision of a doctor, especially in the presence of a complicated medical illness and if other medications are also being taken. More information about alternative therapies can be found in Chap. 21.

MY DOCTOR HAS PRESCRIBED MANY DIFFERENT ANTIDEPRESSANTS FOR ME AND I'M STILL FEELING DEPRESSED. WHAT ELSE MIGHT HELP ME?

Individuals who do not respond to antidepressant medications or who are unable to tolerate them because of side effects may be good candidates for *somatic therapies* (Table 17-5). The most common type is electroconvulsive therapy (ECT),

TABLE 17-5 Somatic (Nonmedication) Therapies for Depression

Electroconvulsive therapy (ECT)
Experimental therapies
  Repetitive transcranial magnetic stimulation (RTMS)
  Vagus nerve stimulation (VNS) with neurocybernetic prosthesis (NCP) stimulation

commonly known as *shock* therapy. This involves giving a depressed person a controlled seizure, usually once every other day for 2 or more weeks (generally between 6 and 12 treatments are required). Despite the stigma attached to ECT and its negative portrayal in movies and popular culture, it is, as practiced today, actually a safe and sophisticated treatment that can alleviate depression in more than 90 percent of cases. Side effects of ECT include headaches and short-term memory loss, though these usually abate once the treatment is completed. Keep in mind that even if you have a good response to ECT, you may still need to take an antidepressant afterwards to prevent the depression from returning. You may also be advised to have "maintenance" ECT treatments on an outpatient basis, usually once a month, to prevent relapse.

Experimental somatic treatments for depression also are under development. For example, *repetitive transcranial magnetic stimulation* (RTMS) involves the application of a magnetic field to the head, which may alleviate depression in some individuals. Another treatment, *vagus nerve stimulation* (VNS), involves the surgical implantation of a neurocybernetic prosthesis (NCP), a device similar to a cardiac pacemaker, which stimulates the vagus nerve periodically and may alleviate depression. These treatments are still experimental and are not yet approved for general use; therefore, to receive them, you would have to qualify for a specific research protocol at an academic medical center.

As mentioned earlier, the addition of talking therapies may also help alleviate depression, at least to some degree, in cases where medications have proven unsatisfactory.

ACKNOWLEDGMENT

The author thanks Dr. William F. Pirl for his helpful suggestions and recommendations for reference materials on cancer chemotherapeutics.

CHAPTER 18

New Therapies and Protocols*

Eyal Attar, M.D.

OUTLINE

Acknowledgment: The author expresses his gratitude to the NCI website http://cancer.gov where much of this information was obtained.

WHAT IS A CLINICAL TRIAL AND WHY DO SUCH TRIALS EXIST?

A clinical trial is a research study in which participants help doctors improve health. Cancer clinical trials help doctors find better ways to prevent, diagnose, and treat cancer. Trials represent the final stages of the cancer research process, in which doctors' best possible ideas are tried out on people. Most of the currently available cancer treatments are the products of clinical trials; in fact, the Food and Drug Administration (FDA) will not approve a medication for general use unless it has been studied in clinical trials. Ultimately, these studies help us understand whether promising approaches to cancer prevention, diagnosis, and treatment are safe and effective.

WHAT ARE THE DIFFERENT TYPES OF CLINICAL TRIALS?

There are four broad categories of clinical trials (Table 18-1). *Treatment trials* test new therapies for cancer, and investigate interventions that have the potential to shrink tumors, prolong survival, and improve quality of life. These may include new cancer drugs, new approaches in surgery or radiation therapy, new combinations of treatments, or new techniques (such as gene therapy).

Prevention trials test new approaches to lower the risk of a certain type of cancer in people who have never had cancer, to prevent cancer from coming back in people who have already had cancer, or to prevent the development of a new cancer in people who have already had cancer. Such approaches may include medicines, vitamins, minerals, and other supplements.

Screening trials assess the best way to find cancer in its early stages, when the cancer is still potentially curable. These trials also identify a population in

TABLE 18-1 Categories of Clinical Trials

Type of Trial	Description
Treatment trials	Test new therapies for cancer, and investigate interventions that have the potential to shrink tumors, to prolong survival, and to improve quality of life.
Prevention trials	Test new approaches to lower the risk of a certain type of cancer in people who have never had cancer, to prevent cancer from coming back in people who have already had cancer, or to prevent the development of a new cancer in people who have already had cancer.
Screening trials	Assess the best way to find cancer in its early stages, when the cancer is still potentially curable.
Quality-of-life trials	Explore ways to improve the comfort and quality of life of cancer patients.

whom the prevalence of cancer is high and in whom screening is thus appropriate.

Quality-of-life trials are also called *supportive care trials*. These trials explore ways to improve the comfort and quality of life of cancer patients.

This chapter focuses mainly on treatment trials; however, the principles enunciated can apply to any trial.

WHAT ARE THE PHASES OF CLINICAL TRIALS?

Treatment trials that test a new drug proceed in an orderly series of steps known as *phases* (Table 18-2). This systematic approach provides reliable information for investigators and also protects patients. Clinical trials are categorized into one of four phases, as outlined below.

Phase I Trials

These are the first studies used to evaluate a drug in human beings; they ask basic questions regarding drug delivery and toxicity (side effects). These trials evaluate the best route to deliver a drug: by mouth, by injection into the blood, or by injection into muscle or skin. They also determine how often a drug should be given (the frequency): for example, daily, weekly, every 2 or 3 weeks, or monthly. Often, a participant's blood is drawn to measure the blood levels of the study drug in order to as-

TABLE 18-2 Phases of Clinical Treatment Trials

Trial Phase	Number of People	Objectives
I	5 to 75	Determine drug dose, route of delivery, frequency of administration, and side effects.
II	50 to 300	Continue to test a drug's safety but also evaluate its spectrum of efficacy; evaluate how well a new drug works on a particular type of cancer.
III	Hundreds to thousands	Continue to test a new treatment's efficacy but compare the new treatment to the current standard for treatment in a specific cancer. Side effects continue to be assessed.
IV	Variable	Postmarketing surveillance studies—evaluate a drug after the FDA has approved it and while it is being used in the general population; look for rare side effects and efficacy in people with cancers.

sess whether the route and frequency are adequate. Last, phase I trials evaluate what medication dose is safe. In doing so, some phase I trials enroll patients in groups called *cohorts*, giving each successive cohort a higher dose of the drug and regularly (every week or two) monitoring for the presence of side effects to determine the maximally tolerated dose (MTD). Phase I trials generally enroll only small numbers of patients (5 to 75 people) and frequently include people with a variety of different cancers. The main purpose of these trials is to evaluate drug delivery and toxicity, not to determine how well a treatment will work for a particular type of cancer (although it is always exciting to see a cancer shrink in response to a phase I drug).

Phase II Trials

These trials continue to test a drug's safety, but they also evaluate its spectrum of efficacy—for example, how well the drug works in shrinking a tumor or in improving a patient's outcome. Using information from a phase I trial, doctors can sometimes predict the types of cancer in which a particular drug may be useful. Phase II trials evaluate how well a new drug works on a particular type of cancer in a larger number of people (typically 50 to 300 participants) than in a phase I trial. Most phase II trials are noncomparative, meaning that a drug is given to a single group of patients with a certain type of cancer, and this group is not evaluated relative to another group receiving standard therapy for that cancer. However, some phase II trials compare groups receiving different doses of a new medication or compare a group of patients receiving a new medication to a similar group that was treated with standard therapy in the past (called a *historical control group*).

Phase III Trials

These trials continue to test a new treatment's efficacy (such as a new drug, a new combination of drugs, or a new surgical procedure), but they compare the new treatment to the current standard of treatment in a specific cancer. This "head-to-head" comparison is made most effectively when patients are assigned to the standard treatment group or to the new treatment group at random. The results of phase III trials are evaluated statistically and, to improve their statistical "power" (the ability to show a difference between two types of treatments), these trials often enroll large numbers of people, sometimes as many as thousands of participants. To achieve this goal, patients from many doctors' offices, clinics, and cancer centers nationwide may be enrolled and their results analyzed collectively. Side effects continue to be assessed in this large group, and it is within these trials that unusual side effects begin to emerge.

Phase IV Trials

These studies are also known as postmarketing surveillance studies. They evaluate a drug after the FDA has approved it and while it is being used in the general population. These trials look for rare side effects and efficacy in people with cancers other than the one examined in the phase III trial.

SHOULD I TAKE PART IN A CLINICAL TRIAL?

Before you consider whether to participate in a clinical trial, you should learn as much as possible about your condition, the standard treatment options, and the clinical trials available. Begin by discussing your cancer and its prognosis with your doctor. Both general and cancer-specific information may be obtained at the CancerNet website of the National Cancer Institute (NCI) at http://cancer. gov. Use the *Finding Clinical Trials* site to learn about current clinical trials that might be appropriate for you. Determine what is right for you by discussing this information with your doctor and/or nurse in addition to family and friends with whom you feel comfortable. Remember, only you can make the decision about whether to participate in a clinical trial, and this decision must be made freely and with full information.

A couple of points are worth emphasizing. It would be unethical to deny a person any therapy that has been demonstrated to prolong survival substantially. Thus, a person participating in a clinical trial will receive therapy that is approximately as good as the standard of care. The investigators conducting the trial are hoping that the therapy will be much better than the standard of care, but it also may be no different or, in rare cases, slightly worse than the standard of care. Also, no person can be forced to participate in a clinical trial. Entering a trial and even remaining as a participant in a trial is completely voluntary; no member of a health care team should think less of a person for not participating in a trial.

WHAT ARE THE POTENTIAL BENEFITS AND RISKS OF CLINICAL TRIALS?

Participation in cancer clinical trials provides many potential benefits (Table 18-3). Involvement in a trial allows a person to make a valuable contribution to cancer research. In addition to receiving access to new drugs before they become widely available, you may be among the first to benefit if the approach being studied is found to be helpful. Every year, clinical trials in a variety of different cancers demonstrate that a new drug, either alone or in combination with other drugs, is more effective than what had been the standard of care. Trial participants play a more active role in their own health care and frequently have contact with leading physicians in the field of cancer research. Last, the trials process requires careful monitoring of your health and possible treatment side effects; this ensures that a participant will have increased contact with medical professionals.

On the other hand, participation may also expose you to potential risks. New drugs and procedures may have side effects (toxicities) or risks that have not yet

TABLE 18-3 Risks and Benefits of Participating in Clinical Trials

Benefits
You will be making a contribution to cancer research.
You will receive access to new drugs before they become widely available.
You may be among the first to benefit from new therapies.
Trial participants play a more active role in their own health and frequently have contact with leading physicians in the field of cancer research.
Trials require careful monitoring of your health and possible treatment side effects and thus guarantee increased contact with medical professionals.

Risks
New drugs and procedures may have substantial side effects or risks.
Such side effects may be worse than those experienced with standard treatments.
A new approach may lack benefit or may benefit people other than you.
You may have to make extra visits to a clinic or hospital or have extra blood draws or radiology examinations.
Health insurers and managed care providers do not always cover all the care costs in a clinical trial.

been identified by doctors. Furthermore, such side effects may be worse than those experienced by people receiving standard treatments. A new approach may lack benefit or may benefit people other than you. Certain trials require that a person make extra visits to a clinic or hospital or have extra blood draws or radiology examinations, and some people do not appreciate the additional contact with medical professionals. Last, health insurers and managed care providers do not always cover all the care costs in a clinical trial. You should discuss this with your insurer or a care coordinator or social worker affiliated with the oncology clinic.

HOW WILL I BE PROTECTED?

Participants in clinical trials are referred to as *human research subjects*. For participants in government-funded trials, the government has a system designed for patient protection, called *human research subject protection*. Before a government-funded clinical trial can begin, the trial plan, or protocol, must be approved in a series of steps involving review committees that make sure the plan is reasonable, based on solid preclinical information, and that patients are not being denied a therapy proven to prolong survival substantially. During the trial, these committees make sure that the plan is being followed and that participants are being protected. In certain trials, other committees, called *data monitoring committees,* might actually stop a trial prematurely if a significant benefit or harm is associated with a given therapy.

For trials sponsored by other institutions, such as universities, an institutional review board (IRB), or a committee that serves the identical function of reviewing the plan prior to its initiation, ensures that the plan is being followed and that patients are protected. In both instances, regulations require that researchers performing studies thoroughly inform patients of the study's treatments, tests, possible benefits, and risks, in a language that can be understood by a person not in the medical field. This is presented to patients for review before they decide whether to participate in the study. This process is designed to ensure *informed consent.*

WHAT IS INFORMED CONSENT?

In the informed consent process, you learn the facts, including the potential risks and benefits, about a clinical trial before deciding whether to participate. These facts are presented to you by a research doctor or nurse in language that can be understood by a person not in the medical field, and you are encouraged to ask questions and to voice your concerns.

In addition, information about the study and your rights as a study participant will be included in a written consent form that you may take home to read and discuss (Table 18-4). Included in the consent form are details about the study approach: the justification to perform the study, the nuts and bolts of how the study will be conducted and how long it will last, the intervention given in the trial (for example, information about the experimental drug), possible risks and benefits, confidentiality, tests that may be performed, rights as a study participant, and telephone contact numbers in the event of an emergency or if additional questions arise. Do not hesitate to ask questions until you are satisfied you have all the information you need before deciding whether you wish to participate.

The informed consent process begins before you agree to participate in a trial and continues as long as you are in the study. Therefore, you should feel free to ask your doctors and nurses any questions you have at any time. Your signature on the consent form only grants the study personnel permission to enroll you in the protocol. You can change your mind and leave the study whenever you want, before the study starts or at any time during the study or follow-up period.

TABLE 18-4 **Information Included in a Consent Form**

The scientific justification for the study
The nuts and bolts of how the study will be conducted
How long the study will last
The intervention given in the trial (for example, information about the experimental
  drug)
Possible risks and benefits
The nature of confidentiality
Tests that may be performed
Your rights as a study participant
Telephone contact numbers in the event of an emergency or if additional questions arise

WHAT IS A PLACEBO AND COULD I RECEIVE ONE?

A placebo is a dummy pill or therapy that contains no active ingredient; it is sometimes called a sugar pill, though it is designed to look, taste, and even smell like the active drug. However, placebos are rarely used in cancer treatment trials. Most treatment trials are designed to compare a standard treatment, based on the results of past clinical trials, with a new treatment, in order to determine the best way to treat patients with a certain cancer. As mentioned above, patients are randomly assigned to one group or another. If no standard treatment exists, a trial may compare a proposed new treatment with a placebo. However, you will be told of this possibility during the informed consent process before you decide whether to participate in the study.

WHAT HAPPENS DURING A TRIAL?

If you decide to participate in a clinical trial, you will work with a research team comprised of doctors, nurses, social workers, study coordinators, dieticians, and other health care professionals. They will provide your care, monitor your health carefully, and give you specific instructions about the study. To make trial results as reliable as possible, it is important to follow the research team's instructions. These may include keeping all appointments for doctor visits and undergoing tests, taking medicines on time without skipping doses, and completing logs (a method of recording on paper the number of pills taken, your symptoms, your diet, and other factors), or filling out questionnaires. Participation in a trial may mean you have more tests and doctor visits than you would have had if you were not in the study. Certainly, you will have close contact with team members during the time you are involved with the treatment and follow-up portions of the protocol. Team members may also continue to stay in contact with you after the trial ends, either to obtain follow-up information about how you are doing or, more commonly, to continue as members of your health care team.

In general, before receiving treatment as part of a trial, you will undergo a series of tests to determine the full extent of your disease. These may include radiographic studies, such as computed tomography (CT) scans to measure the size of your tumor, and blood tests to measure the levels of tumor markers; they are referred to as *baseline* tests.

Then, you will enter a treatment period that may involve several trips to the doctor and several treatments with the modality being studied, such as chemotherapy or radiation therapy. After this period (which can last weeks to months), your tests will be repeated and the results compared to the baseline tests obtained before you entered the treatment study. This comparison allows investigators to determine whether or not the treatment is having an effect on the tumor.

For example, if you have a lung tumor nodule that measures 5 centimeters in diameter (about 2 inches) on a CT scan before enrolling in a treatment protocol studying a new lung cancer drug and this nodule shrinks to 2.5 centimeters in diameter (about 1 inch) after a treatment period (that is, it has become smaller), you might be benefiting from the drug. Alternatively, you may have colon cancer and a blood level of 1400 of a colon cancer–specific tumor marker [carcinoembyronic antigen (CEA)] before treatment with an experimental drug for colon cancer. If, after a treatment period, your blood level then increases to 2000, this might suggest treatment failure. The specific tests and response criteria used to determine treatment benefit or failure are unique to each protocol. In most trials, patients who have not responded to a treatment (i.e., the tumor does not shrink or the level of the tumor marker in the blood does not decrease following therapy) are discontinued from a protocol. For patients who respond to a treatment, most protocols allow continued treatment until the cancer disappears or the treatment stops working.

WHO IS ELIGIBLE TO PARTICIPATE IN A CLINICAL TRIAL?

Each clinical trial has its own guidelines for who can participate, called *eligibility criteria.* Because participants in a trial are alike in key ways, including the type and stage of cancer (to what extent the cancer has spread) and previous treatments, eligibility criteria are included in the study plan. Most trials also have strict criteria for the age of participants (many will not include people over the age of 65 years) and require that a person not have heart, kidney, or liver disease. The best way to find out whether you are eligible for a particular study is to talk to the doctor or nurse in charge of patient enrollment.

WHERE ARE TRIALS CONDUCTED?

Depending on the type of study and on the treatment questions being studied, the clinical trial may be treating participants at one or two highly specialized centers or at hundreds of locations at the same time. Therefore, if you decide to participate in a trial, you could receive your therapy at a large cancer center, such as the National Cancer Institute (NCI) on the campus of the National Institutes of Health (NIH) in Bethesda, Maryland; a university hospital; a local medical center; or your physician's office. You would participate in the trial under the guidance of a team that includes your physician and other health care professionals, who would report your experience with the treatment back to the center responsible for the trial's overall coordination. Experts then use the information from all the participants to evaluate the treatment being tested.

WHO PAYS FOR THE PATIENT CARE COSTS OF A CLINICAL TRIAL?

Even if you have health insurance, your coverage may not include some or all of the costs associated with a clinical trial. This is because some health plans define clinical trials as *experimental* or *investigational* procedures. Alternatively, some health plans will pay only for those portions of a clinical trial that they consider to be part of your routine care (for example, doctor's visits and radiology tests) but will not pay for the portions they feel are being performed specifically for the study (for example, some blood tests or the cost of the experimental drug itself). In these cases, often the sponsor of the trial (the government or a pharmaceutical company) will pay costs not covered by an insurance company. Contact your health insurance carrier to obtain their guidelines. Your doctor may be able to help you communicate your need to your insurance carrier to obtain support.

WHAT QUESTIONS SHOULD I ASK MY DOCTOR BEFORE PARTICIPATING IN A TRIAL?

Anyone considering a clinical trial should feel free to ask questions or to bring up issues concerning the trial at any time. The following suggestions may give you some ideas as you think about your own questions.

About the Study

1. What is the purpose of the study?
2. Why do researchers think the approach may be effective?
3. Who will sponsor the study?
4. Who has reviewed and approved of the study?
5. How are study results and the safety of participants being checked?
6. How long will the study last?
7. What will my responsibilities be if I participate?
8. If this is a treatment study, what is the current standard of treatment for patients with my type of cancer in its current stage (i.e., the degree to which the cancer has spread)?

About Possible Risks and Benefits

1. What are my possible short-term benefits?
2. What are my possible long-term benefits?
3. What are my short-term risks, such as side effects?
4. What are my possible long-term risks?

5. What other options do people with my risk of cancer or type of cancer have?
6. How do the possible risks and benefits of this trial compare with those options?

About Participation and Care

1. What kinds of therapies, procedures, and/or tests will I have during the trial?
2. Will they hurt, and if so, for how long?
3. How do the tests in the study compare with those I would have outside of the trial?
4. Will I be able to take my regular medications while in the clinical trial?
5. Where will I have my medical care?
6. Who will be in charge of my care?

About Personal Issues

1. How could being in this study affect my daily life?
2. Can I talk to other people in the study?

About Cost Issues

1. Will I have to pay for any part of the trial, such as tests or the study drug?
2. If so, what will the charges likely be?
3. What is my health insurance likely to cover?
4. Who can help answer any questions from my insurance company or health plan?
5. Will there be any travel (getting to and from the treatment center and/or paying for parking) or child-care costs that I need to consider while I am in the trial?

Tips for Asking Your Doctor about Trials

When you talk with your doctor or members of the research team,

1. Consider taking a family member or friend along, for support and for help in asking questions or recording answers.
2. Plan ahead what to ask—but don't hesitate to ask any new questions you think of while you're in the medical clinic or office.
3. Write down your questions in advance, to make sure you remember to ask them all.
4. Write down the answers, so that you can review them whenever you want.

5. Consider bringing a tape recorder to make a taped record of what's said (even if you write down answers).
6. Consider scheduling a follow-up appointment with the doctor or members of the research team after the trial details have been presented to you but prior to starting on the trial. You will need time to assimilate all the information that has been presented to you, and new questions probably will arise.

WHERE DO THE IDEAS FOR TRIALS COME FROM?

The ideas for clinical trials often originate in the laboratory. Researchers develop a clinical trial protocol after scientific laboratory experiments indicate that a new drug or procedure is promising. These scientists first develop a theory of how a type of cancer can be incapacitated and what specific drug can cripple the tumor cells. Next, they perform experiments that demonstrate the drug can kill tumor cells in a test tube. Following this, scientists give the drug to animals with cancer, and prove that the drug being studied shrinks tumors in these animals. Finally, the drug can be tested in humans. The first trials of a particular drug or procedure are focused on safety, and subsequent trials focus on whether the drug or procedure works and what types of patients are most likely to benefit.

THE PLAN FOR A TRIAL: WHAT IS A PROTOCOL?

Every trial has a person in charge called the *principal investigator* (PI). The PI is usually a doctor. He or she prepares a plan for the study, called a *protocol*, which explains what the trial will do, how it will be carried out, and why each part of the study is necessary.
The protocol includes the following:

The *reason* for doing the study
How many people will be in the study
Who is *eligible* to participate in the study
What study *drugs* participants will take
What medical *tests* they will have and how often
What *information* will be gathered

In order to collect and compare results from different centers participating in a given study accurately, every doctor or research center taking part in the trial uses the same protocol. This ensures that patients receive identical treatment no matter where they are enrolled in the study and that the information from all the participating centers can be combined and compared.

WHO SPONSORS CLINICAL TRIALS?

Clinical trials are sponsored by organizations or individuals who are seeking better treatments for cancer or better ways to prevent or detect cancer (Table 18-5). *Individual physicians* at cancer centers and other medical institutions can sponsor clinical trials themselves. Alternatively, *pharmaceutical companies* or companies that make diagnostic equipment (like x-ray machines) sponsor trials of their products, hoping to demonstrate that their products are safe and effective. The FDA will permit companies to sell a product only after it has been proven safe and effective in clinical trials.

However, the greatest number of trials are conducted under the sponsorship of *The National Cancer Institute* (NCI), a branch of the National Institutes of Health (NIH) under the United States Department of Health and Human Services. In order to make clinical trials widely available throughout the United States, the NCI has designed a program that makes possible the participation of thousands of investigators at over a thousand sites. The *Cancer Centers Program* represents more than 45 research-oriented institutions designated *NCI Comprehensive or Clinical Cancer Center* sites for their scientific and clinical excellence. These institutions are located throughout the country and play a vital role in cancer research, patient care, public outreach, and education for the public and professionals.

The *Cooperative Clinical Trials Program* brings together groups of researchers, cancer centers, and community physicians into a national NCI-supported network. There are several *Cooperative Groups*, generally organized geographically, that define the key unanswered questions in cancer and then conduct high-quality clinical trials at many sites around the country to answer these questions. The Cooperative Groups enroll about 20,000 new patients in treatment trials each year and, through their involvement in phase III trials, are instrumental in helping establish the state-of-the-art for cancer therapy and prevention. The *Community Clinical Oncology Program* (CCOP) makes clinical trials available in a large number of local communities in the United States by linking community physicians with researchers in cancer centers.

By affiliating with a cancer center or cooperative group, local hospitals throughout the country offer patients participation in clinical trials without having to travel long distances or to change from their usual caregivers.

TABLE 18-5 **Sponsors of Clinical Trials**

Individual physicians or hospitals
Pharmaceutical companies
Medical device companies
The National Cancer Institute or another government agency

WHAT HAPPENS WHEN A CLINICAL TRIAL IS OVER?

Clinical trials accrue a certain number of patients, usually decided upon before the trial even starts. The number varies from trial to trial and generally is based on the number of patients required to give the trial enough information to be convincing—that is, to prove that a new cancer drug, for example, either works or does not work. The concept of having enough patients in a trial to answer the study question is known as *statistical power*.

The type of analysis conducted after a trial is completed depends on the type of trial. After a phase I or II trial is completed, researchers look carefully at the data collected and decide whether to move on to the next phase of trial, such as from a phase I to a phase II or from a phase II to a phase III, or whether to stop testing the treatment because it is neither safe nor effective. As described above, the safety of a drug is tested in phase I, while both safety and effectiveness are tested in phase III.

When a phase III trial comes to an end, researchers look at the data and decide whether the new treatment tested was better than the standard treatment; for example, did the new cancer drug shrink a given tumor better than standard cancer therapy? Researchers then inform the medical community and the public of the trial results, particularly if the new treatment proves to be better. This can occur through several mechanisms.

Sometimes, trial results are published in scientific or medical journals. Other times, they are presented at scientific or medical meetings for discussion. Keep in mind that there are many studies done every year and many do not get published. To find out whether the results of a study in which you participated were published, ask the doctor or nurse in charge of your treatment or find out the official name and protocol number of your study and search for the study in the CANCERLIT or PubMed databases of medical publications. If you have trouble locating the study or searching for it, the research librarian at a university or medical library may be able to help.

Most medical and scientific journals have in place a process called *peer review*, in which experts critique the report of a trial's results before it is published to make sure that the analysis and conclusions are sound. Particularly important results are likely to be featured by the print or electronic media and to be widely discussed at scientific meetings and by patient advocacy groups. Once an intervention is proven safe and effective in a clinical trial, and usually in a series of clinical trials, it may become the new standard of practice. In this way, the development of better interventions for prevention, treatment, detection, and diagnosis is an ongoing, continuous process that builds progressively on itself to improve the quality of cancer care and prevention available to us all.

CHAPTER 19

Psychological Interventions and Support Groups

Lisa F. Price, M.D.

WHY MIGHT PEOPLE WITH CANCER NEED PSYCHOLOGICAL OR SOCIAL SUPPORTS?

A cancer diagnosis often brings up issues never considered previously (Table 19-1). Now, you are faced with learning about your form of cancer, along with treatment options and resources available for treatment. This process of learning by itself can be intimidating for a variety of reasons; people feel overwhelmed by the large body of information to be learned and uncertain about making treatment decisions. Furthermore, many related questions arise with a cancer diagnosis: What will happen to me? How will this affect my body? How will this affect my relationships? Will I be able to do everything I want to do? Will I die before my dreams have been realized? These questions and many others are common among people with cancer, although each person experiences them in his or her own way.

Unfamiliar feelings also may arise. Recurrent worries, feelings of hopelessness and helplessness, and feelings of isolation are experienced frequently. Anxiety and depression may develop in mild or more serious forms. For example, one investigator reported that some form of emotional distress was found in 80 percent of women with newly diagnosed breast cancer. These feelings can arise at any point, from the time of diagnosis through later stages of adjustment, and may remain for months, with periods of alleviation and aggravation along the way. Generally, these feelings wane slowly with time; typically, there is a low incidence of significant distress 1 to 2 years after diagnosis. These distressing emotions, however, can in and of themselves become obstacles to continuing with the routine of one's life.

Thus, people seek additional psychological and social supports (also called *psychosocial interventions*) both to find answers to the many new questions that have arisen and to relieve the troublesome feelings that may develop. People also seek additional help to cope with the problematic side effects of medications; to obtain information about their disease, its treatment, and its prognosis; and to develop contacts with others going through similar experiences. A variety of psychosocial interventions have been developed over the past 20 years to help people cope with

---

TABLE 19-1 Reasons People Seek Additional Psychological and Social Supports

To find answers to the many new questions that have arisen concerning their cancer diagnosis
To relieve difficult feelings that develop
To cope with the problematic side effects of medications
To obtain information about their disease, its treatment, and its prognosis
To develop contacts with others going through similar experiences
To decrease feelings of alienation by talking with others in similar situations
To reduce anxiety about the treatments
To assist in clarification of misperceptions and misinformation
To lessen feelings of isolation, helplessness, and neglect

the emotional aspects of their cancer diagnosis. These interventions aim to decrease worry about medical treatment, to dispel myths and misunderstandings regarding medical care, and to reduce feelings of hopelessness and isolation by allowing people to talk with each other as they undergo similar experiences. These interventions also support heightened efforts to improve health and thereby increase compliance with medication regimens.

WHAT IS THE BENEFIT OF ADDITIONAL HELP?

A significant amount of cancer research has been dedicated to evaluating the impact of additional interventions on cancer patients' outcomes. These interventions involve a focus on psychological concerns and on social/behavioral issues; thus, they are referred to as *psychosocial interventions*. Several researchers have shown that psychosocial interventions can benefit both psychological and physical health. Psychological benefits of interventions include decreased feelings of alienation, lower levels of anxiety and depression, and fewer complications caused by misinformation about illness and its treatment. Physical benefits include decreased physical discomfort, fewer treatment side effects, increased treatment compliance, and a reduction in rates of illness and death. Research into the basis for these positive outcomes is ongoing. While debate continues about the degree of impact psychosocial interventions can have, care providers generally agree that additional support at this time is beneficial. Such assistance is of help not only for the person with cancer but also for family members, who need to adjust to the many changes introduced by cancer.

WHAT KIND OF HELP IS AVAILABLE?

Fortunately, a variety of useful psychosocial interventions exist (Table 19-2). These interventions may be placed in four major categories: group psychotherapy, individual psychotherapy, behavioral interventions, and educational interventions. Each of these interventions has been studied in disparate groups with various forms of cancer. Some studies have introduced these interventions early in a person's treatment, while others have studied their impact later in the course of the illness. Each has particular benefits and, correspondingly, each has areas of weakness.

A group of researchers who conducted a comprehensive evaluation of these techniques concluded that, ideally, a combination of these methods would be most beneficial. They noted that structured interventions comprised of anxiety reduction, health education, behavior modification, problem-solving methods, and group support provide the most aid to newly diagnosed patients or patients in early stages of treatment. While such a multimodal approach may not be developed yet, individuals can create their own adjunctive interventions to suit their interests and needs.

TABLE 19-2 Types of
Psychosocial
Interventions

Group psychotherapy
Individual psychotherapy
Behavioral interventions
Educational interventions

WHAT IS GROUP PSYCHOTHERAPY?

Group psychotherapy is the intervention most available and most familiar to care providers and to the public (Fig. 19-1). Group therapy can be a helpful addition to medical therapy for a number of reasons. In a group, people find others with similar concerns, share information, and help each other along the way. The process of sharing and relating to others decreases feelings of aloneness and relieves some of the concerns that may not have been shared yet with loved ones. In the book *The Human Side of Cancer*, Jimmie Holland and Sheldon Lewis describe some of the topics that arise within groups; these include treatment decisions, opinions about care providers, family responses to cancer, and anger that permeates the adjustment process.

Groups are organized in a variety of ways. Some groups welcome people with all forms of cancer, while others focus on those with a particular form of cancer. Groups may be oriented to individuals with a new cancer diagnosis or to people who have been living with cancer for years. They may focus on cancer at a particular stage, with attention paid to the corresponding issues that arise with localized versus widespread cancer. Some groups invite people of all ages, while others may be oriented to certain age groups, such as children. Groups may be geared toward friends and family of someone with cancer. Some are structured to run for a specific amount of time (with a set start and finish date for all members), while others are ongoing (in which people can join the group at any point).

Groups are based on a variety of theoretical orientations. Some groups (e.g., groups oriented toward cognitive-behavioral therapy) focus on learning particular skills in dealing with cancer over a limited number of sessions. Other groups (e.g., psychodynamically oriented groups) are more interested in the emotional and psychological issues that arise. Various terms are used to describe the group's work, such as *support group* or *group therapy*. These terms may be used in a variety of circumstances; the best way to determine the nature of the group is to ask about its organization.

Given the variety of groups that exist, you can gain the most from the experience by determining your interest and then looking for a group that serves your particular needs. For example, if you are a woman with newly diagnosed breast cancer, you may want to meet with other women with a new breast cancer diagnosis—with women who are facing the same challenges. Alternatively, you may

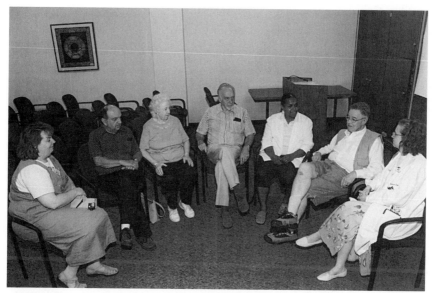

FIGURE 19-1 *Topics that arise in group therapy include treatment decisions, opinions about care providers, family responses to cancer, and the anger that may permeate the adjustment process.*

want to join a group with a mixture of women with a new cancer diagnosis and women who are cancer survivors, so you can learn from those who have made it through what you are experiencing. Care providers can help connect you to the kind of group you desire. On the other hand, there may be limited types of groups within a given geographic area. Even if a group is not tailored to your specific interests, a group may still provide you with significant support.

WHAT IS INDIVIDUAL PSYCHOTHERAPY?

Individual psychotherapy involves meeting with a trained mental health professional in one-on-one sessions to focus on particular concerns. While many people enjoy and benefit from the shared experience found in group therapy, others feel more comfortable in a private setting in which they can communicate their concerns to one person. People turn to individual therapy for the same reasons they seek group therapy: to address fears, anxiety, depression, aloneness, helplessness, and anger as well as specific life struggles.

Individual therapy exists in many forms and is described by various names. *Psychotherapy, therapy,* and *counseling* all are terms used to describe the process of meeting with a mental health professional. As with group therapy, a wide spectrum of approaches to therapy exists. Cognitive-behavioral therapy (CBT) involves reviewing your ways of thinking and developing new skills that will better aid you in coping with your concerns. Psychodynamic therapies focus on your internal emotional and psychological experience, with a similar goal of improving the way you cope with the struggles in your life. Both of these types of therapy may be conducted for as long as the treater and the person seeking help find the therapy useful; therapy also may be conducted for a specified length of time. Other therapies, such as crisis counseling, in which the focus is getting through a particular crisis, are inherently time-limited.

Some specially trained therapists work only with people who have cancer. Many others are trained to work with people at all stages of life and can help manage any of a number of distressing matters. These professionals include social workers, nurses, psychologists, and psychiatrists. Finding a therapist who routinely works with people who have cancer may be particularly important for some people because of the confidence that comes from working with a therapist who is familiar with the particulars of cancer-related issues. On the other hand, many therapists have worked with people who have a wide spectrum of medical illnesses as well as a wide spectrum of related life struggles that affect work, relationships, and one's view of oneself. Most importantly, in beginning individual therapy, strive to find a therapist with whom you feel at ease. The positive relationship between a person with a problem and his or her therapist is the best predictor of successful treatment; it may be more important than the type of therapy employed.

WHAT ARE BEHAVIORAL INTERVENTIONS?

Behavioral interventions encompass a variety of methods developed to decrease the distress related to a diagnosis of cancer (Table 19-3). These interventions include progressive muscle relaxation (PMR), hypnosis, biofeedback, meditation, guided imagery, and deep breathing. These techniques may be taught in individual sessions, as with therapist-guided hypnosis, or they may be taught in groups. They have also been used to decrease generalized stress and anxiety. In addition, they have been used to target specific physical discomforts (such as pretreatment and posttreatment nausea and vomiting) due to chemotherapy.

The techniques are taught for a discrete period of time with the goal of enabling a person to use them on his or her own. These methods may be used simultane-

TABLE 19-3 Types of Behavioral
Interventions

Progressive muscle relaxation (PMR)
Hypnosis
Biofeedback
Meditation
Guided imagery
Deep breathing

ously, and some programs teach multiple behavioral interventions. They are particularly useful for people who would like to use a specific tool in addressing their stress or discomfort.

WHAT ARE EDUCATIONAL INTERVENTIONS?

Educational interventions provide information to people with cancer. Researchers have found that simply providing information to individuals decreases their feelings of helplessness. These feelings are then replaced with an improved sense of control over the decisions that must be made. Educational interventions often involve the use of reading materials, videotapes, audiotapes, and lectures to better inform a person about his or her cancer. Topics discussed include information about the cancer itself, treatment options, coping strategies, and the physical, emotional, and social consequences of cancer. Conveniently, educational interventions can be used easily by people in their own homes as well as through formal programs.

HOW CAN I FIND PSYCHOSOCIAL INTERVENTIONS IN MY AREA?

The best first contact for any of the above services is your own medical care team. Your doctor, nurse, or social worker may be generally familiar with group therapists, individual therapists, or behavioral and educational programs and may work closely with these caregivers. Some people even receive care in centers where such interventions are an integral part of cancer treatment programs. One advantage of consulting your medical care team is that you are more likely to be referred to someone with a history of successful treatment.

For group therapies, the following are respected organizations that can be contacted to find meetings in a given area: American Cancer Society, Wellness Community, Gilda's Clubs, Cancer Care, Y-Me, and Us Too. They can be reached by telephone or via the Internet. Additional sites include the National Cancer Institute, Oncolink, QuitNet Online, and the Cancer Resource Room at your hospital.

For individual therapy, your doctor, nurse, or hospital social worker all may be able to provide names of individual therapists. The department of psychiatry, psychology, and social work at the hospital in your area also would be particularly able to provide names of qualified individuals. They also may be able to provide information about behavioral interventions and educational interventions. Cancer support organizations (including those listed above) may provide such techniques themselves or the means to enter treatment. In addition, a significant body of writing regarding cancer and coping with cancer exists and may be accessed through these resources.

CHAPTER 20

Bone Marrow Transplantation

Corey Cutler, M.D., M.P.H., F.R.C.P.C.

OUTLINE

WHAT IS BONE MARROW?

The bone marrow is a large liquid organ found inside most long and flat bones of the body, such as the pelvis, the femur (thigh bone), and the breastbone (sternum). Bone marrow can be thought of as the body's factory for the production of all the blood components (red blood cells, white blood cells, and platelets), which are produced continuously to meet the body's ongoing requirements. Red blood cells provide oxygen to the body's organs and tissues, white blood cells fight infections, and platelets help stop bleeding. These mature cells and cellular components all derive from a single *grandfather* cell, called a *stem cell*. This stem cell still evades precise identification, though it can be identified by certain proteins found on its surface.

Analogous to the transplantation of a kidney, a liver, or a heart, transplantation of bone marrow is a commonly practiced procedure at many cancer centers. The first report of transplantation of human bone marrow dates as far back as a century ago. Since then, major advances have been made in transplantation technology and, as a result, the reasons for receiving for transplantation have expanded; bone marrow transplantation (BMT) is now used for cancers of the blood (hematologic malignancies—e.g., leukemias, lymphomas, and multiple myeloma) and for some noncancerous conditions and solid tumors, such as cancer of the kidney.

WHAT IS BONE MARROW TRANSPLANTATION?

The first step in a BMT involves taking bone marrow from a donor (in a procedure known as a *harvest* or a *collection*). The *marrow*, or *graft*, as it is often termed, is then given to a person with cancer, also known as the *recipient* or *host*. The recipient receives the bone marrow only after he or she has been treated with high doses of chemotherapy and sometimes also radiation therapy, which kills any residual cancer cells.

When physicians discuss a BMT, they divide the procedure broadly into two large categories, termed *autologous BMT* and *allogeneic BMT. Autologous* (derived from the Greek word *autos*, or "self") refers to a BMT procedure in which the person with cancer is both the donor and the recipient of the bone marrow. *Allogeneic* (from the Greek word *allos*, or "other") refers to a BMT procedure in which the person with cancer receives normal bone marrow from a healthy donor. This donor can be either a family member (often a sibling) or someone who is unrelated to the person with cancer.

BMT also is referred to as *stem cell transplantation* (SCT). As the important component of the bone marrow that is transplanted is the stem cell (the grandfather or grandmother cell that gives rise to the components of blood), the two terms are used interchangeably. Bone marrow cells can actually be found in very small numbers in the blood. When these cells are collected using machines designed for this purpose, the collected cells are referred to as *peripheral blood stem cells* (PBSCs), and they are used in place of bone marrow for transplantation.

HOW DOES BONE MARROW TRANSPLANTATION HELP PEOPLE WITH CANCER?

There are two main ways in which BMT can help people with cancer (Table 20-1). The first is by providing a source of healthy stem cells to replace those damaged by high-dose chemotherapy and radiotherapy. This benefit applies to both autologous and allogeneic transplantation.

Prior to receiving bone marrow, all BMT patients first receive "conditioning" chemotherapy. This is generally given over several days and in high doses. Often, it is combined with radiation therapy. High-dose chemotherapy and radiation therapy are given to kill remaining cancerous cells that have not been killed by conventional chemotherapy—i.e., chemotherapy given in lower doses. In addition to killing cancerous cells, the high doses of chemotherapy and radiation therapy damage the normal stem cells of the marrow, rendering them incapable of forming the elements of blood—red blood cells, white blood cells, and platelets. At this point, healthy bone marrow that has been collected is given to a BMT patient (the recipient, or host) to replace the damaged bone marrow. The new marrow is given as an intravenous (by vein) infusion, a process similar to a blood transfusion. The newly infused bone marrow then "homes" to the bone marrow space in the recipient where it grows, producing new red blood cells, white blood cells, and platelets and eventually replaces the damaged marrow cells.

The second method through which a BMT helps people with cancer is mediated through the immune system—the system in the body that ordinarily fights infections. All of the cells involved in the body's immune system are produced in the bone marrow and are collectively known as the *white blood cells*. In addition to recognizing bacteria and viruses as being foreign to the body and then trying to eliminate them, white blood cells are capable of recognizing cells as "self" by reading a unique label found on every cell of the body—a sort of "bar code" specific to you. Each person has a unique label that differentiates him or her from every

TABLE 20-1 How a Bone Marrow Transplantation (BMT) Helps a Person with Cancer

Rationale	Type of BMT
Provides a source of healthy stem cells to replace stem cells damaged by high-dose chemotherapy and radiotherapy.	Autologous Allogeneic
Provides a new immune system which attacks residual tumor cells.	Allogeneic

other person. When bone marrow (or the graft) is transplanted from one individual to another (allogeneic transplantation), a new immune system is also transplanted. This transplanted immune system now recognizes the person receiving the bone marrow (the recipient, or host) as being "foreign." As the new white blood cells encounter residual tumor cells marked with the unique label of the host rather than the label of the donor, these tumor cells will be recognized as foreign. This, in turn, causes the newly transplanted immune system to attack the tumor cells, leading to their destruction. This effect is referred to as a graft-versus-tumor effect, and it occurs only in the setting of an allogeneic BMT.

HOW ARE PEOPLE MATCHED FOR BONE MARROW TRANSPLANTATION?

Every person has a unique combination of chromosomes and genes (the blueprints for cell growth and reproduction, located in the center of every cell in the body) that contributes to his or her individuality. A collection of these genes is found on the sixth chromosome (each person has 23 pairs of chromosomes) and is referred to as the *human leukocyte antigen* (HLA) *complex.* This complex of genes provides the code that produces the unique "self" label found on all cells. A total of six important genes make up the HLA complex. You inherit three of the genes from your mother and three from your father. When white blood cells encounter this HLA gene complex, they know that they should not destroy that "self" cell. Foreign cells, such as bacteria, do not possess the specific HLA complex recognized as self, and thus are destroyed.

In trying to determine whether someone is a suitable candidate to be a bone marrow donor (termed a *match*), blood is taken for analysis of that person's unique set of six genes. Ideal matches share all six of the coding genes (and are termed "six out of six," or 6/6 matches). When no 6/6 match is available, consideration is given to lesser degrees of matching (such as 5/6 matches). Since genes of family members most closely resemble each other, the highest likelihood of finding a "perfect match" is within a patient's own family. In fact, mathematically, the chance that a brother or sister of a patient will be a perfect match to the patient is about 1 in 4, or 25 percent.

Children and parents of patients are unlikely to be perfect matches, as these family members have either received or passed on only three of the six genes necessary for a perfect match. Sometimes, however, children or parents of patients can match; this usually occurs in the setting of specific ethnic groups in which both parents are members of the same ethnic group and the diversity of the coding genes is more limited. Unfortunately, spouses of patients are no more likely than are members of the general population to be a match for a patient, because spouses are not blood relatives.

When a perfect match cannot be found within your family, a search for an unrelated donor must be performed. In the United States, a registry of volunteers has been collected and maintained by the National Marrow Donor Program (NMDP).

This program maintains a large database of potential donors (with their genetic information) and provides matches for patients in whom no suitable family member is available. The NMDP has cooperative relationships with similar organizations in Canada, Europe, and Asia. Many patients who do not have a suitable donor within their families will find a match in the national registry, though the percentage varies significantly with ethnicity.

WHO CAN RECEIVE A BONE MARROW TRANSPLANT?

A BMT is an effective treatment for only certain types of cancer. The major indication for BMT is a cancer of the bone marrow itself. Examples of cancers of the bone marrow include the acute and chronic leukemias, multiple myeloma, and some forms of malignant lymphoma (see Chap. 3 for more information about these cancers). In these conditions, the bone marrow cells have become cancerous (or malignant) and cannot be eliminated with standard chemotherapy and/or radiotherapy. Transplantation in these conditions can occur either at the time of diagnosis, after standard (regular-dose) chemotherapy has brought about a complete remission (in which the cancer cannot be detected anywhere in the body), or when a person relapses and the cancer returns following standard chemotherapy.

In addition to the medical indications, you must meet other specific requirements before proceeding to transplantation. A BMT is a dangerous and often life-threatening procedure. Allogeneic transplantation is more risky than autologous transplantation and therefore is generally reserved for people under the age of 55 years who are otherwise in good physical and psychological health. Autologous transplantation can be performed in people even in their seventies provided that they are in excellent physical condition.

The decision to use autologous or allogeneic sources of marrow stem cells is generally made on an individual basis. Some disorders (such as lymphoma) are typically treated with autologous bone marrow, while others (such as acute leukemia) are treated with allogeneic bone marrow. Factors that influence this decision include the age and overall health of the person with cancer, the type of cancer that is being treated, the availability of a suitable allogeneic donor, and the advantage of using the immune system to help eradicate the cancer (which is achievable only with an allogeneic BMT).

Other indications for BMT include rare hereditary or genetic defects that can cause profound anemia, or immune deficiencies. Some solid tumors (such as breast cancer and cancer of the kidney) also are treated with BMT, though many of these approaches remain experimental and are not considered standard therapy.

WHAT HAPPENS DURING A BONE MARROW TRANSPLANT?

The actual BMT (including treatment with chemotherapy and radiation therapy, the bone marrow infusion, and the recovery period) occurs in a hospital BMT unit

TABLE 20-2 **Steps in Undergoing Bone Marrow Transplantation**

Step		Duration
1.	Chemotherapy +/- radiation therapy is given to kill any tumor cells that remain in the body and to prepare the marrow space in the bones to receive the new marrow.	2–7 days
2.	The bone marrow is given to the recipient as an intravenous infusion.	Minutes
3.	The recipient enters a waiting period until the new marrow takes root. During the period when there is no functioning marrow, blood cell counts will be low.	1–4 weeks
4.	Limitations are placed on activities and lifestyle because of the risk of infection.	1 year

(Table 20-2). This is a floor in the hospital with dedicated BMT rooms (one per person) and staff who are experts in caring for people receiving BMTs.

To begin, you will receive high doses of chemotherapy and possibly radiation therapy to kill any tumor cells that remain in the body and to prepare the marrow space in the bones to receive the new marrow. The chemotherapy and radiation therapy can last between 2 and 7 days, but the precise regimen used varies among transplant centers and physicians.

The side effects of the chemotherapy and radiation therapy are similar to those experienced during standard chemotherapy and radiation therapy. They include nausea and vomiting, anorexia (a lack of desire to eat), alopecia (hair loss), and a series of side effects related to each unique drug that can be used. Some of the side effects, such as nausea and anorexia, can last for weeks after the transplant. The chance of experiencing these side effects, along with the potential risks and benefits of the transplant, will be explained by a member of the transplant team prior to hospitalization (see Chap. 18).

Once the chemotherapy and radiation therapy is completed, you will receive the transplanted bone marrow. The marrow, similar in composition to blood, is given as an intravenous infusion over a few minutes. If the bone marrow is harvested from a family member, he or she usually will undergo the procedure on the same day, in the same hospital in which the transplant will occur. If the bone marrow is harvested from an unrelated donor, the bone marrow may be driven or flown to the transplant center from anywhere in the country or even the world. Unfortunately (or fortunately), the actual transplant procedure is far less exciting than people expect! Many refer to the transplant day as their new birthday.

Once the transplant has occurred, you enter a waiting period until the new marrow takes root in your bones and grows. During the period when there is no functioning marrow (i.e., a person's old marrow has been killed by chemotherapy and the new marrow has not yet grown), you will have low blood counts. Most people will become anemic due to decreased production of red blood cells and will require transfusions to feel more energetic and less tired. You also may develop low platelet counts that place you at risk for bleeding complications, and which necessitate platelet transfusions. Last, you will probably have a low white blood cell count, which puts you at risk for serious infections.

Because of this risk of serious infection, most transplant procedures are performed in sterile environments (often with high-efficiency air filters to remove bacterial contaminants). Most transplant centers employ strict isolation (to prevent the spread of infection) for people undergoing allogeneic transplant; for the same reason, all visitors must wear sterile masks and gloves while visiting. Most centers also prohibit fresh flowers and fruit from a person's isolation room, as these may contain infectious organisms.

Despite all of the precautions, the risk of infection is quite high. At this point, the body's natural defenses against infection are essentially nonexistent, and even seemingly minor infections can become life-threatening. Most BMT patients develop a fever at some point following the transplant, necessitating the use of powerful intravenous antibiotics for several days to weeks. Most also will develop sores (which can be quite uncomfortable) in their mouths and throats; pain control may require the use of morphine. These sores are due to a condition called *mucositis*, as it involves the mucous membranes which line the mouth and throat. These membranes are sensitive to the high-dose chemotherapy and to radiation therapy.

The "danger period" is the time during which the various cell counts are low (a condition called *cytopenia or neutropenia*). This critical period after transplantation can last anywhere from 1 to 4 weeks, depending on the type of BMT (autologous or allogeneic) a person receives and the source of the stem cells (marrow or peripheral blood). On average, the recovery time after autologous transplantation is between 7 and 14 days. After allogeneic transplantation, the cytopenic period is more variable, ranging from 14 to 28 days.

Generally, people who have a peripheral blood stem cell transplant will *engraft* (the term used to describe the regrowth of marrow cells) a couple of days earlier than those who have traditional bone marrow used as the source of stem cells. The white blood cells usually are the first cells to recover to adequate numbers, followed a couple of days later by the platelets, and, last, by the red blood cells. Commonly, however, the platelets and red blood cells take a longer time to recover fully, sometimes even months. This delayed recovery often does not impede discharge from the hospital, as transfusions can be given in outpatient clinics when needed. You will not be discharged from the hospital prior to engraftment of the white blood cell line, particularly the subtype of white blood cells called *neutrophils*, which must reach a level (the absolute neutrophil count, or ANC) of 500 per cubic millimeter.

WHAT ARE SOME OF THE IMPORTANT RISKS OF BONE MARROW TRANSPLANTATION?

A BMT is a high-risk, rigorous medical procedure that should be undertaken only by individuals who are both physically and psychologically up to the challenge. This point cannot be emphasized enough, as a BMT is considered more dangerous than most chemotherapy regimens and is often reserved for people who have no other reasonable chance to be cured of their cancer. While estimates vary depending on the reason for the transplant and on some patient characteristics, up to one in five people (20 percent) undergoing a BMT procedure will have a fatal complication as a result of the procedure (Table 20-3).

One of the most important risks that people undergoing allogeneic transplantation need to be aware of is a disorder called *graft-versus-host disease* (GVHD). Earlier in this chapter, the role of the transplanted immune system in eradicating residual tumor cells was discussed. The newly transplanted immune system (the graft) recognizes protein labels on the remaining tumor cells and destroys these cells; that is, the graft does not recognize these cells as "self." As the same "label" is carried by all cells in the recipient's (the host's) body, it is possible that the new immune cells will recognize not only residual tumor cells as foreign but also the rest of the body's cells.

When this occurs, the new immune system (or graft) attempts to reject the host; that is, the immune cells try to destroy the host cells. This is termed GVHD. GVHD is a clinical disorder characterized by any of the following: skin rash, profuse diarrhea, abnormalities in liver function, and an increased risk of serious infection. Almost any organ can be involved by GVHD, and the risk of GVHD increases when the donor and recipient are not perfect HLA matches (i.e., the donor and recipient have only five out of six identical HLA genes). GVHD may be a more common occurrence when peripheral blood stem cells are used as the stem cell source.

GVHD can be prevented to some extent, and it can be treated. Prevention of GVHD is brought about through the use of medications that suppress the immune system. Once the immune system is suppressed, the newly transplanted immune cells (the graft) will be unable to attack host cells with the wrong cell "label." Medications are given around the time of transplantation and for several months afterward to prevent GVHD. If GVHD does occur, stronger doses of these immunosuppressive medications are used. Examples of these medications include steroids (prednisone, cortisone), tacrolimus (FK 506), and cyclosporine (and similar drugs).

Another alternative to preventing GVHD is to modify the graft prior to transplantation by removing some of the immune cells that can cause GHVD. The immune cells involved in GVHD are a subset of white blood cells, called T cells. These can be removed using specialized machines and techniques in a process known as

TABLE 20-3 Potential Complications of Bone Marrow
Transplantation

Infection
Bleeding
Graft-versus-host disease (GVHD)
Veno-occlusive disease (VOD) of the liver
Diffuse alveolar hemorrhage (DAH) or idiopathic pneumonia syndrome (IPS)

T-cell depletion of the graft. As these T cells also are important in killing residual tumor cells, T-cell depletion is associated with a higher risk of tumor relapse.

A second important complication of a BMT is a disorder called veno-occlusive disease (VOD) of the liver. VOD can occur after both autologous and allogeneic transplantation, though it is more common after allogeneic transplantation. This disorder is caused by toxic destruction of the small and large veins of the liver and is typified by abdominal pain (from a congested liver), by weight gain, and possibly by liver dysfunction or failure. There are only experimental treatments for VOD. When this disease is mild, the liver repairs itself and no long-term sequelae develop. However, in a significant proportion of people who develop severe VOD, the disease can be fatal.

Another complication of a BMT is a disorder called diffuse alveolar hemorrhage (DAH) or idiopathic pneumonia syndrome (IPS), often characterized by bleeding within the lungs. Alveoli are the smallest segments of lung tissue. Like VOD, DAH probably occurs as a result of lung exposure to toxic substances such as those administered during chemotherapy. This clinical disorder is typified by bleeding from the small airways of the lungs; people suffering from DAH will therefore complain of shortness of breath and may even cough up blood. DAH occurs anywhere from 10 to 180 days following the transplant; when severe, it can be life-threatening and may require the use of a breathing tube (ventilator). Steroids are the only known effective treatment.

Infections are an important cause of sickness and death following transplantation. Despite the transplantation of a seemingly healthy, new immune system into the host, this new immune system is functionally immature and does not provide complete protection against infection. Transplant patients are even more susceptible to infection because of the immunosuppressive medications required to keep GVHD at bay. Infections may be similar to the common illnesses (such as pneumonia) seen in the general population, or they may be uncommon and unique to the transplant population. Infections that fall into the latter category include viral infections with cytomegalovirus (CMV), PCP pneumonia (caused by the organism *Pneumocystis carinii*, as seen in the AIDS population), and infections caused by invasive fungi and molds.

WHAT ARE THE PHYSICAL AND PSYCHOLOGICAL EFFECTS OF BONE MARROW TRANSPLANTATION?

The transplantation of any organ, including the bone marrow, is not an easy procedure to tolerate. Screening prior to undertaking the procedure is mandatory. Those people who are not well enough physically or not prepared psychologically to undergo the rigors of transplantation should delay the procedure until they are ready.

Most people feel unwell during the process of transplantation, despite the liberal use of effective methods at controlling nausea, vomiting, and pain. Those undergoing allogeneic transplantation generally have a tougher transplant course than people receiving autologous transplants because of their longer period of cytopenia (i.e., having low cell counts) and a longer length of stay in the hospital. The length of stay in the hospital is quite variable; it can be as short as 2 weeks for some undergoing autologous transplantation and as long as a month or more for those receiving an allogeneic BMT.

After transplantation, it usually takes several months for you to feel like yourself again. It may even take up to a year for those who have undergone allogeneic transplantation to feel "normal." This length of time depends highly on your physical condition prior to BMT and on the types of side effects experienced during transplantation.

Common complaints after transplantation include a lack of appetite, a lack of energy, low libido, and at times, a state of depression. Psychologically, many people have a difficult time confronting transplantation. The prospect of facing a real risk of serious physical complications and even death is difficult. Furthermore, the knowledge that, after BMT, things are unlikely to be as they were beforehand makes some people uneasy. It often is helpful, prior to undertaking the procedure, to speak with those who have undergone BMT successfully. Experienced BMT patients can often provide a different set of perspectives that physicians, no matter how experienced, cannot.

WHAT IS MINITRANSPLANTATION?

Minitransplantation (also termed *nonmyeloablative transplantation*) is a relatively new advance in the field of BMT. The *mini* in minitransplantation refers to the conditioning regimen (the chemotherapy and sometimes radiation therapy) used in these procedures. In contrast to the high-dose chemotherapy and radiotherapy used in traditional allogeneic and autologous BMTs, minitransplantation uses reduced-dose regimens that are not designed to kill all remaining tumor cells in the body. These regimens, however, are extremely immunosuppressive and allow the new donor marrow to take residence in the recipient's bones (to *engraft*), even when the old recipient marrow is still present. This technique relies on the immune function of the newly transplanted marrow to eradicate remaining tumor cells. Because high doses of chemotherapy are not given to kill remaining tumor cells, autologous minitransplantation cannot be attempted, since autologous marrow does not elicit any immune responses against remaining tumor cells.

Several months are required following the minitransplant to determine whether the newly transplanted bone marrow will be able to kill remaining tumor cells. The new marrow must be allowed to grow and to replace the old marrow in order for it to establish enough of a stronghold within the bone marrow space to produce normal blood cells and destroy tumor cells. Sometimes, however, the new marrow fails to engraft or does not engraft fully: it does not take over the recipient's bone marrow space completely. When both marrows coexist, the condition is termed *mixed chimerism* (from the Greek mythologic creature called the *chimera,* which possessed body parts from several different beings).

This situation may not be desirable if residual tumor cells are allowed to live and to grow in the marrow space. To convert the recipient from a mixed chimera to a full donor marrow state, several therapeutic maneuvers can be attempted. The first involves decreasing your immunosuppressive medications, which allows the new marrow to step up its attack on the old and diseased marrow. The other therapeutic maneuver is called *donor lymphocyte infusion* (DLI). In this process, a subset of white blood cells (or *lymphocytes*) are collected from the bone marrow donor and given to the recipient in the form of a blood transfusion. This provides a boost to the struggling donor bone marrow and increases the chances of the marrow engrafting completely. This approach also is used when BMT patients relapse (the cancer returns) after a seemingly successful minitransplant.

Although the name is deceiving, the only thing "mini" about a minitransplant is the conditioning regimen. Due to its relatively less severe nature, these procedures can often take place outside of a hospital, with chemotherapy and the transplant itself being given in a hospital clinic. In addition, because the conditioning regimen is easier to tolerate, people who would otherwise not be candidates for traditional transplantation may be eligible for minitransplantation—particularly those over the age of 55 years who are otherwise healthy.

The risk of graft-versus-host disease (GVHD) is as significant as in a traditional BMT. Approximately half of all patients undergoing minitransplantation will experience some degree of GVHD. The minitransplant approach has not yet replaced conventional transplantation for many indications and is still considered experimental.

WHAT TYPE OF BONE MARROW TRANSPLANT DO I NEED, AND WHERE SHOULD I GO TO GET IT?

There are many choices to be made prior to undertaking a BMT; most people rely on their physicians to guide them through this decision-making process. People with cancer should seek second opinions actively when they are not comfortable about the advice they receive or in making decisions related to transplantation, and they should consider visiting a nationally recognized transplant center before committing to a procedure.

Large centers with worldwide reputations are found throughout the United States. In fact, the majority of allogeneic transplants in the United States are performed at only a handful of transplant centers. The decision to undergo a transplant in one of these centers should be tempered by the hardship of being away from family (during the transplant and for several weeks after it), when you need to stay close to your transplant center and to your physicians (for follow-up visits and exams).

Many of the technicalities regarding the type of BMT (autologous versus allogeneic) and the type of stem cell to be used (marrow versus peripheral blood stem cell) should also be discussed with a transplant physician. That being said, most physicians often make these types of decisions on behalf of patients based on an understanding of the patient's cancer type and their own years of experience in the field.

LIFE AFTER BONE MARROW TRANSPLANTATION

Life before and during transplantation is difficult, but life after even a successful transplant can be just as arduous. Limitations imposed by physicians, coupled with physical limitations imposed by a deconditioned body, can make adjusting to post-transplant life challenging. Keeping up with medication schedules and physician visits alone can be quite draining!

After transplantation, BMT patients are instructed to be careful to avoid any type of infection. You cannot remain in public places for extended periods of time, and when you do go out in public, you must often wear masks and gloves to protect yourself from the viruses and bacteria that are abundant in the outside world. Your diet, too, must be modified to prevent food-borne illnesses; in general, fresh fruits, raw eggs, raw fish, and raw meats must be avoided.

Most people will also experience a decrease in sexual desire after a BMT, and certain restrictions are placed on sexual activities. Despite all of these limitations, most people gradually regain the quality and enjoyment of life that they experienced prior to the procedure. Some may not feel "normal" for a full year following the transplant, but there are others who feel well in as little as 3 months.

All of these issues need to be discussed in detail prior to transplantation. The decision to undertake this procedure is important, because transplantation is a life-altering event; you and your caregivers must be emotionally ready to make sacrifices for the chance of a cure from your cancer. Dedicated transplant physicians, nurses, pharmacists, and counselors are available to help transplant patients make decisions on their way toward a cure.

CHAPTER 21

Alternative and Complementary Therapies

HAROLD J. BURSTEIN, M.D., PH.D.
DAVID MISCHOULON, M.D., PH.D.

OUTLINE

WHAT IS "ALTERNATIVE MEDICINE"?

Complementary or alternative therapy or medicine (sometimes called *integrative* or *nontraditional therapy*) refers to a large number of health-related behaviors and practices that are, by definition, considered outside the realm of traditional western "allopathic" medicine. The number, variety, and extent of these practices defies easy categorization. Practices typically considered to be alternative therapies include herbal remedies, traditional Chinese medicine, acupuncture, natural or homeopathic treatments, relaxation techniques, spiritual or faith healing, unusual diets, chiropractic medicine, megadose vitamin therapy, massage, healing (or therapeutic) touch, Reiki (Fig. 21-1), aromatherapy, as well as the use of specific agents such as shark cartilage or hydrazine sulfate (Table 21-1). Some people even consider supportive group therapy or other forms of counseling to be "alternative" treatments.

Thus, the expression *alternative therapy* captures an enormous spectrum of health-related behaviors and interventions, and these therapies differ in many ways from each other (Table 21-1). Some, like traditional medicines, are ingested and are marketed to look like normal pills, while others have their foundation in distinct spiritual theories or lifestyles; still others are embodiments of whole philosophical or religious schools or cultural traditions.

Because of the heterogeneous practices encompassed within "complementary or alternative therapy," these terms do not have a standard definition. There have been attempts, however, to define these health practices by their relationship to

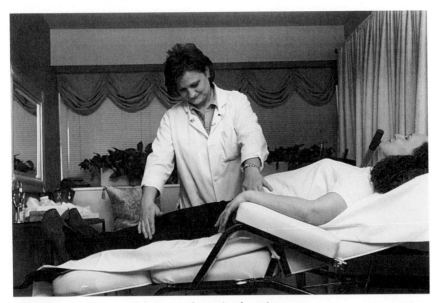

FIGURE 21-1 Reiki is one of the many alternative therapies.

TABLE 21-1 Types of Alternative Therapies

Acupuncture	A Chinese practice that dates back 2500 years. Fine needles are inserted into acupoints—specific areas along the body that, when stimulated, help rebalance the natural energy flow within the body.
Acupressure	A Japanese practice also known as *shiatsu massage*. Finger pressure is used instead of needles to stimulate specific points along the body to restore the body's life energy and bring it into balance.
Aromatherapy	The use of highly concentrated plant extracts to balance and restore the body, mind, and spirit.
Chi Kung	Developed in China, this mind/body technique uses different body positions (lying, sitting, standing still, and moving) to facilitate using the body effortlessly, and in so doing uniting the body and mind.
Vitamins	Their use may help the body repair normal cells and destroy damaged cells.
Yoga	From India, these exercises help balance and harmonize the body and mind to create a sense of well-being.
Guided imagery	This process of relaxed-focused concentration uses memories, dreams, or fantasy visualization to refocus attention away from a stressful situation.
Massage therapy	The use of touch and techniques of stroking or kneading the body's muscles to improve body structure and function.
Reiki	This Japanese technique involves the laying on of hands as a conduit for the "life force energy" that flows through the body. It promotes relaxation, stress reduction, and the immune system.
Therapeutic touch	A process of energy exchange in which the practitioner holds his or her hands a few inches from the body to correct the energy imbalance caused by disease.

standard medicine. Thus, "alternative" treatments are those that people might choose instead of traditional western medicine, while "complementary" suggests that these practices are pursued alongside traditional medicine. Despite this distinction, surveys have consistently demonstrated that the vast majority of people who seek out complementary or alternative medicine are simultaneously engaged in traditional medicine. Thus arose the term integrative medicine, reflecting the integration of both nonstandard (alternative or complementary) and standard (western or allopathic) medical treatments.

One predominant feature shared by complementary or alternative therapies is that they are rarely offered or endorsed by providers of traditional medicine; these therapies tend to flourish outside the confines of conventional clinics, hospitals, and pharmacies. Often, alternative therapies are recommended by nontraditional medical practitioners. Over the past few years, it has been recognized that many patients are interested in nontraditional health practices even as they are visiting allopathic providers.

WHAT TYPES OF ALTERNATIVE MEDICINE ARE AVAILABLE?

An innumerable variety of alternative medicine practices are available. There are no real data as to why people choose one type over another. Studies do suggest that cultural traditions dramatically alter alternative medicine behaviors. One study of women with breast cancer in San Francisco found that the rate of use of alternative therapies in four different cultures (white, African American, Hispanic, and Asian) was quite similar but that the particular types of alternative therapy varied enormously from culture to culture. For instance, use of spiritual therapies was more common among African Americans, while Chinese Americans were more likely to use herbal remedies and Latino and Caucasian populations tended to use dietary supplements and vitamins.

Over the past 15 years, a growing literature has documented the prevalence (the fraction of people engaging in an activity at a given point in time) of alternative therapy use among people in general and among people with cancer in particular. Studies consistently show that large percentages of cancer patients pursue alternative therapies. The actual prevalence varies depending on how one defines alternative medicine. However, it is clear that at least half of all cancer patients are engaged in some sort of alternative health behavior—that is, a practice designed to improve their health and well-being that is outside the realm of traditional (western) medical recommendations. For cancer patients, then, alternative medicine is the norm, not the exception.

HOW SAFE ARE ALTERNATIVE MEDICINES?

There are no data on the safety and efficacy (i.e., how well treatments work) of most alternative therapies. In the United States, a drug that is approved by the Food and Drug Administration is subject to extensive testing to define the precise contents of the drug, its safety, and its efficacy. This information is publicly available. By contrast, most alternative medicines are sold as nutritional supplements and are not subject to the scrutiny of any regulatory agency. Thus, neither the contents nor the safety of most alternative medicines is well documented. Similarly, there are few if any data on the use of alternative medicines in combination with traditional medicines. People using alternative therapies must be aware of the genuine lack of information on their safety and efficacy.

While most alternative medicines are probably safe, there are case reports of toxic, even life-threatening side effects from the use of some alternative medicines. Fortunately, these serious reactions are rare; however, they do underscore the point that "natural" remedies may not be free of side effects.

There are, on the other hand, many alternative health practices that do not require exposure to, or ingestion of, unusual substances. These methods—including relaxation techniques, visualization, and spiritual practices—undoubtedly

TABLE 21-2 Criteria to Use in Selecting an Alternative Care
Practitioner

What is the practitioner's level of experience?
Is he or she recommended by others?
Is he or she willing to communicate with your doctors?
Have the claims associated with any treatment been evaluated critically?

---

pose little threat to health, and can be considered "safe." Other alternative treatments, such as acupuncture, may in principle pose health hazards through the communication of infection or bruising/bleeding. The safety of such practices depends in large part on the experience, skill, and sterile techniques practiced by the provider. Generally speaking, there are no standard regulations for the licensing, inspection, or certification of such practitioners. Commonsense questions and observations can help, as can discussion with other patients and providers. The level of experience, recommendations of others, and willingness to communicate with orthodox physicians are all important in selecting an alternative care provider (Table 21-2).

WHAT STUDIES HAVE COMPARED ALTERNATIVE MEDICINES TO TRADITIONAL CHEMOTHERAPY?

In treating cancer, oncologists rely upon well-designed clinical trials to determine the usefulness of a cancer treatment (see Chap. 18 for a more detailed description of clinical trials). These trials have specific eligibility criteria to ensure a uniform patient population, standardized treatment plans and measurements of side effects, and predefined endpoints (which are agreed upon in advance) to demonstrate whether a treatment works.

In general, clinical trials examining the efficacy of alternative medicines are either inadequate or nonexistent. Such practices simply have not been studied in the same way as have more traditional cancer treatments, such as chemotherapy or hormonal therapy. Most reports on the use of alternative therapy, when such reports exist at all, have included small numbers of patients with different types and stages of cancer receiving nonuniform treatments and without objective measures of the success of treatment or the side effects associated with treatment. There are almost no studies that have compared alternative treatments with standard treatments. With few exceptions, there are no data that any specific method of alternative therapy cures, treats, or changes the natural history of specific cancers. A limited number of studies have, however, raised the possibility of clinical activity for some treatments, such as PC-SPES in prostate cancer. The National Institute of Health is sponsoring many active trials of alternative therapies.

If you are interested in alternative treatments, you should critically evaluate the claims associated with any given treatment. Many alternative therapies make statements about potential benefits. It is often difficult for consumers to know the basis for any such benefits if they exist. You can write to manufacturers to discuss specific claims.

WHY DO PEOPLE USE ALTERNATIVE THERAPIES?

Traditional allopathic or western treatments for cancer are often intense, debilitating, and associated with side effects. Many times, traditional therapies are inadequate at treating cancer. Under such circumstances, it is not surprising that many people prefer treatments that may have fewer side effects and may help relieve the fatigue, anxiety, and discouragement that can be associated with cancer or allopathic cancer treatments.

Studies have examined the motivations underlying interest in alternative therapy among people with cancer. These surveys consistently show that people appreciate the more "natural" or holistic emphasis in alternative therapy and like the opportunity to participate actively and directly in their health care. People like making their own decisions, and alternative therapy is an area in which they may be able to "take control" of their lives and their therapy. Additionally, people who are interested in alternative therapy often report feeling discouraged, anxious, uncomfortable, tired, or in pain. People who turn to nontraditional therapies are more likely to report symptoms of psychosocial distress. These are problems that can sometimes be addressed effectively with standard medical interventions. In fact, it is possible that an interest in alternative therapies may be sparked when an oncologist fails to ask his or her patients about these symptoms, so that the potential of treating these symptoms with western medicines is not even raised. Finally, people with cancer may look to alternative therapy as a way to fulfill needs that are not, or cannot be, met by doctors alone.

CAN I USE BOTH ALTERNATIVE MEDICINES AND CHEMOTHERAPY?

Surveys of cancer patients receiving both routine and experimental treatments reveal that a large fraction of people are also taking alternative medicines. It is not known whether it is safe to take most alternative medicines, nor is it known (for most alternative therapies) whether there are interactions between conventional cancer treatments and the alternative medicine. These types of interactions could result in either the conventional medicine (i.e., chemotherapy) or the alternative medicine reaching levels in the bloodstream that are either too high, and thus potentially dangerous, or too low, and thus potentially ineffective. You should talk with your doctor and discuss specific alternative practices or medicines that you are taking and how they might affect your regular cancer treatments.

A number of major cancer institutes have recognized the widespread interest in alternative therapies and have therefore established clinical centers specializing in alternative care. Such centers can be valuable resources for information on alternative and complementary therapy, including referrals to local providers. They may also have up-to-date information on the safety of many alternative practices and may be participating in clinical trials of alternative treatments.

The costs of most alternative therapies are not covered by traditional insurance. However, some health plans or insurance carriers will cover consultations with certain alternative providers. You should speak with representatives familiar with your particular health care coverage in order to understand the financial implications of alternative treatments.

SHOULD I TELL MY DOCTOR THAT I'M USING AN ALTERNATIVE MEDICINE?

It is important for you to talk with your oncologist about your use of alternative or complementary medicine. Most doctors understand the widespread interest people, and particularly people with cancer, have in alternative medicine and will be neither surprised nor offended to hear of your interest. First, you should make sure that the alternative health practices you are pursuing are safe and will not interfere with your conventional cancer treatments (if you choose to pursue both modalities of therapy). Second, you should discuss with your doctor the feelings or concerns that prompted you to use alternative therapy. You may have symptoms that your doctor can address with changes in your regular medical regimen. Finally, talking about alternative therapy may be a way of forging a stronger relationship between you and your doctor. It helps your doctor better understand your state of mind, priorities, and physical and emotional well-being. Sharing in the experience of cancer is part of what makes doctors valuable partners in treating your cancer. The relationship you have with your physician can be enriched when you talk about alternative health practices.

WHAT "ALTERNATIVE" OR NATURAL MEDICATIONS ARE AVAILABLE FOR DEPRESSION AND ANXIETY?

Depression and anxiety are common in people with cancer, a topic covered in detail in Chap. 25. If you have symptoms of either of these conditions, your first step should be to tell your doctor. Traditional medications or therapy sessions may relieve your suffering. There are several natural medications available for psychiatric conditions. Most of them fall into the category of antidepressants and antianxiety medications. Some of the more popular ones are reviewed here and are summarized in Table 21-3. The efficacy of most of these medications has not been studied formally.

St. John's wort, derived from the plant *Hypericum perforatum,* is the most popular mood-altering medication worldwide. As mentioned in Chap. 17, there is a

TABLE 21-3 Popular Natural/Alternative Medications for Psychiatric
Conditions

Medication	Putative Indication	Suggested Dose	Possible Adverse Effects
Ginkgo biloba	Dementia	120–240 mg/day taken in divided doses two or three times a day	Mild stomach upset, headache, irritability, dizziness
Homeopathy	Various disorders	Variable	Transient worsening of symptoms
Kava (*Piper methysticum*)	Anxiety	60–120 mg/day	Stomach upset, allergic reactions, headaches, dizziness, imbalance, hair loss, visual problems, respiratory problems, and skin discoloration
Melatonin	Insomnia	0.5–5.0 mg/day	Sedation, confusion, decreased fertility, decreased sex drive, low body temperature, retinal damage, and weakening of the immune system
Omega fatty acids	Mania, depression, psychosis	200–3000 mg/day	Stomach upset
SAM-e (S-adenosyl methionine)	Depression	200–1600 mg/day	Stomach upset
St. John's wort (*Hypericum perforatum*)	Depression	900 mg/day taken in divided doses	Dry mouth, dizziness, constipation, easy sunburn, and toxic reactions when combined with certain other medications
Valerian (*Valeriana officinalis*)	Insomnia	450–600 mg/day	Blurry vision, muscle dystonias, liver toxicity, and possibly cancer

fair amount of research-based evidence to suggest that it is effective for mild-to-moderate depression, but less so for more severe depression. It usually is dosed on a twice- or thrice-daily schedule; the recommended therapeutic dose is about 900 milligrams per day. Although side effects are mild and uncommon, potentially dangerous interactions may occur with other medications. For example, people who are taking antiretroviral medications (e.g., protease inhibitors) used to combat HIV infection should not use St. John's wort, as it may decrease the blood levels of these medications. Likewise, St. John's wort may reduce blood levels of cyclosporine, which is used to prevent transplant rejection and may also be used in the setting of bone marrow transplantation. Transplant recipients who are taking these medications should avoid using St. John's wort.

SAM-e (S-adenosyl methionine) is a compound made in the human body. It is involved in the synthesis of neurotransmitters (chemicals in the brain), such as serotonin and norepinephrine, which are thought to be involved in depression. SAM-e has been studied extensively, and research supports its effectiveness for depression, particularly in individuals with medical illness who may have trouble with side effects from conventional medications. SAM-e is available in capsule form and in some cases in an injectable form. Recommended doses for the treatment of depression can be quite high (up to 1600 milligrams per day), which can, for some, render the cost of treatment prohibitive.

Omega-3 fatty acids, derived primarily from fish oils, are thought to function as mood stabilizers for individuals with bipolar disorder. There also is some evidence that they may function as antidepressants and antipsychotics. They seem to have a benign side-effect profile, with stomach upset being the only significant complaint reported. Doses may vary from 200 milligrams per day to 3 grams (3000 milligrams) or more per day. There are several different types of omega-3 fatty acids, including docosahexaenoic acid (DHA) and eicosapentaenoic acid (EPA). Preparations may include combinations of the different oils in varying ratios. It is not yet clear which specific oils may be most responsible for the psychiatric effects.

Kava, derived from the plant *Piper methysticum,* is a popular medication believed to be useful for mild anxiety. It is available in several forms, including a capsule, a tincture that can be diluted with water, or as a "tea bag" used to prepare a hot drink. The usual dose varies between 60 and 120 milligrams per day. Kava is not as effective for more severe anxiety or panic attacks. There is evidence of long-term side effects, including a yellow discoloration of the skin. Therefore one should not use kava for more than a few months.

Valerian, derived from the plant *Valeriana officinalis,* is a medication used for the treatment of insomnia. It is generally recommended as a means of restoring normal sleep in "poor sleepers" over a few weeks, as it does not work immediately. The dose commonly used is 450 to 600 milligrams per day to be taken 1 to 2 hours before bedtime. Valerian has a benign side-effect profile and does not seem to cause daytime sedation. Preparations of valerian made in India and Mexico have been shown to contain high levels of carcinogens and therefore are not recommended.

Melatonin is a hormone manufactured in the human brain. It regulates, among other processes, the sleep cycle, and is therefore popular as a treatment for insomnia, especially among people who travel across time zones. Recommended doses may range from 0.5 to 5 milligrams per day at bedtime. Individuals who have weakened immune systems—for example, people with AIDS or transplant recipients—should avoid melatonin, as it may compromise their immune systems even further.

Ginkgo biloba, derived from the seeds of the ginkgo tree, is popular in the treatment of memory loss and cognitive difficulties, often encountered in Alzheimer's disease and other types of dementias. There is some evidence that this supplement is effective, but it may take several months or even up to a year of treatment before results are seen. Some preliminary reports suggest that Ginkgo may also help to ameliorate the sexual dysfunction caused by antidepressants. Doses recommended are between 120 to 240 milligrams per day, usually divided in a thrice-daily regimen. Although side effects are rare, *Ginkgo* may increase the risk of bleeding and therefore should not be used if you have a bleeding disorder, a low blood count, or are taking blood thinners (anticoagulants).

Homeopathy often involves a combination of small quantities of herbal and/or mineral-based medications specifically tailored to your symptom(s). Homeopathy has been used for many psychiatric conditions, including depression, attention deficit disorder, and different types of anxiety disorders. However, there is little scientific evidence to support its effectiveness in these cases. Homeopathic remedies may worsen your symptoms upon initiation of treatment and alleviation may take several weeks or months. If you choose to pursue homeopathy as a treatment, you may be better off doing so under the supervision of a trained homeopathic practitioner.

As emphasized in Chap. 17, natural psychiatric medications may be useful for the treatment of mood and anxiety disorders. However, they should be used with care (preferably under the supervision of a doctor), especially if you have a complicated medical illness and are taking other medications. Patients with symptoms of severe psychological distress or psychiatric illness should be referred for evaluation by a trained mental health professional.

CHAPTER 22

The Management of Pain

SCOTT SHAPIRO, M.D.
MENEKSE ALPAY, M.D.

OUTLINE

CAN MY PAIN BE MANAGED EFFECTIVELY?

If you ask people with cancer and those close to them what their biggest fear about cancer is, many will say that it is a fear of pain and discomfort. Most worry that their pain will neither be addressed nor relieved. However, cancer and pain specialists generally agree that cancer pain can be treated in up to 90 percent of people. Despite the many effective treatments that are available, however, pain is often addressed inadequately. There are a host of reasons for this. Health care providers, people with cancer, and their families fear the use of potentially addictive medications. They have concerns about side effects, and they minimize the impact of psychological factors that contribute to pain. This chapter discusses several different types of pain, reviews how pain can best be treated, and considers how psychological factors affect the perception of pain.

HOW DOES CANCER CAUSE PAIN?

Cancer causes pain in a variety of ways (Table 22-1). Because the mechanisms by which cancer induces pain are varied and the treatments of various types of pain differ, it is crucial to understand the source of pain. The underlying cause of the pain also affects how a person experiences the pain and which treatments will be most helpful. Cancer causes pain by pushing on bodily organs or bones, by stretching the capsule that surrounds organs, by invading nerves, by causing inflammation, by blocking hollow organs (such as the intestines), or by releasing chemicals that create a sensation of pain.

WHAT TYPES OF PAIN ARE THERE?

Cancer pain is categorized by its type, duration, severity, and location. The causes of pain can be divided broadly into four categories: somatic (related to solid organs such as skin, bone, and muscle); visceral (related to hollow organs such as the intestines); neuropathic (related to nerves); and other types of pain (Table 22-2). Each of these types of pain can be divided further by its duration (either acute or

TABLE 22-1 **How Cancer Causes Pain**

Pushes on bodily organs or bones
Stretches the capsule that surrounds an organ
Invades nerves
Causes inflammation
Blocks hollow organs (such as the intestines)
Releases chemicals that create a sensation of pain

TABLE 22-2 **Types of Pain**

Type	Description
Somatic	Related to solid organs, e.g., skin, bone, and muscle
Visceral	Related to hollow organs, e.g., the intestines
Neuropathic	Related to nerves, e.g., as in shingles

chronic), severity (often quantified on a scale that stretches from "0," meaning no pain, to "10," meaning the worst pain a person has ever experienced), and location (where in the body the pain is experienced).

Somatic Pain

Pain signals travel along nerves. Nerves course through the body (from the most superficial organ, the skin, to deeper structures and organs, such as the brain), carrying messages from the outside world to the brain. In addition to pain, nerves carry messages about touch, temperature, and vibration. Nerves also send information about the inside of the body to the brain. Pain that comes from the skin, bones, or muscles is called *somatic pain.* Often, these pains are experienced as aching, sharp, squeezing, stabbing, or throbbing. Common examples of somatic pain include the pain experienced when you are struck by an object, when your joints ache from arthritis, or when you experience a headache.

Visceral Pain

Another type of pain arises from injury or pressure on organs. Another name for organs is *viscera;* hence pain from organ injury is called *visceral pain.* When visceral pain is due to blockage of a hollow organ (such as the intestine), the pain usually feels crampy or gnawing. Visceral pains are experienced when a person has a gallstone or when the colon has a blockage. When the pain is due to the capsules or linings that surround organs, it often is experienced as aching, stabbing, or throbbing. This is the pain experienced by people with hepatitis.

Another type of visceral pain is called *referred pain.* This type of pain occurs at a site distant from the part of the body involved with cancer, in the absence of spread of the cancer to that distant body area. It occurs because of the way nerves are hard-wired together. For example, cancer that is limited to the pancreas (located near the lowest rib in the center of the abdomen) can actually produce pain in the shoulder blade. However, the cancer has not spread from the pancreas to the shoulder blade. Rather, the cancer in the pancreas is pressing on nerves that connect to the area around the shoulder blade.

Neuropathic Pain

The types of pain discussed above assume that the nervous system is normal and functioning properly. However, cancer (such as a lymphoma) and cancer treatments (particularly radiation therapy or chemotherapy drugs such as cisplatin, carboplatin, and paclitaxel) (see Chap. 14) can affect the nervous system directly. This type of cancer-related pain is called *neuropathic pain* and is unrelated to actual tissue damage. You might already be familiar with this type of pain. Some examples of neuropathic pain include the pain related to carpal tunnel syndrome (in which nerves are entrapped) or to chickenpox or shingles (in which nerves get infected with a virus and become inflamed). Neuropathic pain is often difficult to describe because it may be unlike any pain the individual has previously experienced. It may also feel as though one's skin were burning, like an electric shock, or might be experienced as numbness, tingling, or moving from one location to another (i.e., shooting pain).

Acute Pain

Frequently, the first question that must be addressed is whether the pain is new in onset or has been experienced for a long time. New-onset pain (or pain that reflects a change from a person's baseline pain) usually develops over hours or a day and is called *acute pain*. Often, it is related to a tissue injury.

Typically, pain is a signal that a body part is not functioning properly. It usually improves when the underlying injury or chemical abnormality is corrected. Acute pain is always accompanied by physical signs of pain (such as sweating, an increase in blood pressure and heart rate, or facial grimacing).

Chronic Pain

Pain that is present for more than 6 months is called *chronic pain*. Unlike acute pain, chronic pain is not accompanied by the physical signs described above. Health care providers and their support systems may underestimate and undertreat this kind of pain, and this can frustrate the person experiencing it; it also may lead to feelings of not being understood. Chronic pain takes a toll on the body, both physically and emotionally.

HOW DO PSYCHOLOGICAL FACTORS AFFECT THE PERCEPTION OF PAIN?

For centuries, people have discussed the relationship between the mind and the body. The more we learn about cancer pain, the more we increase our understanding of the interrelationship between the perception of pain and psychological factors.

Even though medicine has a long way to go to understand why pain and emotions affect one another, we do understand that the part of the brain that is responsible for our emotions, the limbic system, interacts closely with the pain pathways and receives pain signals. Thus, pain affects how we feel, and how we feel affects the severity of our pain. It is believed by most pain specialists that the most effective way to treat someone with cancer pain is to address the physical, psychological, and social issues that may be playing a role in pain perception. At times, this is difficult for any given health care provider to do; a coordinated approach from an array of professions—including cancer doctors (oncologists), psychiatrists, psychologists, nurses, social workers, and pastoral care providers—may be necessary (see Chap. 26).

WHAT TYPES OF PAIN MEDICATIONS ARE THERE?

Medications that treat pain are called *analgesics*. However, many types of medications that are not classified as analgesics are still useful as enhancers (adjuvants) of the effects of analgesics. These medications include anticonvulsants (antiseizure medications), cardiac medications (medications for the heart), antidepressants, and stimulants (Table 22-3).

The type of painkillers (analgesics) prescribed depends on several factors: the type, severity, and location of pain; the duration of the pain; the potential side effects of the medications; other medications used; and illnesses experienced by the person with cancer. People with cancer and their doctors often become frustrated because there are no "tests" or "studies" to determine the severity of a person's pain. You should feel comfortable explaining your pain to the doctor, feel that you are being taken care of, and feel that your complaints are being taken seriously. You are the only one who knows how severe the pain is and whether the medication is relieving the pain.

WHICH TYPES OF PAIN RESPOND BEST TO ANTI-INFLAMMATORY AGENTS, ANTICONVULSANTS, NARCOTICS, ANTIDEPRESSANTS, AND OTHER CLASSES OF MEDICATIONS?

Anti-inflammatory Medications

Anti-inflammatory medications [such as salicylic acid (aspirin) and ibuprofen (Motrin, Advil)] are useful for mild to moderate pain. They can help reduce inflammatory reactions to cancer that cause pain by direct invasion or compression of body tissues, or they can diminish the impact of chemicals that cancers can release. In addition, these agents help alleviate bone pain, which might occur with cancer that has spread to the bones.

TABLE 22-3 Major Classes of Pain Medications and Adjuvants

Medication	Typical Dose Range, (mg/day)	Common Side Effects
Anticonvulsants		
Valproate (Depakote)	500–2000	Sedation, weight gain, nausea, vomiting, diarrhea, liver toxicity
Carbamazepine (Tegretol)	400–1600	Dizziness, nausea, sedation, liver toxicity, bone marrow toxicity
Gabapentin (Neurontin)	300–5400	Sedation, dry mouth
Antidepressants		
Selective serotonin reuptake inhibitors (SSRIs)		
Paroxetine (Paxil)	10–50	Nausea, diarrhea, sedation, sexual dysfunction
Fluoxetine (Prozac)	10–60	Nausea, diarrhea, sexual dysfunction
Citalopram (Celexa)	20–60	Nausea, diarrhea, headache
Escitalopram (Lexapro)	10–30	Nausea, diarrhea, headache
Sertraline (Zoloft)	50–150	Nausea, diarrhea, headache, sexual dysfunction
Tricyclics		
Amitriptyline (Elavil)	100–300	Dry mouth, sedation
Monoamine oxidase inhibitors		
Tranylcypromine (Parnate)	30–60	Sedation, dizziness, significant interaction with certain foods and medications
Opioids		
Morphine	60–400	Nausea, itching, sedation
Oxycodone (Percocet, Percodan)	5–20	Nausea, itching, sedation
Methadone (Dolophine)	10–40	Nausea, itching, sedation
Nonsteroidal Anti-Inflammatory Drugs (NSAIDs)		
Naproxen (Naprosyn)	750–1100	Abdominal distress
Ibuprofen (Motrin)	1600–2400	Abdominal distress
Acetaminophen (Tylenol)	1000–2000	Liver toxicity (at higher doses)
Aspirin	1200–2600	
Diflunisal (Dolobid)	500–1000	
Ketorolac tromethamine (Toradol)	10–40	(For short-term use only)

A host of anti-inflammatory medications are currently available. They include both prescription and nonprescription agents (including aspirin and ibuprofen). Some newer anti-inflammatory medications, such as rofecoxib (Vioxx), are believed to be better tolerated and to have a longer-lasting effect than previously prescribed agents. Some people with cancer who do not respond to one medication (i.e., the medication does not improve their pain) may still respond to another medication.

Another commonly used analgesic for cancer pain is acetaminophen (Tylenol). It is not truly an anti-inflammatory medication (i.e., it does not reduce inflammation the way aspirin does) and is not very effective for bone pain. Acetaminophen does provide relief from mild to moderate pain without the risk of irritating the digestive system. However, acetaminophen does not diminish the inflammation that is commonly associated with cancer pain. In addition, acetaminophen can be harmful to the liver if taken in doses higher than prescribed, and it may interfere with the blood levels of other medications, such as the blood thinner warfarin (Coumadin).

Opioids

Opioids are a class of drugs with a chemical structure similar to morphine. Opioid medications differ in their potency, their side-effect profile, and their duration of action. Many painkillers, such as Vicodin or Percocet (including hydrocodone or oxycodone and acetaminophen), are combinations of opioids and anti-inflammatory medications. Opioids can be habit-forming; thus, working closely with one doctor (as opposed to multiple physicians each prescribing an analgesic) is essential. Together, you and your doctor can develop a plan to maximize pain control and to minimize the risk of addiction.

Often, people with cancer, their family members, and even physicians are reluctant to use opioids because of a fear of addiction and the propensity of these drugs to cause side effects. However, when opioids are used prudently, they can improve an individual's quality of life and help to avoid needless suffering; remember, the risks involved with the use of opioids can be minimized. Most pain can be treated with traditional painkillers (analgesics). The World Health Organization (WHO) has offered recommendations for the type of pain medication that should be used, depending on the severity and type of the pain. If the pain is mild, ibuprofen (e.g., Motrin, Advil) or acetaminophen (e.g., Tylenol) should be used first. If the pain is moderate or severe, medications such as codeine or morphine can be used along with ibuprofen or acetaminophen.

Anticonvulsants

Anticonvulsant medications [such as valproic acid (Depakote), carbamazepine (Tegretol), gabapentin (Neurontin), and clonazepam (Klonopin)] have been used to treat seizures for many decades. In addition, many studies and a vast clinical experience have shown that these medicines can be helpful in the treatment of neuropathic pain. They may be used alone in cases of mild pain and in combination with nonsteroidal anti-inflammatory drugs (NSAIDs) and opioids in cases of more severe pain. In many people, they can eliminate or reduce the intensity of neuropathic pain. In people with severe pain, they are good adjuvants to opioids. Gabapentin has been shown to be more effective than the other anticonvulsants and is the most commonly prescribed medication in this class for this indication. It also appears to have fewer side effects than other anticonvulsants.

Antidepressants

Antidepressants, including the tricyclic antidepressants (TCAs), have also been used to relieve pain. The exact mechanism by which these medications help alleviate pain is unclear. Antidepressants can also be helpful in treating cancer pain, particularly neuropathic pain. In general, they are not helpful for acute pain, but they can diminish pain when it is chronic. Tricyclic antidepressants, such as amitriptyline (Elavil, Endep) and desipramine (Norpramin), have been well studied in chronic pain. When they are used for chronic pain (and not for depression), the doses are often much lower than when these medications are used for their antidepressant effects.

SHOULD I CONSIDER HAVING TREATMENTS (SUCH AS ACUPUNCTURE, NERVE BLOCKS, HYPNOSIS, AND MASSAGE) OTHER THAN MEDICATIONS FOR PAIN RELIEF?

Many other types of treatments are helpful when used either alone or in conjunction with analgesic medications (Table 22-4). Some examples within the medical field include nerve blocks, electrical stimulation treatments (transcutaneous electrical nerve stimulation, or TENS), neurosurgery, the use of implantable devices, and acupuncture.

Nerve Blocks

Among their many functions, nerves carry pain signals to the brain. Thus, when pain is well localized (i.e., it occurs in a specific organ or part of the body), injecting chemicals into the nerves that carry these signals can block them. Depend-

TABLE 22-4 Ways to Control Pain without Medication

Nerve blocks
Electrical stimulation treatments (transcutaneous electrical nerve stimulation, or TENS)
Neurosurgery
Implantable devices
Acupuncture
Psychological therapies
Alternative and complementary therapies

ing on the anatomy of the pain, the pain signal can be blocked at any point along the path of the nerve: either from where it originates, where it travels (e.g., within the spinal cord), or where it is received in the brain.

Transcutaneous Electrical Nerve Stimulation

TENS involves the administration of low-voltage electrical currents. The current produced travels through the skin and interferes with the pain signals that are being carried by nearby nerve fibers to the brain, thus diminishing the intensity of the sensation. It is safe and can be helpful in the treatment of neuropathic pain.

Neurosurgical Treatments

When medications are neither tolerated nor effective for the treatment of cancer pain, neurosurgical procedures can be helpful. Several different types of neurosurgical treatments exist. One type interferes with pain transmission mechanically by surgically cutting the nerve that transmits the pain. A second type of procedure involves implanting a device in the body, typically near the spinal cord. This device, called an intrathecal pump, can either deliver medications to a specific area or send out electrical signals that interfere with a pain signal.

WHAT PSYCHOLOGICAL TREATMENTS ARE HELPFUL?

Addressing the psychological well-being of a person with cancer and his or her family can help ease suffering. Individual and group therapy provides such people and their families with emotional support and with coping skills to address a range of issues. It is common to worry about the unknown, about whether you will survive, about the possibly terminal nature of your illness, and about how your illness will affect family members. In addition, problems that existed prior to the onset of cancer still have to be addressed.

Cognitive-behavioral therapy (CBT) is a specific type of therapy that focuses on the interactions among thoughts, feelings, and behavior. CBT can reduce anxiety and depression, as well as give you a renewed sense of control. Frequently in CBT, the therapist teaches relaxation techniques, meditation, or imagery.

Hypnosis is another technique that can reduce pain. Hypnosis works by placing a person in a state of "heightened and focused concentration," thus allowing him or her to redirect attention away from the pain and to diminish fear and anxiety

Another key treatment modality involves the use of medications. A person with cancer may have a preexisting psychiatric illness; if this is untreated, his or her pain, in turn, will be more difficult to treat. In addition, research shows that there is an increased risk of having a psychiatric illness, such as depression or anxiety, when one has chronic pain.

HOW SHOULD MY CANCER PAIN BEST BE MANAGED IF I HAVE A HISTORY OF DRUG OR ALCOHOL USE?

Many individuals with a current or past history of drug or alcohol use are concerned about how their cancer pain is going to be treated. Some are concerned about whether their pain is going to be taken seriously and whether the medications they will receive will lead to relapse (if they are former users of drugs or alcohol). Doctors and nurses, too, are confronted with difficult decisions and concerns. They may ask themselves: "Is my patient's pain real? Will I cause my patient to become an addict or to relapse?"

The first rule in treating pain in a person with cancer is: "All people with cancer deserve the same attention and respect." Thus, the relationship between you and your doctor must occur in an environment of trust. Otherwise, the treatment is doomed. Here are several tips to ensure the effective treatment of cancer pain: You and your doctor should agree that there will be only one provider writing medication prescriptions. This allows your doctor to know what is helping and enables him or her to monitor any potentially dangerous drug interactions. Your doctor must discuss treatment goals with you. If you have chronic cancer pain, the pain will not disappear completely. Thus, the goal of treatment is to diminish your pain to a tolerable degree, allowing you to function at your highest level. There must be an ongoing discussion not only about pain control but also about your work, family relationships, sexual functioning, sleep, and appetite. Frequent follow-up appointments are helpful in building an effective relationship and understanding how you are coping.

NONMEDICAL TREATMENTS

Many people find nonmedical treatments (such as yoga, tai chi, massage, herbal remedies, and relaxation techniques) helpful in the treatment of chronic pain (see Chap. 21). The precise explanation of how these techniques help is unclear; in addition, it is difficult to determine ahead of time who will benefit from them. However, as we learn more about the connection between the mind and the body, we are realizing that addressing and treating stress, anxiety, and depression can alleviate pain as well as improve quality of life. Many cancer centers even have integrative or complementary therapy centers that combine these therapies with traditional chemotherapy or radiation therapy.

CHAPTER 23

The Role of Faith in the Lives of People with Cancer

OLIVIA OKEREKE, M.D.

OUTLINE

WHAT ROLE DOES FAITH HAVE IN THE LIFE OF SOMEONE WITH CANCER?

Learning that you have cancer is a pivotal and life-changing event. Faith may help you navigate the often stormy seas of cancer's aftermath. Many turn to their established religion; others find it for the first time.

HOW CAN THE ROLE OF RELIGION IN A PERSON WITH CANCER BE EVALUATED?

Religion is a sensitive matter for most people. However, a number of key questions can help you or your physician evaluate the role of faith as you face cancer.

Several authors have described the basic elements of taking a "spiritual history." Taking a spiritual history involves determining not only religious beliefs but also spiritual values. Either you or a member of your health care team can assess whether you were raised in a certain religious faith or denomination, what role your parents played in the conveyance of religious ideas, and whether that upbringing involved extended exposure or study (e.g., parochial school, Sunday school, or religious retreats). You might also review your current religious practices and reflect on your idea of God and whether you find religion supportive, comforting, or frightening; as a follow-up, you can ask yourself how these ideas have evolved over time.

You may realize that you attended services regularly as a child but practice religion less regularly as an adult. Or you may have abandoned religion altogether only to return to it during a time of crisis. Regardless of how much time you have spent in actual spiritual observance, it is essential to know how those religious beliefs affect the conduct of your everyday life.

Ned Cassem (former Chief of Psychiatry at the Massachusetts General Hospital, a Professor of Psychiatry at Harvard Medical School, and a Jesuit priest) for years has encouraged physicians to take a comprehensive spiritual history that incorporates developmental aspects. He has advocated asking about the details of *cognitive* childhood memories (e.g., service attendance, daily prayer, home rituals, holidays, and community activities). Then, inquiries about the quality of *emotional* memories with which these events are associated (e.g., joy, expectation, tedium, guilt, dread, warmth, isolation, mystery, anger, resentment, confusion, and disbelief) should follow.

You can also reflect on the impact of religious leaders (e.g., pastors, priests, rabbis) on your notion of organized religion and whether those figures were considered to be role models or mentors. Recognizing that adolescence and young adulthood are periods of tremendous and rapid spiritual and intellectual change, you can ponder whether a growing intellect created a challenge to your faith or a deepening of it. You can also wonder if you were drawn further to religion or drifted away—deliberately or gradually, by defiance or by neglect.

HOW SHOULD I THINK ABOUT MY RELATIONSHIP TO GOD?

Let's start with the concept of God. Do you view God as stern or gentle? Forgiving or punitive? Rigid or flexible? Demanding or lenient? Detached or interested? From there, let's consider how your relationship with God has evolved over time. You can ask whether your relationship has become characterized by love or fear, by intimacy or distance, by judgment or acceptance, by presence or abandonment.

After considering God's attributes and the nature of the relationship, attention can be turned to communication. Assessment of communication involves issues of how you "talk to God" and whether this talk is perceived as one-way (a monologue) or two-way (a dialogue). Furthermore, you can think about how often and under what circumstances [e.g., daily, occasionally, rarely, or only during times of crisis—(also called "foxhole religion," as in, "there are no atheists in foxholes")] you communicate with God. You can reflect on whether you have any sense that God is communicating something back. Finally, you can consider your sense of God's presence (e.g., vague or vivid, rare or constant) and what you think about the strength of that relationship. A question to ask might be: "Have you ever turned to God during another time of trouble or during the illness of a loved one or yourself? If so, what was your experience and how would you describe the outcome?"

WHAT IF I DON'T BELIEVE IN GOD?

Spirituality is not confined to a religious experience with God. Spirituality has been described by Clifford Kuhn as a capacity that enables you to transcend any experience and to seek meaning and purpose beyond present circumstances.

As soon as you are diagnosed with cancer, you invariably will attach some meaning to the diagnosis, a meaning that is informed by your prior experience. Zbigniew Lipowski has described eight frames of reference through which we view illness: (1) as a challenge, (2) as an enemy, (3) as a punishment, (4) as a weakness, (5) as a relief, (6) as a strategy, (7) as an irreparable loss or as damage, and (8) as something of value (Table 23-1). Susan Sontag would probably encompass all of these with the notion of "illness as metaphor." Spirituality plays a key role in how we synthesize the meanings and metaphors of our diagnosis.

HOW CAN I ASSESS MY SPIRITUALITY?

Cassem also outlined nonreligious elements of the individual's spiritual history that are vital for understanding the person as a whole and his or her philosophy of life. Descriptions of several of these elements follow.

TABLE 23-1 **Eight Frames of Reference of Viewing Illness**

Illness as challenge
Illness as enemy
Illness as punishment
Illness as weakness
Illness as relief
Illness as strategy
Illness as irreparable loss or damage
Illness as value

Self-Description

Consider how you would describe yourself. Some questions that may reveal additional information include: "How do you like to be thought of? How would you like to be remembered (by friends, parents, spouse, children, peers, pupils, or mentors)? How do you perceive yourself at your best and at your worst? Do you view your life as evolving in any particular direction?"

People

It is critical for you to know who the most important people are in your life. Furthermore, you can ask whether there are special roles that you have played in the lives of others or that other individuals or organizations have played in your life (e.g., as heroes, identified groups, or causes).

Goals

Knowledge of any dreams and aspirations in your life will help shape your understanding of the meaning of illness. You can determine if there are goals that you want to achieve or if there is anything you wish to improve upon or resolve. If not, you may ask yourself, "Why not?"

The Past

How should you evaluate your past? Do you consider past events as triumphs or failures, as achievements or disappointments? You can inquire about their meaning and assess whether you have learned from these events or feel proud of them.

Philosophy of Life

All people have certain ethical codes by which they live. You can contemplate your virtues—for example, loyalty, honesty, love, or courage—and determine how they rank. Do you identify anything as being worth taking a stand for or even dying for?

Humor

Having or retaining the capacity for humor and laughter is essential when one is facing cancer or another serious illness. You can determine how much laughter and fun you have each day and the times when you have had the most laughter or fun.

WILL FAITH HELP ME FACE THIS ILLNESS?

Rabbi Harold Kushner emphasized that religious faith has often been used poorly in situations of tremendous loss or illness. What many people need most in these situations is consolation, not explanation. Pastors, rabbis, and other religious leaders often try to explain to those who are suffering that "This will make you stronger in the end," or "God has a purpose for everything." These statements often make a person with cancer feel worse! You, like others living with cancer, need comfort and hope, not empty reassurances. Rarely do people expect miracles; however, they do look to their faith for enough hope, courage, and strength to do whatever needs to be done. Statements such as "Don't take it so hard," or "It's all for the best," or worst yet, "It could be worse" should be avoided. Most people do not want to be told how to respond. Instead, a person with cancer appreciates those who visit as often as they can and who are prepared to listen.

HOW DOES SPIRITUALITY FACTOR INTO MY LIFE?

When affected by a chronic illness, such as cancer, six principal elements of spirituality operate (Table 23-2). They are *hope* (or a will to carry on), *trust* (in one's religious practices or in whatever one holds dear), *courage* (to face daunting obstacles and adversity), *faith* (in one's beliefs), *peace* (inner strength), and *love* (from God, a spiritual being, or for and from those with whom you have contact). Health care providers can help facilitate the integration of spiritual beliefs into your ability to cope. Providers can listen to your discussion of your own spiritual concerns, pray with you if you desire, read spiritual material to you if appropriate and if requested; and refer you to a member of the clergy.

TABLE 23-2 Six Principal Elements of Spirituality

Hope (or, a will to carry on)
Trust (in one's religious practices, or in whatever one holds dear)
Courage (to face daunting obstacles and adversity)
Faith (in one's beliefs)
Peace (inner strength)
Love (from God, a spiritual being, or for and from those with whom you have contact)

An essential aspect of spiritual care is being connected, whether to God, family, or church. These connections are vital; they create a stabilizing matrix of spiritual support and prevent you from feeling truly alone.

I AM ANGRY ABOUT HAVING CANCER. WHY SHOULD I CONTINUE HAVING FAITH?

While we often ask what role faith plays in the setting of cancer, the prevailing issue for many is that *faith is tested* during times of crisis. You may ask questions like "If there is a God, how can this be happening?" or "How can I continue to believe in God's goodness and fairness?"

You may make sense of your misfortune by seeing it as a punishment for past wrongs. This can leave you feeling angry with God but unable to voice or admit your anger and disappointment for fear that you will be punished further. In this unfortunate scenario, religion may simply help to make you feel worse.

Ever since the Bible and the story of Job, writers of nonmedical literature have grappled with the question of why people suffer. Anger at God is futile and counterproductive; it should be directed at a more appropriate target, thus preserving your faith and your relationship with God.

Whether you see misfortune as punishment or as an opportunity for self-improvement, these viewpoints share a basic idea: God is responsible for what is happening. Whether your God is punitive or kind, attempt to comfort yourself with a sense of an *order to all things* as you hold God responsible. However, what if God is not in control of all accidents, injuries, deaths, or illnesses? What if His purpose is to be there, ready to help you through whatever problem randomly occurs? Nonetheless, the frequently cited concept, "God helps those who help themselves" prompts positive action. When you have experienced suffering, you should avoid the self-destructive but all too human impulse to compound that suffering with additional damage. This may occur through drinking and smoking excessively, by not taking medicine, by not going to appointments, by having poor nutrition and exercise regimens, or by other passively suicidal or self-destructive behaviors.

WHAT ARE THE ADVANTAGES OF RELIGIOUS FAITH AND OBSERVANCE FOR ME AND MY FAMILY?

One of the unifying faith activities of all world religions is prayer. Regardless of creed or denomination, prayer plays a central role in observance. You can pray for wellness, a cure, or for just enough time to see to important business. You can pray for peace of mind and for the alleviation of pain and suffering.

The advantages of faith and prayer are numerous. Prayer returns a sense of control and of active participation. Prayer and religious observance may decrease stress and help you to feel more balanced. Prayer can provide needed assurance and comfort for you, as well as for your family and friends. Finally, prayer offers time and the opportunity for reflection on your life, on the lives of your loved ones, and on your achievements—moments and accomplishments for which you can be grateful.

HOW CAN I PRAY?

There is no right or wrong way to pray. You can pray for yourself; you can pray on behalf of others. You can pray by reciting a well-known religious verse, by speaking spontaneously, or by engaging in deep, quiet meditation.

Nevertheless, there are a few examples of what have been considered improper prayers, such as praying for something that cannot be changed or that would require someone else to suffer. For example, if you hear news of a shooting at your child's school and that a student has been reported dead, you might pray that it is not *your* child. Praying that someone else's child is dead, however, would seem to be an improper prayer. Also, attempting to "bribe" God appears inappropriate: "Just grant this prayer, God, and I'll do X, Y, or Z good thing." Many believe that God does not grant things—money, winning a ballgame, or good health. But He can offer courage, strength, hope, grace, peace—and the chance to remember that you are not alone.

CAN FAITH HELP ME GET BETTER OR HEAL FASTER?

Herbert Benson, the well-known proponent of the "relaxation response" (a technique, like meditation, used to induce or facilitate a state of calm), described the healing virtues of the "faith factor," which can be summarized as the combination of relaxation and the repetition of a religious or spiritually meaningful belief or concept. Benson and others have written widely about the effects of meditation, of spiritual mindfulness, and of guided imagery on physical symptoms (such as pain, which is a major concern for people with cancer).

Some researchers have looked beyond the benefits of spiritual mindfulness and meditation and have formally examined whether religious prayer can provide better health outcomes. Studies of prayer and health focus on *intercessory* prayer; one must distinguish this type of prayer from *petitionary* prayer. *Intercessory* prayer refers to prayer on behalf of others, while *petitionary* prayer refers to praying for oneself. This distinction has methodologic importance because it would be impossible to study effects of petitionary prayer scientifically. One would never be able to tell whether given results were due to a person's actual prayers or to other mental effects, such as the "placebo effect" (whereby a person feels better when he or she takes a pill or participates in an intervention, even if that pill or intervention is useless).

In one of the most famous and controversial experiments of intercessory prayer, Randolph Byrd (a cardiologist at University of California at San Francisco School of Medicine) randomized (placed people into groups in no particular order or with no preference) 393 patients in the coronary care unit. These people were placed into one of two groups: the first received intercessory prayer; the second, a control group, received no religious intervention. Intercessory prayers were offered by groups outside the hospital, and these people were not instructed on how to pray or how often to pray—only to pray as they saw fit. The study had a double-blind design (i.e., the groups had no idea for whom they were praying and patients, physicians, and nurses did not know who was receiving prayer).

In spite of some methodologic problems (such as the possibility of "extraneous prayer" from family and friends, the unknown effects of quantity versus quality of prayer, and the use of an unvalidated outcome measure), the study was able to demonstrate trends of improved outcome on major variables (such as survival, rate of requiring a breathing tube and ventilatory support, incidence of infection and heart failure, and need for cardiopulmonary resuscitation). In all these areas, prayed-for patients did better. Nevertheless, this study has been highly controversial and the accuracy of its results has been hotly debated. Many are still reluctant to accept that prayer can achieve such results.

The bottom line is that research tends to show that prayer works. In the end, the question of whether one finds this research credible is probably irrelevant. What seems to matter most to people with cancer is the meaning of the act of prayer (whether done by themselves or by others) and the feelings derived from it.

ARE THERE ANY DOWNSIDES TO RELIGIOUS FAITH FOR THOSE WITH CANCER?

The problems associated with faith during cancer treatment are similar to those seen in other settings. You should always be on the lookout for professed faith-based groups that are actually cults looking to extract time and money from you and your family. Also, caution is needed in situations in which your strong adherence to religious beliefs works against a literal understanding of your cancer diagnosis or treatment.

WHAT RELIGIOUS RESOURCES ARE AVAILABLE TO ME AND MY FAMILY?

Resources vary depending on the setting—e.g., hospital inpatient (acute and chronic), outpatient, home, or hospice environments. Hospital chaplains are crucial in maintaining basic feelings of serenity and well being. Chaplains can provide such services as prayer, counseling, last rites, and blessings; often they are most helpful by merely sitting quietly and listening. You and your family can attend church, synagogue, or mosque (as available) together. Many individuals have a strong desire for access to holy men and women (e.g., pastors, rabbis, and imams).

WHAT IS THE ROLE OF FAITH WHEN FACING DEATH?

No discussion of the role of faith in the life of a person with cancer would be complete without addressing spiritual concepts of death and dying. Sadly, many people with cancer battle their disease in its terminal stages or in the face of a grim prognosis. Thus, it is important to recognize the views on death and dying of many of the world's religions, as they may influence your experience.

Judaism

Attitudes are influenced by belief (or nonbelief) in an afterlife. There are several major categories of Jewish faith: Orthodox, Conservative, Reform, and Reconstructionist. For some, the focus is on the importance of resurrection upon the coming of the Messiah. For others, it is of primary importance to focus on the fundamental value of life as a gift from God; efforts to preserve a productive life and to remember that the good deeds of the individual live on in his or her loved ones are encouraged. For Orthodox Jews, friends and relatives may establish a *Bikkur Cholim*, whose purpose is to visit and provide comfort to the person who is ill. Events following the death of an Orthodox Jew may be supervised by a Jewish Burial Society. Mourning prayers (*kaddish*) are recited by a rabbi or by a family member; a specific period of mourning (*shiva* and *sh-loshim*) follows.

Christianity

The three major traditions of Christian faith—Eastern Orthodox, Roman Catholic, and Protestant—approach the rituals of attending to the sick and dying in different ways. However, common to all is a belief in the afterlife. As death approaches, many Christians and their families request visits from a priest or minister (either their own or a hospital chaplain); Eastern Orthodox, Catholic, and some Episcopalian Christians will request anointment or a "sacrament of the sick." The death itself is usually followed by a wake (a period during which family and friends may gather together to pray, talk, and view the body) and then burial. For secular humanists, specific religious traditions are less important. They emphasize instead the importance of life and life's accomplishments, which may be remembered at a formal nonreligious memorial service.

Islam

Death is viewed as a spiritual transition to eternal life with Allah (God). Friends and family are encouraged to view the death as the will of Allah and as a temporary loss, or in terms of resurrection after a final judgment—similar to the doctrines of Christianity. As death approaches with sickness, family members or an imam read from passages of the Qur'an and pray. After death, burial almost always takes place within 24 hours (as is the case in Jewish custom).

Eastern Traditions of Hinduism and Buddhism

The concepts or death and dying for the Hindu are greatly influenced by the concept of reincarnation. While most Hindus recognize a pantheon of many lesser gods, they generally believe in the existence of a singular Supreme Being. The time of imminent death is a time of reflection upon how one has lived in the world and how he or she may return in the next life in accordance with karma. Hindus usually prefer to die at home, where they can be more certain of the presence of a knowledgeable Hindu priest.

Unlike Hindus, Buddhists do not subscribe to a belief in any Supreme Being or God. However, they do believe in the concept of rebirth. Death is recognized as a part of the cycle of life, the goal of which is to follow the "eightfold path" of right *belief, intent, speech, conduct, endeavor, mindfulness, effort,* and *meditation.* A Buddhist monk may chant prayers for a fellow dying, devout Buddhist in order to encourage peace of mind at the time of death.

SUMMARY

Faith in spirituality or in God offers meaning. It gives us the opportunity to see misfortune not as "something for the best"—an empty denial of the tragedy—but as part of an overall context of life, a reminder not only of what we have lost but also of what has enriched us. Faith is a source of strength, hope, and, most importantly, inspiration and love.

CHAPTER 24

Fertility and Cancer

WOLFRAM GOESSLING, M.D., PH.D.

OUTLINE

Having cancer had made me appreciate life more than I even thought possible—not only do I appreciate the life I have but the ability I have to give life. Though I've always wanted to have children, I believe that my experience with cancer has deepened this desire. I feel that the cancer has prioritized my life, which in turn could give me the opportunity to be a wonderful mother by understanding that each moment of every day is important—more so than material items.

—A YOUNG SURVIVOR OF COLON CANCER

WHY IS FERTILITY SO IMPORTANT AND INFERTILITY SO DIFFERENT IN PEOPLE WITH CANCER?

As is apparent from the statement quoted above, people with cancer are often faced with issues of death and dying. In general, this leads to a profoundly different appreciation of life and the ability to give life. While most cancers, such as prostate and lung cancer, are diseases of older adults, many cancers affect children or young adults in their reproductive years, before they have had a chance to have a family or to complete their family plans.

Today, 180,000 to 220,000 survivors of childhood cancer are living in the United States. Each year, 17,000 men between the ages of 15 and 45 years are diagnosed with, and treated for, Hodgkin's disease, lymphoma, sarcomas, testicular cancer, and leukemia, while 35,000 women in the same age group are diagnosed with breast cancer, Hodgkin's disease, lymphoma, and leukemia. Many of the treatments for these cancers can cause decreased sperm production in men or premature menopause in women, thereby making it impossible for couples to conceive a child naturally (Table 24-1). The incredible emotional pain of infertility is then increased by the heightened appreciation of and hunger for life, as well as by the incentive to give life.

HOW CAN CANCER AFFECT MY FERTILITY?

While cancer treatment (certain types of chemotherapy, radiation therapy, and surgery) certainly can cause infertility, the cancer itself can disturb both sexual and reproductive function. The gonads (i.e., testes and ovaries) can be the origin of the cancer, as with testicular or ovarian cancer; or they can be involved with a cancer that originated in another organ, as in the case of gastric cancer that spreads to the ovaries. Other organs or structures of the reproductive tract (including the penis, the fallopian tubes, and uterus) may also have impaired function because of cancer involvement. Some cancers can interfere with the centers of reproductive hormonal control in the brain or the pituitary gland, resulting in a lack of stimulation of the gonads and in reduced levels of the hormones estrogen, progesterone, and testosterone, which are required for reproduction.

Finally, a person with cancer may be concerned about the possibility of genetic disease and the chance of passing the susceptibility for cancer on to children. For this

TABLE 24-1 Cancer Therapies That Can Affect a Person's Fertility

Therapy	Mechanism
Chemotherapy	Can cause prolonged absence of sperm in the semen (azoospermia) or a permanent lack of ovulation (ovarian failure).
Hormones	Block the effects of estrogen or testosterone.
Radiation therapy	Can damage gonadal cells in the testes or ovaries through direct radiation exposure.
Surgery	Infertility results from removal of testes or ovaries or through nerve damage from removal of, for example, lymph nodes.

reason, some couples may decide that they do not want to have children even in the absence of physical infertility. This issue is addressed in more detail in Chap. 8.

WHAT MAKES SPERM AND EGG CELLS SO VULNERABLE TO CANCER TREATMENT?

Both chemotherapy and radiation therapy are effective cancer treatments because they predominantly attack the rapidly dividing cancer cells. Ordinarily, they do not affect "resting" cells in the liver, heart, or lungs to as great an extent. However, some body cells—such as hair follicles, intestinal and bone marrow cells, as well as sperm and egg cells—divide and turn over rapidly and may therefore be more affected by chemotherapy than are "resting" cells.

In men, sperm develop from primitive cells in the testes called *spermatogonia*. These cells mature through different stages of development—as spermatogonia, spermatocytes, and spermatids—to finally become sperm. The differentiating spermatogonia are the most actively dividing cells and therefore the most vulnerable to the effects of chemotherapy, while in the later stages of sperm development—as spermatocytes, spermatids, and sperm—cells are fairly resistant to being killed by chemotherapy but may still suffer DNA damage, rendering them nonfunctional. Therefore, although the sperm count normally does not drop for about 2 months after chemotherapy, those sperm may carry mutations in their DNA and may thus be dysfunctional.

The "helper cells" in the testes—the Leydig cells, which produce testosterone, and the Sertoli cells, which produce support factors—are also quite resistant to cancer therapy, explaining the normal testosterone levels in men after chemotherapy. The recovery of the sperm count and fertility is ultimately dependent on the survival of the primitive spermatogonia.

The characteristics of gonadal cells in women are quite opposite to those in men. In women, germ cell proliferation takes place before birth and then stops until a woman reaches puberty, at a stage of maturation called the *oocyte stage*. Most of the oocytes never develop into fertile eggs. At birth, there are about 1 million oocytes; 300,000 remain at puberty, but only about 500 mature to the mature follicle state and progress to ovulation. During menstrual cycles, the stromal cells, the "tissues" of the ovary, interact with the oocytes, producing the estrogen necessary for oocyte maturation and ovulation. Cancer therapy may affect both the oocytes and the surrounding cells, resulting in a failure to ovulate and a lack of estrogen, with subsequent premature menopause. As the ovaries require a minimal number of follicles that can mature in order to function and as this number decreases through the reproductive years, women in their late thirties and forties are more likely to experience ovarian failure after cancer treatment than women in their late teens and twenties. Some women may be able to ovulate after receiving chemotherapy or radiation treatment, but their reproductive life span may be shortened by the loss of follicles in the ovaries, leading again to premature menopause.

HOW CAN TREATMENT FOR CANCER AFFECT MY FERTILITY?

Generally, there are three different cancer therapies that can affect a person's fertility: chemotherapy, radiation therapy, and surgery.

Chemotherapy

Chemotherapy can affect both the testis and the ovary, but not every chemotherapeutic agent has the same impact. In fact, many anticancer drugs do not affect fertility. Alkylating agents—such as cyclophosphamide, melphalan, busulfan, and chlorambucil, as well as cisplatin (see Chap. 14 for a more detailed explanation of these drugs)—are typically the drugs that cause prolonged absence of sperm in the semen (*azoospermia*) or a permanent lack of ovulation (ovarian failure). In general, the cumulative treatment dose (the total amount of drug given over weeks or months) is more important than the single dose given each cycle. Most often, combinations of several drugs, as given in the treatment of Hodgkin's or non-Hodgkin's lymphoma or in testicular cancer, cause more damage to the gonads than single chemotherapeutic drugs. Some of these regimens, such as MOPP [mechlorethamine, vincristine (Oncovin), procarbazine, and prednisone], which is used in the treatment of Hodgkin's disease, can cause a prolonged or permanently diminished sperm count in 50 to 100 percent of men and ovarian failure in up to 85 percent of women. Therefore infertility after chemotherapy in certain cancers is not just a theoretical concern and should be discussed with the treating physician in great detail prior to treatment.

Besides chemotherapy, hormones and biological agents also are used to treat cancer. The most widely used agent is tamoxifen, a drug that blocks the effect of estrogen and prevents the ripening of the follicles in the ovaries, inducing amenorrhea (a lack of menstruation) in women. These effects, as with antiandrogens in men, are generally reversible after discontinuation of the drug.

Radiation Therapy

Radiation also has effects on both the testis and the ovary, which react differently to radiation than do most other tissues in the body. Ordinarily, radiation is given in several small doses (fractions) over the course of several weeks, depending on the cancer, to reduce side effects and damage to the internal organs (see Chap. 16). However, in the gonads, this pattern of fractionation causes more damage than when the radiation is given as a single dose. In most instances, when cancers are being treated with radiation therapy, the gonads are shielded as much as possible.

In men, relatively small doses of radiation to the testes (as scattering from radiation being given to other body parts) can cause decreased sperm counts approximately 6 weeks after therapy has been initiated. Recovery of the sperm counts may take up to 18 months. When radiation is given directly to the testes at high doses, the Leydig cells can also be damaged, leading to a decreased testosterone level and loss of libido (sex drive).

In women, the ovaries are sometimes radiated directly—for example, as part of the lymph node radiation for Hodgkin's disease or as part of pelvic irradiation for cervical cancer. Occasionally, the ovaries can be moved out of the way surgically prior to the treatment so they will not be damaged as much by direct radiation and so that a greater reserve of follicles can be ensured. As with chemotherapy, younger women generally are more likely to be fertile after the completion of radiation treatment. In contrast, the high doses of radiation given during total-body radiation in preparation for a bone marrow transplant (see Chap. 20) permanently impair the ovarian function in all women, including younger women.

Surgery

Surgical treatment also may impair fertility. Naturally, removal of the ovaries, uterus, or testes renders a person infertile. In addition, nerve damage during the removal of the prostate gland or the removal of lymph nodes in the retroperitoneum (i.e., as treatment for testicular cancer), can interfere with a man's ability to have an erection and to ejaculate, rendering him infertile.

CAN I PROTECT MY TESTES OR OVARIES DURING CANCER TREATMENT?

For the most part, it is difficult to protect the gonads from the side effects of cancer treatment. With radiation therapy, shielding is used as much as possible; occasionally, in women, the ovaries can be moved out of the radiation beam field by surgery, reducing the dose to the ovaries in pelvic irradiation to approximately 10 percent of the original dose.

Based on the observation that chemotherapy in prepubertal boys causes some-what less infertility, several studies have been conducted trying to suppress testicular function and sperm production in men through the use of hormones. However, to date no hormonal regimen given during chemotherapy has been successful in lowering the likelihood of infertility after chemotherapy or radiation.

Similar hormone studies have been conducted in women, and some recent results suggest a protective effect of hormones acting on the pituitary (gonadotropin-releasing hormone agonists)—hormones that put the ovaries in a prepubertal state again. However, these hormones are not yet routinely used in young women receiving chemotherapy.

WHAT OPTIONS DO I HAVE TO PRESERVE MY GERM CELLS (SPERM AND OOCYTES) AFTER CANCER TREATMENT?

Sperm Banking

The idea of freezing sperm so that a man can father a child at some time in the future is more than 200 years old. It became a reality over 50 years ago with the discovery that the sugar compound glycerol, when added to sperm cells, protects them from the damage of rapid deep-freezing. Soon thereafter, the first babies conceived with the frozen sperm were born. Sperm banking is now routinely available in the United States and most countries in the world in order to preserve sperm prior to the initiation of chemotherapy or radiation treatment (Table 24-2). Generally, three sperm samples are obtained by masturbation at least 48 hours apart and then stored (frozen at very low temperatures) for decades without loss of quality. It costs approximately $1200 to $1500 for three sperm samples to be banked for 5 years.

There are different ways the frozen sperm can be used to fertilize an egg. The first is *intrauterine insemination*, in which sperm are inserted into the uterus after ovulation, which is often induced by hormones. This is the least costly method; at about $250 per cycle, and it is effective in 30 percent of cases. *In vitro fertilization*

TABLE 24-2 Options for Preserving Sperm and *Oocytes*

Method	Cost
Sperm banking	$1200–$1500 for three sperm samples to be banked for 5 years
Fertilization methods	
Intrauterine insemination	$250 per cycle
In vitro fertilization	$10,000 per cycle
Intracytoplasmic sperm injection	$11,000–$12,000 per cycle
Freezing oocytes or ovarian tissue	Not widely available/experimental
Freezing embryos	$800–$1000

(IVF) brings egg and semen (approximately 100,000 motile sperm) together in a test tube, and the fertilized egg is later implanted in the uterus. This costs approximately $10,000 per cycle. The most expensive technique ($11,000 to $12,000 per cycle) is *intracytoplasmic sperm injection* (ICSI), in which a single sperm is injected directly into an egg cell under the microscope and later implanted in the uterus.

Both IVF and ICSI have a success rate of approximately 33 percent per cycle; ultimately 80 to 100 percent of couples achieve pregnancy. These recent advances in reproductive technologies have changed the criteria of what is considered a good sperm sample suitable for storage. In the early 1980s, some 5 to 10 million motile sperms per milliliter were considered necessary for successful fertilization; in the early 1990s, this number had dropped to 2 million per milliliter. However, with the development of ICSI, theoretically only one live sperm is needed for fertilization.

Discussions of sperm banking may be difficult for you and your physician, as they force you and your doctor to think and talk about the possibility of infertility after treatment as well as the possibility of death. While this discussion may be uncomfortable, it is necessary: some studies have shown that people with cancer were surprised by finding that they were infertile after treatment, as they had never talked about these issues with their physicians or could not recall having talked about them. Because sperm banking is so easy and is universally accessible, it should be discussed with and offered to any man who has not had children or completed his family plans as well as to teenage boys. With certain cancers, such as lymphoma or leukemia, treatment must generally be started soon after diagnosis. Therefore this topic should be brought up as soon as the possibility of radiation or chemotherapy arises. It is important to recognize, however, that some people may be infertile because of their cancer at the time of diagnosis and thus may be unable to participate in sperm banking.

Sperm Banking in Adolescents

Sperm banking is also available for adolescent boys during puberty, even if they have not yet had spontaneous emission of sperm. However, discussing the issues of potential infertility and sperm banking may be even more difficult with adolescents than with adults. Parents who see their children as children only and not yet as future parents may be forced to discuss issues of sexuality and parenting with their teenaged sons. Adolescents with cancer need to understand the impact and risk of infertility even if they are not yet sexually active.

Freezing Oocytes

Female eggs are much larger than sperm; in fact, they are among the largest cells in the human body. Therefore it is much more difficult to successfully freeze, thaw, and then fertilize eggs, and only about one out of five eggs can be fertilized after thawing, with even fewer resulting in pregnancies. While some babies have been born after in vitro (outside the body) fertilization from frozen eggs, this technique is not widely available yet. In a person with cancer, it may not even be feasible, as it takes time to stimulate the ovaries to ovulate and harvest the eggs. This process may take too long if treatment must be initiated quickly. No successful pregnancy has been reported to date using frozen eggs from a person with cancer.

Freezing Ovarian Tissue

This technique is still at an experimental stage. Essentially, a part of an ovary is removed prior to the initiation of cancer treatment and kept frozen. After the completion of therapy, this tissue is transplanted back into the body, with the expectation that ovulation will occur and that the egg can subsequently be harvested for IVF. However, this therapy is not offered routinely. There is also the concern, especially with cancers that have entered the bloodstream, such as leukemia or lymphoma, that some cancer cells may be transferred back to the body by the transplanted tissue, putting a person at risk of cancer recurrence.

Freezing Embryos

Another option for women who want to have children after cancer treatment and have a partner at the time of a cancer diagnosis is *embryo cryopreservation* (which costs approximately $800 to $1000). This technique is more successful than the freezing of eggs, with approximately 75 to 85 percent of embryos remaining alive after freezing and thawing, and up to 20 to 30 percent of implanted embryos resulting in successful pregnancies. The embryos can be stored for several years, and there is no increased risk of birth defects. As with the preservation of eggs, it takes time to stimulate ovulation and harvest the oocyte—a process that may not be possible if cancer treatment must be initiated quickly.

CAN I BANK SPERM EVEN IF THE CANCER AFFECTED MY SPERM PRODUCTION BEFORE TREATMENT?

Cancer can affect sperm quality indirectly; the illness can cause fevers, weight loss, and malnourishment, all of which can contribute to inadequate sperm production. Many studies have shown that, at the time of a cancer diagnosis, some men have such low sperm counts that they would not be able to father a child naturally even prior to receiving treatment. Therefore, in the past, some physicians have not encouraged sperm banking by these people. However, as mentioned above, just one live, nondeformed sperm, even if it cannot move, is enough for ICSI and a subsequent successful pregnancy. The rates of successful pregnancies are lower if the sperm quality is poor.

HOW LONG SHOULD THE SPERM BE KEPT?

This may at first sound like a trivial issue, as sperm can be kept frozen at very low temperatures for many years without loss of quality. However, men who undergo sperm banking should discuss with their partners and their physicians whether the sperm should be kept in the case of the donor's death. Emotionally, this is a difficult issue to consider, as it requires a conversation about the possibility of death even in the case of highly curable diseases, such as Hodgkin's disease. This is an important conversation to have, however, as it will provide guidance to loved ones left behind about whether they should discard or keep the sperm. These concerns also apply to frozen eggs and embryos. In the latter case, the ethical concerns and legal aspects are even more difficult to resolve.

SHOULD I CONSIDER ADOPTING A CHILD?

Adoption is another way for an infertile couple to have a family, and this is no different for families in which one person has cancer. The one caveat to this statement is that public agencies may be hesitant to consider cancer survivors as parents because of the fear of a shortened life span due to cancer recurrence. Thus, in order to be considered as parents for adoption, people with a history of cancer may need to be free of cancer for several years and to have their physician attest to an extremely good prognosis for prolonged survival.

HOW CAN THE CANCER TREATMENT AFFECT MY UNBORN CHILD?

As mentioned above, cancer therapy is meant to attack rapidly dividing tumor cells. During pregnancy, the cells of the developing embryo are dividing just as fast; therefore all cancer therapy can affect the embryo at all stages of pregnancy. Currently, knowledge regarding the effect of chemotherapy in pregnancy is incomplete. Theoretically, during the first 2 weeks of pregnancy, chemotherapy should not affect the fertilized egg, as the egg has not established its placental blood supply with the mother. Radiation treatment during this time, however, generally results in the loss of the fetus. Both radiation therapy and chemotherapy should be avoided during this period.

The most crucial period for organ development is the second half of the first trimester, during weeks 5 through 10. In general, if the mother is receiving chemotherapy or radiation during this time, 10 to 20 percent of fetuses will have major congenital malformations, a rate 2.5 to 5 times higher than in the general population. The second and third trimesters of pregnancy tend to be safer, as by then the major steps of organ development have been completed. If you are pregnant and have just been given a cancer diagnosis, you should ask your physician whether it is feasible to delay cancer treatment until this stage. If possible, chemotherapy should be avoided a few weeks prior to the expected due date, as there is an increased risk of infection and bleeding for the mother if her blood counts are low at delivery. After delivery, breast-feeding should be avoided, as many chemotherapeutic agents enter the breast milk.

HOW DANGEROUS IS IT TO ATTEMPT A PREGNANCY OR TO BECOME PREGNANT WHILE RECEIVING CANCER TREATMENT?

In general, no one should attempt to become pregnant while being treated for cancer. Sexual intercourse in itself may be dangerous in cancer patients who have low blood counts from chemotherapy, as it exposes a person to risks of infection and bleeding. If a woman is undergoing cancer treatment, the cautions about the risks of chemotherapy during pregnancy mentioned in the above section apply. If a man is being treated, his sperm may carry DNA mutations, placing a developing fetus at a higher risk for congenital malformations or for a blighted pregnancy. You should discuss these issues with your doctors and use contraception up to six months after the completion of cancer treatment. The treating physician should be consulted by women who have a hormone-sensitive cancer, such as breast cancer, as a pregnancy in such a woman may increase the risk of cancer recurrence.

HOW WILL THE CHEMOTHERAPY OR RADIATION THERAPY AFFECT MY CHILDREN IN THE FUTURE?

Many people who are planning to have children after cancer treatment and who regain or keep their fertility fear possible congenital diseases caused by the treatment. As noted above, chemotherapy and radiation treatments damage the DNA in both sperm and egg cells. One way to assess damage prior to conception is to look at the genetic material in sperm. Several laboratory techniques have been developed to detect genetic abnormalities. There is no precise information regarding the risk of congenital abnormalities following treatment, but the estimates based on calculations from experiments in animals suggest that the risk would be increased by less than 2 percent even with the highest possible doses of chemotherapy.

The best information, which is generally reassuring, stems from several reports looking back at the previous experience with chemotherapy as well as at the children of people who survived the atomic bombs in Japan. These studies suggest that the risk of birth defects or genetic diseases in children of cancer survivors is not increased compared to the 4 percent baseline risk in any pregnancy in the rest of the population. However, these risks may differ from treatment to treatment; a geneticist should be consulted if there are any concerns about future childbearing. During a pregnancy, the embryo can be monitored with frequent ultrasounds as well as with amniocentesis to screen for genetic malformations.

SUMMARY

Infertility caused by cancer treatment can occur fairly frequently and should be discussed with the treating physician early; that is, prior to starting therapy. There are no established methods to prevent infertility during cancer treatment, but several options are available that can make it possible to have a child after treatment. Sperm banking is the best-established technique available for men. It is fairly inexpensive and can be used later with intrauterine insemination, IVF, or ICSI. In women, the options are more limited and experimental; they range from the preservation of eggs and ovarian tissue to the freezing of embryos. Pregnancy should be avoided during active cancer treatment, as it poses a risk of congenital malformations. People with cancer and their physicians should discuss all issues regarding infertility prior to treatment.

CHAPTER 25

Depression and Anxiety Associated with Cancer

LISA F. PRICE, M.D.

OUTLINE

WHAT ARE NORMAL FEELINGS IN RESPONSE TO A CANCER DIAGNOSIS?

The diagnosis of cancer is a life-changing event, with emotional distress as a normal and predictable response. In modern times, Erich Lindemann first described the constellation of symptoms associated with acute (sudden-onset) grief after the 1944 fire in the Coconut Grove nightclub in Boston, Massachusetts. Survivors of the fire were found to have somatic (or bodily) complaints, guilt, anger, intrusive thoughts, and a diminished ability to function normally. Similar symptoms develop following a cancer diagnosis, in addition to general feelings of anxiety and depression. Crucial points at which symptoms arise include the times of initial diagnosis, the initiation of treatment, the recurrence of cancer, the period after a failed treatment, and upon the termination of treatment.

Initially, you may feel stunned and doubt the information given to you; next, you may enter a period of mixed feelings that include depression, anxiety, irritability, and impaired sleep. These feelings and symptoms can last up to several weeks. The degree of distress at these junctures varies from person to person; it depends on a number of factors, including your medical condition (e.g., the site and stage of the disease at the time of diagnosis, available treatments, cancer progression, and symptoms), psychological issues (e.g., coping skills, maturity, severity of disruption of life), and social factors (e.g., financial and emotional supports).

WHAT WILL HELP ME COPE WITH MY ILLNESS?

Undoubtedly, before your diagnosis of cancer, you faced difficult experiences. How you dealt with those experiences reflected the coping strategies you developed over your lifetime (Table 25-1). Unfortunately, some strategies that may have been helpful with certain experiences in your life may be less helpful now as you face cancer. On the other hand, skills that you do have may aid you in your adjustment.

Good copers are confident of their ability to find solutions. Rather than focusing on a distant future or an unrealistic wish, good copers focus on present challenges. In addressing such challenges, these people identify a number of options for themselves, so that they always have an acceptable course of action. They educate themselves about the range of potential results. They are willing to consider new ideas and thus are flexible in their stance. At the same time, good copers maintain their position as the ultimate decision maker in their care. Finally, good copers are in general emotionally even; they avoid extremes of emotion that could bias their opinion.

Bad copers have greater difficulty living with cancer because of their approach to illness. They tend to have unrealistically high or rigid expectations for themselves and for others. They are stubborn and unwilling to consider a variety of stances. Correspondingly, they may not ask for assistance in times of need. They

TABLE 25-1 **Coping Strategies**

"Good" copers . . .
Are confident in their ability to find solutions
Focus on present challenges
Identify a number of options for themselves, so they always have an acceptable course of action
Educate themselves about the range of potential results
Are willing to consider new ideas and thus are flexible in their stance
Maintain their position as the ultimate decision maker in their care
Avoid extremes of emotion that could bias their opinion

"Bad" copers . . .
Have greater difficulty living with cancer because of their approach to illness
Tend to have unrealistically high or rigid expectations for themselves and for others
Are stubborn and unwilling to consider a variety of stances
May not ask for assistance in times of need
Are less likely to come to a decision after careful consideration and, instead, may make sudden decisions
Are prone to denial and to rationalization
Are unable to advocate for themselves

---

are less likely to come to a decision after careful consideration and, instead, may make sudden decisions. Bad copers are prone to denial and to rationalization. They are unable to advocate for themselves. People with poor coping skills are not inherently flawed. They simply have not learned more helpful skills.

Coping skills can be improved. By reflecting on your own approach to coping, you can determine which attitudes are helpful to you and which are not. Being familiar with good coping strategies allows you to adapt those skills that will be more useful to you. Coping skills evolve over a person's lifetime, particularly with repeated self-reflection. Coping skills are relevant in this discussion of depression and anxiety because good coping skills mitigate the difficult feelings each person with cancer experiences. However, even people with good coping skills may experience distress.

HOW WILL I KNOW IF MY FEELINGS OF DEPRESSION AND ANXIETY REQUIRE TREATMENT?

When depression or anxiety interferes with your life and persists beyond a few weeks, it should be treated (Tables 25-2 and 25-3). A *major depressive episode* merits treatment when at least five of the following symptoms (including depressed mood) have been present for 2 or more weeks:

A depressed mood (most of the day, nearly every day, either as described by the person experiencing a depressed mood or as observed by others)

A significantly decreased interest or pleasure in activities

A change in appetite or weight

Insomnia or hypersomnia (too much sleep)

Slowed movements or excessive activity observable by others

Fatigue or a loss of energy

Feelings of worthlessness or guilt

Impaired concentration or indecision

Recurrent thoughts of death (not just the fear of dying) or suicidal thoughts

Anxiety that has developed into a *generalized anxiety disorder* (a condition that should be treated) is defined by excessive anxiety and worry for at least 6 months, an inability to control the worry, impairment of daily functioning due to anxiety or depression, and at least three of the following six physical symptoms:

TABLE 25-2 **Symptoms of an Episode of Major Depression**

A depressed mood (most of the day, nearly every day, either as described by the person experiencing a depressed mood or as observed by others)
A significantly decreased interest or pleasure in activities
A change in appetite or weight
Insomnia or hypersomnia (too much sleep)
Slowed movements or excessive activity observable by others
Fatigue or a loss of energy
Feelings of worthlessness or guilt
Impaired concentration or indecision
Recurrent thoughts of death (not just the fear of dying) or suicidal thoughts

A person must have at least five symptoms (including depressed mood) for at least 2 weeks.

TABLE 25-3 **Generalized Anxiety Disorder**

Excessive anxiety and worry for at least 6 months
An inability to control the worry
Impairment of daily functioning due to anxiety
At least three of the following six physical symptoms:
    Restlessness
    Easy fatigue
    Difficulty concentrating
    Irritability
    Muscle tension
    Sleep disturbance

Restlessness

·Easy fatigue

Difficulty concentrating

Irritability

Muscle tension

Sleep disturbance

Anxiety may also manifest itself as panic attacks.

Commonly, people with cancer develop serious mood disturbances, with a mixture of depression and anxiety. If you are concerned that you have developed symptoms that require treatment, you should discuss your concerns with your physician.

Diagnosing depression and anxiety in people with cancer can be challenging for a number of reasons. The physical symptoms of depression and anxiety overlap with the physical symptoms of cancer and cancer treatment. For example, fatigue, sleep difficulty, and altered appetite may be caused by cancer itself, by the side effects of chemotherapy, or be a preexisting mood disorder (e.g., anxiety or depression). Consequently, the identification of a mood disorder in a person with cancer relies more heavily on recognizing psychological symptoms.

Diagnosis also is challenging because both the person with cancer and the physician can mistakenly believe that these debilitating mood states are normal. In such cases, a person may not discuss his or her feelings with the doctor, or the doctor may not know how to treat such symptoms. Again, if a question of a treatable mood disorder arises, consultation with a mental health professional may be beneficial.

WHICH FACTORS WILL PREDISPOSE ME TO ANXIETY OR DEPRESSION?

It helps to know about factors that are associated with increased rates of depression and anxiety (Table 25-4). These factors include a history of psychiatric illness, a poor early adjustment to cancer, limited social supports, and poor performance status (i.e., the ability to function free of cancer or treatment effects). Mood disorders may be more prevalent with advanced states of disease, though research in this area has not been conclusive.

TABLE 25-4 **Factors Associated with Increased Rates of Depression and Anxiety**

A history of psychiatric illness
A poor early adjustment to cancer
Limited social supports
Poor performance status (i.e., the ability to function free of cancer or treatment effects)

Undertreatment of pain is the leading cause of anxiety in people with cancer; thus, pain must be addressed thoroughly before diagnosing a psychiatric illness. Mood disorders also may be caused by underlying medical conditions (such as respiratory impairment, cardiovascular compromise, endocrine abnormalities, neurologic conditions, metabolic imbalance, infection, medication side effects, and withdrawal from substances). Underlying medical conditions also must be treated prior to concluding that a primary psychiatric disorder is present.

Mood disorders are common among people with cancer. Approximately 25 percent of people with cancer develop a major depressive episode during the course of their illness. These rates are even higher in individuals with involvement of the central nervous system (the brain). Older adults are at greater risk of depression and suicide. Given the potential for a treatable depressive episode or an anxiety disorder, familiarity with the symptoms and risk factors of these disorders is worthwhile.

WHY IS IT IMPORTANT TO TREAT DEPRESSION AND ANXIETY?

As the cornerstone of medical care is to provide relief from suffering, it is imperative that you receive some type of therapy once a mood disorder has been identified.

There are numerous treatments (both pharmacologic and psychotherapeutic) for depression and anxiety. The simple addition of a sedative at night to relieve insomnia or the use of an antidepressant to decrease depression or anxiety can improve a person's quality of life significantly. Addressing symptoms of disordered mood is critical to the success of cancer treatment in general. Pain tolerance decreases in the presence of a mood disorder. People with untreated symptoms are less able to attend to instructions and to daily self-care and are more likely to become hopeless or impatient with themselves and with those around them. They are at risk for decreased compliance with their cancer regimen and may even discontinue treatment. On the other hand, prompt treatment of mood disorders may prevent further progression of symptoms related to those disorders. Improvement of these symptoms enables the person to engage in his or her treatment and, more importantly, in his or her life.

ARE THOUGHTS OF DEATH AND SUICIDE NORMAL?

The fear of a painful death is paramount for people with cancer. Fears of disability, of bodily disfigurement, and of the loss of loved ones also are common. One group of clinicians has noted that once they establish a comfortable relationship with their patients, patients with cancer almost always disclose occasional thoughts of suicide as a way to avoid the inundating fears associated with cancer. This finding contrasts with several studies that report a low incidence of suicidal ideation in people with cancer. In those studies, suicidal ideation tends to be restricted to individuals with extensive cancer, to those who are hospitalized or receiving palliative care, or to those who are insufficiently treated for pain or depression. In either case, people with cancer may find themselves having thoughts of death or even of suicide. As with depression and anxiety disorders, when a person has persistent symptoms or intrusive thoughts, he or she will benefit from an open dialogue about these feelings.

SHOULD I BE CONCERNED ABOUT SUICIDE?

Although people with cancer are at higher risk for suicide (the risk of suicide is twice as high among them as it is among those without cancer), few people with cancer commit suicide. Variables associated with an increased risk of suicide in people with cancer include advanced illness, poor prognosis, depression, hopelessness, delirium, loss of control, helplessness, exhaustion, fatigue, uncontrolled pain, preexisting psychopathology, and a personal or family history of suicidal ideation or attempts (Table 25-5). As a number of these risk factors (depression, delirium, helplessness, exhaustion, and pain) can be treated, psychiatric evaluation of the individual with suicidal thoughts is crucial.

A common myth among the public as well as among some health professionals is that raising the issue of suicide will introduce the idea to the person. In fact, discussing these feelings generally provides relief; isolation, on the other hand, contributes to suicidal thoughts. An open discussion of such thoughts with your physician provides the opportunity to explore the burdens that contribute to those thoughts, to identify any undiagnosed mood disorder, to discuss end-of-life concerns, and ultimately to regain a sense of control.

TABLE 25-5 **Variables Associated with an Increased Risk of Suicide in People with Cancer**

Advanced illness
Poor prognosis
Depression
Hopelessness
Delirium (confusion)
Loss of control
Helplessness
Exhaustion
Fatigue
Uncontrolled pain
Preexisting psychopathology
Personal or family history of suicidal ideation or attempts

HOW CAN I RECEIVE TREATMENT FOR DEPRESSION AND ANXIETY?

Your physician and your medical team are the best resources for exploring additional care options. Your physician may feel comfortable treating your symptoms. However, your treaters may seek consultation with mental health professionals. Use of medication and counseling for people with cancer are discussed in detail in Chaps. 17 and 19.

CHAPTER 26

Multidisciplinary Care

FRED H. MILLHAM, M.D., M.B.A.
LAURA M. PRAGER, M.D.

OUTLINE

WHAT IS MULTIDISCIPLINARY CARE?

Living with cancer is a long journey over difficult and variable terrain; it requires many different guides and companions. Members of a multidisciplinary team function as guides and provide care for people with cancer. The term *multidisciplinary* implies that specialists with many different areas of expertise come together to participate in the complicated aspects of cancer care (Fig. 26-1).

Breast cancer is an excellent example of a condition that benefits from multidisciplinary care. Modern management of breast cancer frequently involves combinations of surgery, chemotherapy, and radiation therapy. Both the disease and its treatment can have physical and emotional consequences that require special attention. A multidisciplinary breast cancer team might include surgical oncologists, medical oncologists, and radiation therapists as well as plastic surgeons, rehabilitation specialists, nutritionists, psychiatrists, and social workers.

Because many forms of cancer and treatments for cancer have well-known side effects and predispose to potential complications, a multidisciplinary team is designed and organized to anticipate, prevent, and recognize these complications and side effects and to intervene in a timely fashion when appropriate. The cancer care journey takes a number of turns and has many peaks and valleys. The multidisciplinary team is designed to provide care specific for each segment of the journey and to help people with cancer anticipate and cope with particularly difficult stages of the trip.

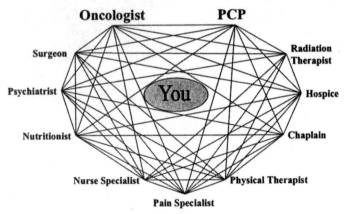

FIGURE 26-1 *The concept of multidisciplinary care: communication-planning and cooperation among the members of the health care team.*

Multidisciplinary teams have the advantage of bringing together experts from many fields to manage difficult problems. The whole in this case is far greater than the sum of its parts. For complicated treatment plans, having all of the specialists organized ahead of time into a team improves communication among team members and between you and your team. The composition of the multidisciplinary team allows you to have access to the latest therapies and the most recent clinical trials. In many cases, you can even meet with more than one specialist during a given visit to the clinic, particularly in designated cancer centers.

After everyone (often including a medical oncologist, surgical oncologist, radiation therapist, and social worker or care coordinator) has gotten the chance to meet and examine you, they gather in a room to review your laboratory data (often with the assistance of a pathologist) and formulate treatment recommendations that will be presented to you before you leave (Fig. 26-2). This also raises the one disadvantage of a multidisciplinary care team: with so many people involved in your care at the same time, visits to your health care center may last a while!

As with any team, multidisciplinary treatment teams have a captain or leader. This person is usually a medical oncologist; the leader may, however, be a surgeon, an internist, or a specialist from another field. The team leader is responsible for the coordination of the different facets of the care plan and for involving other members as needed. Some but not all members of multidisciplinary cancer teams are listed in Table 26-1.

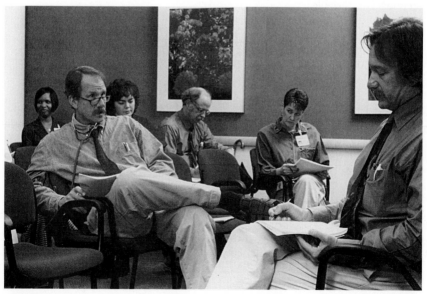

FIGURE 26-2 After all the members of your multidisciplinary team have met and examined you, they gather in a room to review your data and formulate treatment recommendations.

TABLE 26-1 The Multidisciplinary Cancer Team

Primary care physician	Chaplain
Medical oncologist	Physical therapist
Surgeon	Pain specialist
Radiation therapist	Case manager
Medical specialist	Social worker
Psychiatrist	Nurse clinician

IS MULTIDISCIPLINARY CARE RIGHT FOR ME?

Whether multidisciplinary care is best for you depends on the nature of your disease, the environment in which you are treated, and your personal preference. Your primary care doctor or oncologist can help you make these decisions. It is important to stress, however, that the most important member of the team is *you*! You must feel comfortable with other team members and confident that you are receiving the best care possible. You must be able to understand and to agree with the treatment regimen your doctors recommend. You may want to research your condition on the Internet or in the library to see what options exist. However, discussing your disease, its treatment, and your options with a doctor you trust is the best way for you to decide in which direction to proceed. Do not be afraid to ask questions, to look into alternatives, and to seek out treatment settings where *you* are most comfortable.

WHO IS ON A MULTIDISCIPLINARY CANCER TEAM?

Primary Care Physician

Your "regular" or primary care physician (PCP) who has known you for many years will remain involved in your care throughout your treatment. The team leader will ensure that your PCP is kept informed of your progress. Your PCP will be called upon to help with the management of any other medical problems that you may have now or that may develop during your treatment.

Medical Oncologist

The medical oncologist is an internist who specializes in treating your cancer with medications, specifically chemotherapy. The medical oncologist will plan any chemotherapy, adjust medication dosages, and help you to deal with side effects (such as nausea and diarrhea) from your cancer or from the therapy for your cancer. The medical oncologist is frequently the team leader—the person who coordinates the entire treatment plan; he or she is usually involved in your care throughout the entire course of treatment.

Surgeon

The first step in many cancer treatment plans is to confirm the diagnosis by obtaining a tissue sample and to remove all or as much of the cancerous tissue (the "mass" or "tumor") as possible. A surgeon who has special training in cancer management usually performs these procedures. Your surgeon will also manage your postoperative care.

Radiation Therapist

Many cancer treatment plans include the use of radiation therapy. Radiation treatments require careful planning and monitoring. The radiation therapist has special training in radiation physics and in the effects of radiation on bodily tissues. He or she determines the method of administration and dose of radiation that will be used to treat your cancer. This specialist also is skilled at recognizing and managing any side effects of radiation treatment.

Medical Specialist

Sometimes, cancer treatment can lead to other problems (such as infections, cardiac issues, or gastrointestinal problems) that require the help of a medical specialist. For example, intensive chemotherapy treatments can suppress the body's normal immune responses. Consequently, unusual and serious infections can occur. In this setting, an infectious disease specialist may join the treatment team to help choose the medications used to fight infection.

Psychiatrist

Both cancer and the treatment for cancer, including chemotherapy and radiation therapy, can precipitate mood and anxiety disorders, even in individuals who have never suffered from psychiatric symptoms before. Multidisciplinary teams often include psychiatrists who can facilitate the diagnosis of, and initiate treatment for, such problems. The psychiatrist may prescribe medications to relieve symptoms and can arrange for supportive psychotherapy if needed.

Chaplain

Many patients choose to discuss their cancer diagnosis with a member of the clergy of their faith, even if they are not involved in any religious organization. Most multidisciplinary teams offer access to hospital chaplains, who can visit people in their hospital rooms.

Physical Therapist

Cancer and cancer treatment can be debilitating. Physical therapy is an important component of multidisciplinary cancer care; physical therapists can help people with cancer to regain their strength so that they can resume their normal activity level as quickly as possible. Resuming normal activities also can help reduce the likelihood of infections, bed sores, and even of loss of bone density.

Pain Specialist

The treatment of pain is complicated and challenging. Most multidisciplinary cancer teams include doctors who have specialized knowledge of the different medications and even procedures that can minimize both pain and excessive sedation. Pain specialists also may be able to refer patients for other types of pain management (such as acupuncture, meditation, and biofeedback). (See Chap. 22 for a more complete discussion of this topic.)

Case Manager

A case manager makes sure that insurance issues are dealt with promptly; he or she effectively coordinates home services if needed. While you are in the hospital, the case manager may serve as a communication link between you and members of your care team. The case manager is also the link between insurance companies, home health care organizations, and the multidisciplinary team. This is important, as many of the treatments you receive in the hospital will be continued at home. The case manager ensures that you will continue to receive the interventions your caregivers have prescribed as well as other services, such as the help of a home health care aid, after you have been discharged home. The case manager may also serve as your advocate with insurers in the event that issues regarding your coverage arise.

Social Worker

The social worker is an integral member of the multidisciplinary team. His or her responsibilities range from coordinating the same services as a case manager to acting as a therapist. For example, the social worker can arrange for transportation for you or for your family to and from the hospital. He or she can also help family members find a place to stay near the hospital if home is far away and they would like to remain close to you while you are an inpatient. Social workers can help your family members gain access to resources in your area for continuing supportive care or even respite care. Sometimes, social workers provide individual supportive counseling for you or for a family member during your inpatient stay and possibly even after you leave the hospital.

HOW CAN I ARRANGE FOR MULTIDISCIPLINARY CARE?

Your primary care physician may be able to direct you to a multidisciplinary team, which he or she would be a part of, within your present health care system. Or your doctor may be able to refer you to a center where such care is available. You can also learn which institutions offer these types of services from a library or by using the Internet (see Chap. 12). Don't be afraid to be proactive. The idea behind multidisciplinary care is to offer services for all aspects of your condition. You have the right to expect the best and most complete cancer care. You should not be afraid to demand this level of service from your health care system, no matter who you are or where you live.

CHAPTER 27

Stress Reactions in Caregivers

OLIVIA OKEREKE, M.D.

OUTLINE

IS WHAT I AM EXPERIENCING A STRESS REACTION?

Primary caretakers of people with cancer take on new and difficult tasks. Consequently, they are subject to a variety of stresses, both physical and emotional (Table 27-1). Physical responses can include muscle aches, fatigue, and disturbed sleep. Emotional reactions may involve feelings of anxiety, fear, depression, guilt, anger, irritability, detachment, and of being overwhelmed or of having a sense of resignation, hopelessness, or helplessness. In some caregivers, these reactions become intense, prolonged, and complicated; thus, they can be regarded as manifestations of a psychiatric condition.

One well-recognized lay term for prolonged caregiver stress is *burnout.* Burnout can be recognized by its physical, affective, behavioral, and cognitive features (Table 27-2). Physical signs include fatigue, chronic aches (especially headaches), stomach upset, and flareups of preexisting medical problems. Uncharacteristic or unwanted behaviors—such as smoking cigarettes, drinking, using drugs, taking undue risks, or having temper outbursts—may also reflect the effects of prolonged caregiver stress. Changes in a caregiver's usual emotional tone and attitude may also be noticeable. Individuals who are normally friendly, positive, and polite may become distant, paranoid, nervous, angry, tense, cynical, bitter, resentful, or filled with despair. Finally, interpersonal relationships of caregivers may suffer; they may become characterized either by increased distance or overattachment as well as by anger toward, and conflict with, the person being cared for, family members, a spouse, coworkers, or friends.

TABLE 27-1 **Stresses in Caregivers of People with Cancer**

Physical responses
   Muscle aches
   Fatigue
   Disturbed sleep
Emotional reactions
   Anxiety
   Fear
   Depression
   Guilt
   Anger
   Irritability
   Detachment
   Feelings of being overwhelmed
   Resignation
   Hopelessness
   Helplessness

TABLE 27-2 **Signs and Symptoms of Burnout**

Physical signs
  Fatigue
  Chronic aches (especially headaches)
  Stomach upset
  Flareups of preexisting medical problems
Uncharacteristic or unwanted behaviors
  Smoking cigarettes
  Drinking
  Using drugs
  Taking undue risks
  Temper outbursts
Changes in emotional tone
  Distance
  Paranoia
  Nervousness
  Anger
  Tenseness
  Cynicism
  Bitterness
  Resentment
  Despair
Damaged interpersonal relationships
  Increased distance
  Overattachment
  Anger
  Conflict

WHAT EXACTLY CAUSES A STRESS REACTION IN A CAREGIVER?

Under conditions of acute stress, people experience increases in tension, heart rate, and respiratory rate. These changes typically result from elevated levels of certain chemicals in the bloodstream, called catecholamines (such as epinephrine, or adrenaline, and norepinephrine) and cortisol, a glucocorticoid hormone. These chemical responses are normal in situations of acute stress, as when a person encounters an angry tiger in the jungle and must either fight or flee. However, when stress is continuously experienced, these responses begin to produce serious adverse effects.

Stress, according to Hans Selye (the author of numerous publications on the origins and effects of stress), is the result, mental or physical, of a demand on the body. He divided stress into two types: *eustress*, or a sense of pleasant fulfillment (as you might experience after exercise), and *distress*, which may be associated with *burnout*.

WILL I BE AT RISK FOR A CAREGIVER STRESS REACTION?

Whether you are a friend, significant other, spouse, child, sibling, parent, extended family member, or professional health care provider, you are subject to stress and distress. Loved ones tend to feel the stresses of caregiving most acutely, as their bond is strongest.

HOW DO RELATIONSHIPS BETWEEN PEOPLE WITH CANCER AND CAREGIVERS CHANGE?

The major challenge faced by partner-caregivers revolves around role change. The benefits of this role change include an enhanced sense of love, caring, intimacy, and purpose. The downside includes an increase in physical and emotional stress, a decrease in time for oneself, and a less equal relationship than previously experienced. When such situations arise, it is helpful for people with cancer and their partners to *acknowledge openly and directly* the changes that are occurring, to maintain flexibility and sharing in activities (for example, a partner may need to take the responsibility for driving, but the person with cancer learns how to cook), and to allow the person with cancer to continue to do as much as he or she is capable of doing. If role changes are not discussed, the person with cancer may harbor anger and resentment or feel undermined and infantilized.

WHAT ARE COMMON SOURCES OF CAREGIVER WORRY (TABLE 27-3)?

Doing Too Much or Going It Alone

Too often, caregivers of those with cancer take on the burden of caring for the other person entirely on their own. This can compound their stress reaction; distribution of the load among caregivers is likely to alleviate distress. Thus, care-

TABLE 27-3 Common Sources of Caregiver Worry

Doing too much or going it alone
Worries about not having done enough
Uncertainty
New responsibilities and shifting priorities
Fears of one's own mortality and health vulnerability
Lack of support
Dealing with the medical system and understanding medical terms and medications
Communication
End-of-life concerns

givers are well served by a team approach to caring for the person with cancer. A large team, comprised of oncologists, primary care doctors, specialists, nurses, and social workers as well as nonprofessional staff, provides better care and ultimately serves the best interests of the person with cancer.

Worries about Not Having Done Enough

It is common for caregivers to worry about factors (such as disease progression) that they can no longer control. Caregivers may ask themselves: "What could I have done differently?" Whenever the threat of death arises, a change in focus, for all concerned, frequently results. Caregivers may struggle with their new roles as caretakers for those with whom there had been great conflict (e.g., related to infidelity, domestic violence, or abuse). Some rush in to undo the past and to "fix" everything because time appears limited. Such actions can generate further stress.

Uncertainty

Few fears of caregivers are worse than the feeling of uncertainty. Caregivers work arduously, tending to the daily needs of the person with cancer without having a clear sense of whether their loved one will "make it." It is stressful to have to wonder how much time may be left for a person with a serious diagnosis. Caregivers hope that they are not contributing to the distress of their loved one. They must balance the hardship of watching a friend or relative suffer with a desire to avoid abandonment. This conflict creates feelings of guilt.

New Responsibilities and Shifting Priorities

Cancer often brings about changes in the roles of people with cancer, their family members, or their friends. An individual who once was relied on to provide strength and support for others may find him or herself too weakened by the complications of cancer or its treatment to continue in that role. Furthermore, he or she may no longer be able to attend to self-care without help. Caregivers may be forced to balance preexisting obligations, such as child care or work, with new responsibilities to the person with cancer. As priorities change, anxiety, fatigue, or resentment may develop.

Financial expenditures for caregivers (including expenses related to leaving work, traveling, and providing care) can be large. Fortunately, some supports, such as the Family and Medical Leave Act (FMLA), are built into the system. Few employers, however, allow indefinite leave to provide care for a loved one; hiring outside care presents an additional expense. At some point as a caregiver, you may have to consider leaving your job to devote your full attention to the person with cancer.

Fears of One's Own Mortality and Vulnerability

After someone close (particularly, a relative) is diagnosed with cancer, many people contemplate their own risk of cancer; they may even fear having the illness. Epidemiologic data show that certain cancers have a strong genetic component, so this fear is understandable. It is also common for you, as a caregiver, to ponder your own mortality. Furthermore, caregivers and people with cancer may share lifestyles that increase the caregiver's own risk for cancer (e.g., smoking). Some caregivers look for signs and symptoms in themselves that they noticed in their loved ones with cancer. After having seen a physician for an evaluation and being told that there is no evidence of cancer, ongoing feelings of being overwhelmed or persistent overwhelming worries about cancer in oneself may be an indication for further support and counseling.

Lack of Support

Most people rely on the support of friends and family to help them through hard times; employers and coworkers may even pitch in. Nevertheless, caregivers sometimes feel as though they were shouldering the heavy responsibilities of care alone. While in many cases this perception may not be the reality, it is no less distressing. Furthermore, family conflict, lack of financial resources, or poor communication with health care professionals may give rise to inadequate support for caregivers.

Dealing with the Medical System and Understanding Medical Terms and Medications

A barrage of new and tongue-twisting terms confronts the person given a new cancer diagnosis (and his or her caregivers). You may struggle to distinguish the *radiologist* from the *radiation oncologist* and to decipher lengthy names of chemotherapy drugs. All the while, you must cope with long lists of appointments, visits to large hospitals, and navigation of an increasingly confusing and inaccessible health care system. These frustrations and demands can prove overwhelming at times.

Difficulty with Communication

Communication with someone who has cancer is perhaps the most important and challenging charge of the caregiver. While the caregiver's priority is to maintain the best care and wellness of his or her loved one, the priority of the person with cancer is often to maintain as much autonomy and control as possible. Conflicts and communication breakdowns often result. In addition to communication problems involving the person with cancer, caregivers also struggle to see eye-to-eye with medical providers or other relatives of the person with cancer, many of whom may have contradictory views on how that person should be treated.

End-of-Life Concerns

Managing the day-to-day tasks of caregiving is difficult. These challenges must often be met while anticipating end-of-life matters. Caregivers confront the reality that cure may be impossible. Careful attention must be paid to the practical considerations of end-of-life planning as well as to the emotional consequences of losing a loved one. For some, the hardest stage is not at the end of life. It may be after a loved one has passed away, when the caregiver has lost a parent, a companion, or a lover, or when a person may feel as if he or she has lost a sense of purpose.

WHAT ARE SOME OF THE MOST STRESSFUL TIMES AND CONDITIONS FOR CAREGIVERS?

Certain points in time during the struggle with cancer are associated with notable amounts of stress. These include the point when a cancer diagnosis is first received; during a hospitalization; during the adjustment to a new lifestyle, pattern, or activity (necessitated by being a caregiver); after losing the ability to engage in activities one used to share with loved ones; while witnessing the effects of chemotherapy and the progressive effects of the disease on the function of a loved one; while watching your loved one experience pain; during end-of-life decision-making; and at the time of death and during the bereavement period.

WHAT ARE THE CONSEQUENCES OF PROLONGED STRESS ASSOCIATED WITH BEING A CAREGIVER?

Research has demonstrated that depression and anxiety are as common among caregivers as they are among people with cancer. Thus, up to half of all caregivers have symptoms of a mood disorder; such symptoms are severe in up to one-fourth of those affected. It is helpful for the caregiver to be seen by a member of the health care team from time to time, either along with the person who has cancer or alone—perhaps by the primary care physician—to assess how he or she is coping. If necessary, individual referrals can be made to support groups for counseling or for formal psychiatric evaluation and possible treatment with medicines that enhance mood, reduce anxiety, and promote sleep (see Chaps. 17 and 25 for further details.)

HOW CAN THE STRESS OF CAREGIVING BE AVOIDED OR MANAGED?

General Considerations

A variety of avenues are available to caregivers. These include support groups for cancer caregivers and their relatives (in person or on-line), support received from health care providers (including oncologists, surgeons, internists, and psychiatrists already involved in the care of the person with cancer), educational resources, self-care routines (such as time-outs and planned breaks or respites), maintenance of regular diet and exercise, and meditation and relaxation techniques. If needed, physicians can refer caregivers (or caregivers may refer themselves) for psychiatric evaluation to determine whether a treatable psychiatric condition is present.

To the extent possible, oncologists and other medical providers can offer emotional support and reassurance to stressed caregivers. However, physicians must remain mindful of their own potential for becoming overwhelmed by the emotional needs of their patients' caregivers. Consultation with mental health providers and social service agencies is essential in maintaining adequate coping as well as in setting appropriate boundaries on doctors' roles and interventions.

A good way for medical providers to avoid major problems and help caregivers manage stress is to *keep talking about it.* Caregivers often feel enormous pressure to keep their suffering to themselves and away from the person with cancer. This strategy tends not to work. When as much support as possible is provided to caregivers, better outcomes result. Unacknowledged or unspoken grief, by extension, adversely affects the emotional well-being of caregivers.

In addition, practical help, which can be provided by home nurses, visiting nurse associations (VNAs), and care assistants, is available to caregivers. Treatment teams should make prompt referrals for these services when appropriate. Also, respite care and the use of day centers can provide needed breaks for caregivers. Caregivers should be encouraged to take time, no matter how brief, to participate in a pleasurable activity for themselves (e.g., taking a walk, enjoying a hobby, or getting a haircut or manicure).

WHAT DIFFICULTIES ARISE IN CARING FOR CHILDREN WITH CANCER?

Caring for a child with cancer is uniquely stressful; it is one of the heaviest of burdens for any parent. Parents of children with cancer have the additional burden of helping their child get through a maze of medical tests, procedures, and changes at a time in their lives when they are least prepared to understand them. Parent caregivers should learn as much as they can about their child's illness. They should discuss all aspects of it (e.g., feelings about the cancer, the doctors, the treatments, and the hospitals) together, explain decisions, remain open with all children in the family (as their ages permit), and work to maintain the family unit (see Chap. 9 for further details).

ARE THERE ANY PRACTICAL GUIDELINES FOR CAREGIVERS?

General Approach

You will serve the person with cancer and yourself best by working together to solve problems, by enlisting others to help solve problems, by maintaining a positive attitude, and by taking care of yourself. Professional help should be sought when either you or the person with cancer experience severe anxiety or depression, when communication between you has broken down, and when either of you has a history of abuse, addiction, or any other severe conflict.

Plan early, maintain realistic expectations, share feelings, and ask for help *before* you feel overwhelmed.

Take a stance of initiation and action rather than of following the instructions of others. But don't "go it alone." You can regard yourself as a "team player" and coordinate the best care for the person with cancer with family, friends, medical providers as well as with the person who is ill. To whatever extent possible, the person with cancer should be deeply involved in all problem-solving discussions that affect him or her. Take advantage of the multiple roles played by members. For example, health care staff may be able to provide valuable information on nonmedical problems that come with illness, including support and spiritual concerns; friends may be able to share their own stories as cancer survivors or of loved ones with cancer.

Keep a good attitude. Try to see the positive aspects of the caretaking role. Caregiving can have life-enriching benefits. Closer ties can develop, or new and lasting friendships can be forged with other caregivers who are going through similar experiences.

Take care of your own needs. The more you attend to your own vital needs (e.g., rest, relaxation, and pleasurable activities), the stronger you will feel and the more emotionally equipped you will be to face the challenges of caring for someone else.

Maintain Lines of Communication

Maintenance of communication (between a caregiver and a person with cancer) is perhaps the most important concern for those involved in such a relationship. Whenever that communication breaks down—owing to physical, psychological, financial, or spiritual stress—care of the person with cancer may be compromised. If the caregiver and the person with cancer are unable to talk about important issues, professional help from a counselor or clergyman is advised.

Communication may be adversely affected by a history of physical, emotional, or sexual abuse or a history of infidelity or alcohol or drug addiction. Because deep-seated feelings can cloud judgment, these situations call for professional assistance from the outset.

Face the challenges of helping the person with cancer deal emotionally with his or her diagnosis. Support his or her efforts to cope, but be prepared to step in when avoidance or denial of illness gets in the way of proper treatment (e.g., by avoiding appointments or by continuing to engage in potentially harmful activities). You can create a climate that is conducive to sharing feelings by selecting an appropriate time and place for these discussions. Communicate your availability to participate in these discussions, and encourage the person with cancer to take advantage of that availability on his or her own terms and in his or her own time.

Be mindful of different communication styles between men and women. Women may express feelings with a desire for support, rather than for advice, from a male caregiver; men in American society may not talk openly about their feelings, but they will appreciate receiving special attention when they are talking about issues that are important to them.

Realize that communication does not require agreement on every topic. It is important for each person to retain his or her own values and opinions. You may want to share some feelings while the person you are caring for may be more focused on others. Maintaining a flow of communication about what each person values is key.

Remember that communication does not always require talking; nonverbal communication—with gestures, activities, and touching—can be even more powerful than speech.

Be prepared for disagreements. People may not always "be on the same page" about an issue, and this is to be expected. There are a number of ways to address this; one method is to look back to a time when you disagreed on an important issue and recall how it was handled. For example (if the person with cancer is your spouse or partner), how did you manage when your partner was ready to start a family and you were not? Prior solutions and strategies often pave the way to future ones.

Pick your battles wisely. While you and the person you're caring for may differ on a small point, it is important to avoid locking into a decision unnecessarily or fighting stubbornly about a small issue just for the sake of "winning the argument."

HOW CAN I MANAGE MY FEELINGS?

Shock

It is normal to go through a period of feeling numb, overwhelmed, and confused. Whenever possible, defer important decisions; take time to sort out and to talk over major problems with others—friends, neighbors, and family—that is, anyone who can provide perspective.

Anger, Resentment, and Irritation

These also are normal responses; it is crucial to deal with the anger effectively. Anger should be acknowledged and expressed in an appropriate way before it becomes too severe. Techniques to manage anger include seeing matters from the other person's perspective, removing yourself from the situation for a while, having a "safe" outlet for anger (e.g., beating a pillow, yelling in a car or closed room, or exercising), or talking out feelings with someone else ("venting").

Fear

Manage fear of the unknown by learning as much as possible about the diagnosis, its treatment, and its prognosis. Get information from doctors and from other professionals; this can help bring perspective to the situation and alert you to exaggerated risks and fears. Also, anxiety and fear must be talked about with a trusted and understanding person, such as a physician, clergyman, or friend.

Loss and Sorrow

One grieves not only for the loss associated with death but also for the loss of the "normal" or well person as well as for the "normal" life and activities that were once shared. It is especially valuable to talk about feelings of loss with those who have had similar experiences. Support groups can be helpful in this respect and should be sought out.

Guilt

Caregivers may feel guilty for a variety of reasons—for past or present transgressions or negative feelings, for feeling as though they have not done enough, for believing that they are not good enough as caregivers, for being angry, for being well, or just out of habit. Some people learned as children to blame themselves and to feel guilty whenever something went wrong. However, since guilt can be destructive and disabling, talking about these feelings and avoiding injudicious actions is imperative. Don't expect yourself to be perfect and don't dwell on your mistakes. Control repetitive, negative thoughts, such as guilt, by replacing them with constructive, positive thoughts.

CHAPTER 28

The Portrayal of Cancer and the Media

Eugene V. Beresin, M.D.
Sarah Hall, B.A.

HOW DO THE MEDIA PORTRAY PEOPLE WITH CANCER?

When most of us reflect on how cancer is depicted in the media, we think about the dramatic portrayals on television and in the movies. Like most dramas, those concerning cancer are usually presented in an extreme form: either as the "kiss of death" or as a heroic victory over great odds. In short, cancer is generally portrayed as a fatal, or near-fatal illness and shown in such a way so as to breed fear and to produce drama.

No doubt, when most of us go to see our doctor for a routine examination, or because of a symptom of one kind or another, our greatest fear is that we will be diagnosed with cancer. This fear is compounded by the fact that cancer is a relatively frequent diagnosis and highlighted by the media when any major public figure—politician, actor, or sports star—develops this disease or dies of it. The media represent but one source of the sense of dread that is associated with cancer. Many of us have relatives who have cancer, and we have lived through the emotional upheaval that any serious illness brings with it. To be fair, while the media often make hay with the high drama inherent in a cancer diagnosis, they also frequently depict cancer accurately. Unfortunately, we tend to remember best the most theatrical presentations seen in movies and television dramas.

The media can be helpful for those (people with cancer, family members, and friends) facing a diagnosis of cancer. Today, there are countless books, movies, articles, TV shows, and Internet sites on every type of cancer; they cover almost every aspect of this illness. In fact, there is such a wealth of information that it can be both overwhelming and confusing, especially for someone who is facing the reality of cancer. You may find it difficult to wade through this flood of information. How do you know which resources are reliable? How can you find the best answers to your questions? Where do you go if you have cancer or if you are a relative or friend of someone with a cancer diagnosis? This chapter can serve as a guide to help people with cancer, their family members, and friends by sifting through those media resources that will help to answer some of the many questions that arise.

WHAT CAN I LEARN ABOUT CANCER AND COPING WITH CANCER FROM LITERATURE, TELEVISION, AND THE MOVIES?

Literature on cancer spans essentially every topic and every type of cancer. Books have been written by those who have survived cancer, by health care providers, and by and for those whose loved ones have battled cancer. Books about coping (addressing the emotional issues of a diagnosis of cancer); about the different types of treatment and how to decide which course to take; about the mental and physical strains of treatment; about managing the side effects of cancer and its treatment; about the many issues family, friends, and caregivers may face; about how to manage financially; and about countless other topics also exist. So many titles are available that it would not be possible to list and review them all here; however, a selected bibliography including books available from the American Cancer Society is provided at the end of this chapter. Most of the books listed have been rated as being helpful by people who either had cancer or by those who were facing cancer in someone they loved.

When cancer affects children, special issues arise both for the children themselves and for their parents. This area is particularly problematic because of the high levels of emotion an ill child generates within a family. Parents and relatives need resources to help cope with the uncertainty of the cancer course and with the treatment of childhood cancer. Beyond this, helping children understand and cope with their illness needs to be done in a way that is comprehensible to a child at his or her developmental level. Examples are provided of resources that relate to childhood cancer and that can help in discussions with children.

Articles and columns about various topics related to cancer are also found in many popular newpapers. Although they are not resources specifically devoted to cancer, newspapers contain a good amount of information written at an understandable level. Most major newspaper articles focus on current studies and research findings as well as on issues surrounding the newest medical advances and treatment options. A host of articles also report on the politics of cancer and on the health care industry. For those interested in learning about these new advancements, magazines and newspapers are a good place to turn for the most up-to-date information. You can also find information about local and/or national support groups and resource information in most newspapers' calendars or other sections.

Newspapers also feature articles that focus on the lives of cancer survivors. For example, one such story in *USA Today* consisted of installments chronicling the experiences of a journalist who was diagnosed with breast cancer (*USA Today* Online; *http://www.usatoday.com/life/health/cancer/hainer/hainer.htm*, accessed 6/13/01). It is an inspiring and moving series of excepts from her diary, in which she takes a personal look into the many struggles of living with cancer.

Most national and international organizations and foundations devoted to cancer have pamphlets and brochures available on different aspects of cancer. Many are available free of charge and can be obtained either via the Internet or by calling the respective oragnization. They are useful for finding guidance, resources, and information about cancer and its effects. These organizations were created specifically for the purpose of public education about cancer and for support and guidance of those with cancer.

Fact sheets (two-page sheets that give general information about early warning signs of cancer and ways to prevent several cancers) are available from the Cancer Research Foundation of America (CRFA), (e.g., breast, cervical, colorectal, lung, prostate, skin, and testicular cancer). All of this information is available in Spanish, as is a video *[Por Su Salud y Por Su Familia (For Your Health, For Your Family)]* aimed at teaching breast and cervical health to Hispanic women.

The National Cancer Institute (NCI) also has many pamphlets devoted to most types of cancer: treatment options, clinical trials, testing for cancer, coping with cancer, genetics and risk factors, prevention, basic and laboratory cancer research, and statistics. You can view these publications on the Internet (*http://cissecure .nci.nih.gov/ncipubs/*) and print out paper copies. These publications also can be ordered over the phone at 1-800-4-CANCER (1-800-422-6237).

HOW CAN WATCHING OR DISCUSSING CERTAIN MOVIES (SUCH AS BRIAN'S SONG OR TERMS OF ENDEARMENT) OR TELEVISION SHOWS (SUCH AS ER) PREPARE ME FOR WHAT LIES AHEAD?

Many films and videos have been produced with plots involving cancer. Some are based on real-life stories while others are fictional. Movies such as *Brian's Song* and *Terms of Endearment* might be helpful in that they give the viewer a glimpse into the lives and emotions of people facing cancer. Although everyone's experience is unique, movies and television shows may help prepare someone facing cancer by providing examples of the ways people react to and deal with the many facets of diagnosis, of treatment, and of life with cancer.

It is important to remember, however, that movies and television shows are produced primarily for entertainment; they are often glamorized for public consumption. Most are based on fictional stories or have been altered for TV; they are not likely to depict the reality of any individual's experience with cancer. Anyone watching a movie or television program must keep in mind the period in which the movie was filmed. Particularly with cancer, medicine has progressed rapidly over the past few decades; older movies and shows may portray outdated techniques and/or therapies.

WHAT ARE SOME EXAMPLES OF MEDIA RESOURCES THAT DEAL WITH SPECIFIC CANCER SITUATIONS?

For example, consider the following situation:

My husband has just been diagnosed with cancer and has been given only a few months to live. He is a relatively young man and we have just recently started a family. What movies or books might help us to deal with his illness and with his prospect of leaving his family behind?

My Life would be a particularly relevant movie. It is a touching story about a young man whose life seemed picture perfect until he was diagnosed with lung cancer. With the few months he has left, he began to videotape all aspects of his life so that his unborn child could know him and understand what happened to him. The process turned into much more than he expected and took him on a journey of self-discovery and reconciliation with his family and friends. The film presents a good example of how one man dealt with fears, doubts, and other emotions associated with his own impending death and the reality of leaving behind his young wife, family, and friends.

Or the following situation:

> *Our six-year-old daughter developed leukemia, and we are overwhelmed. We need help in finding ways to explain the illness to her in a way she can understand. As parents, we are desperate to find out how other parents have dealt with this problem. While our doctors are wonderful, the amount of time, education and guidance they give us seems limited. Where can we go for help?*

Several books geared to children have been written on a level that will help explain cancer to them. These include *What is Cancer Anyway?; Explaining Cancer to Children of All Ages; Kathy's Hat: A Story of Hope* (this book received very high ratings); and *Let's Talk about when Kids Have Cancer.*

There are also a number of books written for parents, friends, and relatives of children with cancer. Two examples are *Childhood Leukemia: A Guide for Families, Friends & Caregivers (Patient-Centered Guides)*; and *Surviving Childhood Cancer: A Guide for Families.*

The book *Amanda's Gift* was written by a father whose daughter faced a 7-year battle with cancer. It recounts the pain, grief, and many other emotions a parent might experience when facing cancer in a child. The author also offers information on his family's experience with the health care system.

A video entitled *Why Charlie Brown, Why?* also may be helpful for children facing cancer. It is a story about a new girl in the *Peanuts* neighborhood who develops leukemia. Schultz's other characters try to help her as best they can through her chemotherapy treatments (which are experienced as scary).

Some websites also are useful for parents and children as they look for information and support.

The *Never-Ending Squirrel Tale* (*www.squirreltales.com*) is a site written by mothers and fathers who have dealt with cancer in a child or who are currently facing such a diagnosis. It was developed as a place where parents can find practical tips, information, encouragement, and inspiration, and where they can share their story and get advice from others who have walked the same road.

The NCI has a site at *http://cancernet.nci.nih.gov/occdocs/KidsHome.html* (a link called *Kids' Home at NCI: A Web Site for Kids with Cancer and Other Illnesses*) that has information for and by children and some information for parents; *http://www.cancersourcekids.com/* has links for children aged 6 to 12, teens aged 13 to 18, and parents. Children can learn about cancer while having fun with games and art on this site.

Another vignette follows:

I am a mother of two children, ages 2 and 6. Recently I was diagnosed with breast cancer. I hope that my cancer treatment will be successful, but I realize there are no guarantees. Is there a movie or book to help me with my fears and insecurities and to help me cope?

The following books might be helpful: *Your Breast Cancer Treatment Handbook: Your Guide to Understanding the Disease, Treatments, Emotions and Recovery from Breast Cancer; Coping with Breast Cancer: A Practical Guide to Understanding, Treating, and Living with Breast Cancer;* and *Cancer As Initiation: Surviving the Fire: A Guide for Living With Cancer for Patient, Provider, Spouse, Family, or Friend.*

Two examples of documentaries on breast cancer are also relevant. *Three Days Out: A Breast Cancer Odyssey*, profiles four women living with breast cancer. It takes a look at both the hopes and the fears that can arise in people living with the disease. *Between Us* also features real women who have survived the disease and who share their experiences, knowledge, and hope.

Terms of Endearment is a fictional movie that provides a picture of how some people cope with breast cancer. It portrays the lives and relationships of a mother and daughter who, throughout their relationship, have different views of life and living. The daughter is diagnosed with breast cancer and must come to terms with her impending death and with leaving her children behind. Although the film focuses only on end-stage cancer, it takes a look at how two very different people deal with the reality of this illness.

The following example also provides a useful illustration:

My college-aged son was just diagnosed with lymphoma. Where can he go to find information on coping with cancer? Also, what movies or books can he use for inspiration?

Lance Armstrong's book *It's Not About the Bike: My Journey Back to Life* is an inspiring story about one man's fight against a cancer that spread throughout his body and nearly killed him. It recounts, in great detail, the determined approach Armstrong took to beat testicular cancer and includes his setbacks and ultimate triumph over it. Another story of a triumphant fight against cancer can be found in the movie *Champions*. This is a true story about Bob Champion, a steeplechase jockey, who recovers from cancer and returns to racing.

Your son also might want to watch *Brian's Song*, a movie based on the true story of Brian Piccolo, a young professional football player, who was diagnosed with cancer at the height of his career. This movie takes a good look at one man's tenacious will to live and at the inspiring effect his fight had on his family and friends.

WHICH MOVIES/TELEVISION PROGRAMS/DOCUMENTARIES MAY BE HELPFUL?

The number and scope of films and television programs dealing with cancer are vast. While the decision about whether a movie is good or helpful is subjective, we have included a list of dramatic movies that have been rated highly and that other people with cancer and their families have found helpful.

Along with the movies released for the big screen and on videotape or DVD, several documentaries have been produced for television that focus on cancer. HBO produced a 2-hour show entitled, *Cancer: Evolution to Revolution,* which follows several people with cancer and gives the viewer a look into the world of people living with cancer. The program is a documentary-style series broken into five 1/2 hour segments. The segments cover many topics (including an overview of the impact cancer has had in the United States, what it means to be an active patient, a history of cancer, an explanation of clinical trials, a discussion of the biology of cancer, and information on how support groups can help). Personal stories also take an intimate look into the reality of children's cancer, colon cancer, breast cancer, and prostate cancer.

Nova, produced by the Public Broadcasting System (PBS), has presented a series called *The Cancer Warrior,* which aired originally in February 2001. It is available on videocassette and can be found in retail and web-based bookstores. This series portrays Boston researcher Judah Folkman and his exciting breakthroughs in the development of a class of cancer-fighting drugs called *angiogenesis inhibitors.* It is an informative series and facilitates learning about this cutting-edge research and the ongoing clinical trials. An Internet site devoted to this series allows you to download the program and watch it on a home computer. Additional information on cancer, including other Internet links, can be found on the Internet site *http:// www.pbs.org/wgbh/nova/cancer/.*

PBS also produced a 1-hour documentary (originally aired on September 25, 1998) called *Living With Cancer: A Message of Hope.* This documentary recounts the experiences of a group of people who were diagnosed with cancer, underwent treatment, and now live full and healthy lives. The show also features leading cancer experts as they share information on new research and insights on treatment and provides an overview of steps to take to lower one's cancer risk. Information on this program can be obtained by contacting your local PBS station or on the PBS website, *http://www.pbs.org/.*

HOW ACCURATE ARE THE DEPICTIONS OF CANCER IN THE MEDIA?

Unfortunately, the degree of accuracy of cancer depictions by the media varies widely. Within each type of media presentation one can find well-substantiated information as well as some questionable, more opinion-based comments. Most books, magazine articles, and newspaper accounts (distributed by major publishers), pamphlets (published by organizations), and video documentaries (produced by well-known studios) tend to be fairly accurate; they usually require a rigorous process of editing, reviewing, and fact checking before they reach the public eye. The quality and accuracy of movies are more variable, as are books, many of which are based on personal experiences and beliefs. Some serve as excellent guides for people with cancer (especially as they are written by people who have experienced cancer and know what it is like first hand); on the flip side, personal accounts are just that—personal, or one person's experience with cancer, and thus are not necessarily generalizable.

HOW USEFUL IS THE INTERNET?

The Internet contains an almost endless supply of information, sites, and links devoted to all aspects of cancer. Anyone trolling the Internet can find pages on topics ranging from broad, general information to specific data on almost every cancer-related subject imaginable. As the type of information varies widely, so does the accuracy of that information. Although a lot of good information exists, anyone using the Internet must be careful not to believe every fact that has been posted. The Internet is not regulated; similarly, the information on it is not necessarily reviewed by known authorities in the field. Additionally, the Internet is not sorted in a systematic manner. An individual searching for information on one particular type of cancer is likely to find thousands of articles and sites related in some way to a keyword. Many attempts to seek information are fraught with frustration during this time-consuming process, and the results may be filled with inaccuracies or even blatantly false information.

Websites hosted and sponsored by well-known, reputable cancer foundations and organizations are outlined in Chap. 12.

For those who do not have access to the Internet at home, many foundations have phone numbers and addresses where you can contact them. Most local libraries and universities offer free access to the Internet.

In summary, the media supply people with cancer, their families, and their friends with a wealth of resources and styles of presentation for understanding the nature, treatments, courses, and outcomes of cancer.

SELECTED RESOURCES

From the American Cancer Society Booklist

All of these titles can be ordered online at *http://www.cancer.org/eprise/main/docroot/PUB/PUB_1?sitearea=PUB* or by calling 1-888-227-5552.

Ackermann A, Ackermann A: *Our Mom Has Cancer*. Atlanta, GA: American Cancer Society, 2001.

American Cancer Society: *A Breast Cancer Journey—Your Personal Guidebook*. Atlanta, GA: American Cancer Society, 2001.

American Cancer Society: *American Cancer Society's Guide to Complementary and Alternative Cancer Methods*. Atlanta, GA: American Cancer Society, 2000.

Bostwick DG, MacLennan GT, Larson TR: *Prostate Cancer: What Every Man—and His Family—Needs to Know*. New York, NY: Villard Books, 1999.

Eyre H, Lange DP, Morris LB: *Informed Decisions: The Complete Book of Cancer Diagnosis, Treatment, and Recovery*. Atlanta, GA: American Cancer Society, 2001.

Heiney SP (ed), Hermann JF, Bruss KV, Fincannon JL: *Cancer in the Family: Helping Children Cope With a Parent's Illness*. Atlanta, GA: American Cancer Society, 2001.

Houts PS, Bucher JA (eds): *Caregiving-A Step-By-Step Resource for Caring for the Person with Cancer at Home*. Atlanta, GA: American Cancer Society, 2000.

Levin, B: *Colorectal Cancer: A Thorough and Compassionate Resource for Patients and Their Families*. New York, NY: Random House, 1999.

Runowicz CD, Petrek JA, Gansler TS: *Women and Cancer: A Thorough and Compassionate Resource for Patients and Their Families*. New York, NY: Villard Books, 1999.

Wilkes GM, Ades TB, Krakoff IH: *Consumers Guide to Cancer Drugs*. Sudbury, MA: James & Bartlett Pubs., 2000.

For books on specific stages and experiences of cancer in general, below is a list of some of the top-ranked books on these topics.

Coping

Fiore NA: *The Road Back to Health: Coping with the Emotional Aspects of Cancer*. New York, NY: Bantam Books, 1986.

Holland JC, Lewis S: *The Human Side of Cancer: Living with Hope, Coping with Uncertainty*. New York: Harper Collins, 2000.

Moore K, Schmais L: *Living Well With Cancer: A Nurse Tells You Everything You Need to Know About Managing the Side Effects of Your Treatment*. East Rutherford, NJ: The Penguin Putnam Publishing Group, 2001.

Todd AD: *Double Vision: An East-West Collaboration for Coping with Cancer*. Middletown, CT: Wesleyan University Press, 1995.

General Information and Guides for Patients and Family

Anderson G, Simonton C: *Cancer: 50 Essential Things to Do*. East Rutherford, NJ: Plume, 1999.

Babcock EN: *When Life Becomes Precious*. New York, NY:Bantam Books, 1997.

Canfield J (ed), Hanson MV, Aubrey P, Kirkhart BK, Mitchell-Autio N: *Chicken Soup for the Surviving Soul: 101 Inspirational Stories to Comfort Cancer Patients and Their Loved Ones*. Deerfield Beach, FL: Health Communications, 1996.

Girard V, Zadra D (eds): *There's No Place like Hope: A Book of Hope, Help and Inspiration for Cancer Patients and Their Families*. Lynnwood, WA: Compendium, 2001.

Harpham WS, Jones R: *After Cancer: A Guide to Your New Life*. New York: Harper Perennial Library, 1995.

Therapies and Treatments

Cukier D, McCollough VE, Gingerelli F: *Coping With Radiation Therapy: A Ray of Hope.* New York: McGraw Hill, 2001.

Dollinger M, Rosenbaum EH, Cable G: *Everyone's Guide to Cancer Therapy.* Kansas City, MO: Andrews McMeel Publishing, 1998.

Frahm AE, Frahm DJ: *The Cancer Battle Plan: Six Strategies for Beating Cancer from a Recovered "Hopeless Case.* New York, NY: JP Tarcher, 1998.

Zakarian B, Greenspan EM: *The Activist Cancer Patient: How to Take Charge of Your Treatment.* New York: Wiley, 1996.

Diagnosis

Diamond WJ, Cowen WL, Goldberg B: *Cancer Diagnosis: What to Do Next.* Alternativemedicine.com.

Harpham WS, Pilcher AB: *Diagnosis Cancer: Your Guide through the First Few Months.* New York: Norton, 1997.

Levine M: *Surviving Cancer: One Women's Story and Her Inspiring Program for Anyone Facing Cancer.* New York, NY: Broadway Books, 2001.

Children and Cancer

COPING AND LIVING WITH CHILDHOOD CANCER

Adams DW: *Coping With Childhood Cancer: Where Do We Go from Here?* Hamilton, Canada: Kinbridge Publishing, 1993.

Connolly H, Clancy T, Civi C: *Fighting Chance: Journeys Through Childhood Cancer.* Baltimore, MD: Woodholm House Publishing, 1998.

Dorfman EV: *The C-Word: Teenagers and their Families Living With Cancer.* Portland, OR: New Sage Press, 1998.

Ekert H: *Childhood Cancer: Understanding and Coping.* New York: Gordon & Breach Science Publishing, 1989.

Fromer MJ: *Surviving Childhood Cancer.* Washington, DC: American Psychiatric Press, 1995.

Wolford CB, Wolford F, Moscow J: *My Story About Cancer.* Helena, MT: Seven Locks Press, 1999.

General Information and Guides for Patients and Families

Breen DL, Sion M, Mogul M (eds): *Cancer's Gift,* Rock Wren Publishing, 2000.

Keene N, Lamb L (eds): *Childhood Leukemia: A Guide for Families, Friends & Caregivers (Patient-Centered Guides).* Cambridge, MA: O'Reilly & Associates, 1999.

Keene N, Ruccione K, Hobbie W: *Childhood Cancer Survivors: A Practical Guide to Your Future.* Cambridge, MA: O'Reilly & Associates, 2000.

Steen G, Mirro J Jr (eds): *Childhood Cancer: A Handbook from St. Jude Children's Research Hospital.* Cambridge, MA: Perseus Press, 2000.

The following lists include selected titles that are available for some of the more common types of cancer.

Prostate Cancer

COPING AND LIVING WITH PROSTATE CANCER

Phillips RH: *Coping with Prostate Cancer: A Guide to Living with Prostate Cancer for You and Your Family*. New York, NY: Avery Publishing Group, 1994.

Priest MW: *Diary of Courage Coping With Life Threatening Illness*. San Francisco, CA: Strawberry Hill Press, 1990.

General Information and Guides for Patient and Family

Berberich R: *Hit Below the Belt: Facing Up to Prostate Cancer*. Berkeley, CA: Ten Speed Press, 2001.

Marks S, Moul J: *Prostate & Cancer: A Family Guide to Diagnosis, Treatment & Survival*. Cambridge, MA: Fisher Books, 2000.

Walsh PC, Worthington JF: *The Prostate: A Guide for Men and the Women Who Love Them*. New York: Warner Books, 1997.

Walsh PC, Worthington JF: *Walsh's Guide to Surviving Prostate Cancer*. New York: Warner Books, 2001.

Breast Cancer

DIAGNOSIS

Austin S, Hitchcock C: *Breast Cancer: What You Should Know (But May Not Be Told About Prevention, Diagnosis, and Treatment*. Rocklin, CA: Prima Publishing, 1994.

Link J: *The Breast Cancer Survival Manual: A Step-By-Step Guide for the Woman Newly Diagnosed with Breast Cancer*. New York: Holt, 2000.

COPING AND LIVING WITH BREAST CANCER

Bruning N: *Coping with Chemotherapy*. New York: Ballantine Books, 1993.

Greenberg M: *Invisible Scars: A Guide to Coping With the Emotional Impact of Breast Cancer*. New York, NY: Walker and Company, 1988.

Mayer M, Lamb L (eds): *Advanced Breast Cancer: A Guide to Living with Metastatic Disease*, 2d ed.*(Patient-Centered Guides)*, 2d ed. Cambridge, MA: O'Reilly & Associates, 1998.

Muschal-Reinhardt R, Mitrano BS, McCarthy MR, Brinkman-Grinnan J: *Rituals for Women Coping with Breast Cancer*. New York, NY: Prism Collective, 2000.

Phillips RH, Goldstein P: *Coping with Breast Cancer: A Practical Guide to Understanding, Treating, and Living with Breast Cancer*. New York: Avery Penguin Putnam, 1998.

GENERAL INFORMATION AND GUIDES

Braddock S, Kercher JM, Edney JJ, et al: *Straight Talk About Breast Cancer: From Diagnosis to Recovery: A Guide for the Entire Family*. Omaha, NE: Addicus Books, 1994.

Kneece JC, Brown T (ed): *Your Breast Cancer Treatment Handbook: Your Guide to Understanding the Disease, Treatments, Emotions and Recovery from Breast Cancer*. Seattle, WA: EduCare Inc, 2001.

Love SM, Lindsey K: *Dr. Susan Love's Breast Book*. Cambridge, MA: Perseus Publishing, 2000.

Stone B: *Cancer As Initiation: Surviving the Fire: A Guide for Living With Cancer for Patient, Provider, Spouse, Family, or Friend*. Chicago, IL: Open Court, 1994.

Colorectal Cancer

GENERAL INFORMATION

Dunitz M, Rougier P, Wilke H (eds): *Management of Colorectal Cancer*. Malden, MA: Blackwell Science, 1998.

Johnston L: *Colon & Rectal Cancer: A Comprehensive Guide for Patients & Families*. Cambridge, MA: O'Reilly & Associates, 2000.

Marcet JE: *Colorectal Cancer: A Guide for Patients*. Los Angeles, CA: Health Information Network, 1996.

Miskovitz PF, Betancourt M: *What to Do If You Get Colon Cancer: A Specialist Helps You Take Charge and Make Informed Choices*. New York: Wiley, 1997.

Pazdur R, Royce M: *Myths & Facts About Colorectal Cancer, 2nd edition*. Melville, NY: Publisher Research & Representation, Inc. 2001.

Skin Cancer

COPING AND LIVING WITH SKIN CANCER

Bishop B: *My Triumph over Cancer*. Chicago: Keats Publishing, 1986.

Long W: *Coping With Melanoma and Other Skin Cancers*. New York, NY: Rosen Publishing Group, 1999.

Shuck C, Greenway HT: *Saving Face: My Victory Over Skin Cacner*. Forest Dale, VT: Pauls Eriksson, 2000.

General Guides and Information

Kenet BJ, Lawler P: *Saving Your Skin: Prevention, Early Detection, and Treatment of Melanoma and Other Skin Cancers*. New York, NY: Four Walls Eight Windows, 1998.

Poole CM, Guerry D: *Melanoma: Prevention, Detection, and Treatment*. New Haven, CT: Yale University Press, 1998.

Schofield JR, Robinson WS: *What You Really Need to Know About Moles and Melanoma (Johns Hopkins Press Health Book)*. Baltimore, MD: Johns Hopkins University Press, 2000.

Magazine And Newspaper Articles

USA TODAY

Associated Press (accessed 8/5/2001): Colon cancer screening worth the cost. *http://www.usatoday.com/life/health/cancer/colon/lhcco017.htm*

Associated Press (accessed 8/5/2001): Experimental leukemia drug wins praise. *http://www.usatoday.com/news/healthscience/health/2001-07-25-leukemia-drug.htm*

Associated Press (accessed 8/5/2001): Gene test offers better breast cancer treatment. *http://www.usatoday.com/news/health/2001-02-21-breast-cancer.htm*

Associated Press (accessed 8/5/2001): Green tea may not prevent stomach cancer after all. *http://www.usatoday.com/news/health/2001-02-28-green-tea.htm*

Associated Press (accessed 8/5/2001): Lung cancer surgery: Practice makes perfect. *http://www.usatoday.com/news/healthscience/health/2001-07-18-lung-cancer.htm*

Associated Press (accessed 8/5/2001): Women smokers may get more bladder cancer. *http://www.usatoday.com/news/health/2001-04-03-bladder-cancer-women.htm*

Friend T (accessed 8/5/2001): Histamine doubles survival with melanoma. *http://www.usatoday.com/life/health/cancer/skin/lhcsk011.htm*

Rubin R (accessed 8/5/2001): Viral test could aid detection of cervical cancer. *http://www.usatoday.com/news/health/2001-02-20-cervical.htm*

THE NEW YORK TIMES

Altman LK: Chemotherapy before surgery aids bladder cancer. *New York Times* (electronic version), 5/15/2001.

Ames L: Milestones: A father's triumph over cancer. *New York Times* (electronic version), 10/15/2000.

Brody J: Personal health: Lung cancer cure? Try prevention instead. *New York Times* (electronic version), 11/24/2000.

Cancer drug shows promise, but is no panacea, tests find. *New York Times* (electronic version), 11/11/2000.

Christensen J: Scientist at work: John Reed—Running hot in pursuit of cancer treatment. *New York Times* (electronic version), 12/12/2000.

Grady D: New treatment offers promise against kidney cancer. *New York Times* (electronic version), 9/13/2000.

Kirby D: More options, and decisions, for men with prostate cancer. *New York Times* (electronic version), 10/3/2000.

Kolata G: Studies report no links to cancer in cell phones' use. *New York Times* (electronic version), 12/20/2000.

Wade N: Swift approval for a new kind of cancer drug. *New York Times* (electronic version), 5/11/2001.

THE WASHINGTON POST

Applied orally, missile defense technology may work: A new high-tech test can help target early mouth cancers. *Washington Post* (4/24/2001, p T6).

Help yourself: resources for alternative and complementary cancer treatment. *Washington Post* (9/4/2001, p HE06).

Too young to die: media images aside, breast cancer usually hits after 50. *Washington Post* (5/1/2001, p T7).

Who wants to know? A simple biopsy technique can detect more prostate cancers than are usually caught. but is this really useful? *Washington Post* (8/4/2001, p F4).

THE BOSTON GLOBE

Foreman J: When drugs are the only choice for a mother to be. *Boston Globe* (electronic version), 9/26/2000.

Mishra R: Drug found to be effective in 2 cancers. *Boston Globe* (electronic version), 4/5/2001.

Reucroft S, Swain J: Nicotine and cancer. *Boston Globe* (electronic version), 11/28/2000.

Rosenberg R: Vaccines to treat, not prevent, cancer: Products in test phase aim to help patients live longer. *Boston Globe* (electronic version), 10/15/2001.

Saltus R: A new look at cancer treatment. *Boston Globe* (electronic version), 11/14/2000.

Saltus R: Diet no help: A cancer study finds breast risk unchanged by healthy eating habit. *Boston Globe* (electronic version), 2/14/2001.

NEWSWEEK

A cure for cancer? *Newsweek Magazine* (electronic version), May 28, 2001.

Begley S: Made-to-order medicine. *Newsweek Magazine* (electronic version), June 25, 2001.

Cowley G: Can we overcome cancer? *Newsweek Magazine* (electronic version), fall/winter 2001.

Greenberg SH, Springen K: Keeping hope alive. *Newsweek Magazine* (electronic version), fall/winter 2001.

Kalb C: A cancer "smart bomb." *Newsweek Magazine* (electronic version), December 18, 2000.

Laschever A: When the unthinkable happens. *Newsweek Magazine* (electronic version), August 13, 2001.

TIME *MAGAZINE*

Can food fend off tumors? *Time Magazine* (electronic version), July 19, 1999.

Cancer made to order. *Time Magazine* (electronic version), August 9, 1999.

Closing in on cancer. *Time Magazine* (electronic version), May, 21, 2001.

Curing cancer: The hope and the hype. *Time Magazine* (electronic version), May 18, 1998.

Everything you need to know about colon cancer and how to prevent it. *Time Magazine* (electronic version), March 20, 2000.

CANCER RESEARCH FOUNDATION

The Cancer Research Foundation of America (CRFA) has the following educational materials and resources for the general public:

Colorectal Cancer: Preventable, Treatable, Beatable!

Healthy Kids: 7 Steps to Cancer Prevention for Parents

Healthy Men: Self Help for Cancer Prevention

Healthy Women: Self Help for Cancer Prevention

Living Healthy: 7 Steps to Cancer Prevention

The Cancer Research Foundation of America: Breaking the Codes

These brochures are concise yet informative. They list easy lifestyle changes and habits that can help decrease the risk of developing certain types of cancer. All of this can be found through the following website: *http://www.preventcancer.org/educcrfa.cfm*, ordered by phone (1-800-227-CRFA), or requested by e-mail at *info@crfa.org*. The brochures and fact sheets can be downloaded without charge from the website.

Movies That Depict Cancer

Champions, 1984, USA, Embassy Pictures Corporation.
The true story of Bob Champion (John Hurt), a British steeplechase jockey who, in the late 1970s, was diagnosed with cancer.

Closure, 2001, USA, Twenty One Productions.
Based on a true story. A young married couple and their family struggle when the young woman is diagnosed with cancer.

Counting Days, 2000, USA, Emerald City Films.
A young man struggles to bring his estranged family together and face the demons from his own past after his father is diagnosed with cancer.

Daibyonin (The Last Days), 1993, Japan.
A Japanese movie director must come to terms with his terminal cancer. Despite many painful personal struggles and conflicts with those he loves, he realizes he does not want to die in the hospital and spends his last days peacefully at home.

Developing, 1995, USA.

A short film about a single mother with breast cancer who must deal with her young daughter and help her understand what she is going through.

Dying Young, 1991, USA, Twentieth Century Fox Film Corp.

A young woman looking for a new start in life takes a job tending to a man suffering from a blood cancer. They fall in love, knowing that it cannot last, for the man with cancer is destined to die.

Girls' Night, 1998, USA, Granada Film Productions.

Two best friends fly to Las Vegas to fulfill the dream of one, who is dying of cancer.

God Said, "Ha!" 1998, Oh, Brother Productions Inc.

Julia Sweeney talks about the period when her brother fought cancer and she also was diagnosed with a rare cancer.

My Life, USA 1993, Columbia Pictures.

Diagnosed with cancer and with only a few months to live, a young man sets out to document his life and knowledge for his unborn son. The experience leads him on a voyage of self-discovery and reconciliation.

One True Thing, 1998, USA, Universal Pictures.

A young, independent woman is forced to uproot her life to take care of a mother stricken with cancer. She makes discoveries about her parents and about her own life along the way.

The Politics of Cancer (documentary), 1995, USA, Healing Arts Documentary Productions.

U.S. senators, scientists, doctors, pharmaceutical companies, CEOs, wives, and children confront a chaotic epidemic of cancer.

Princes in Exile, 1990, Canada, CBC.

A young boy, angry at his diagnosis of brain cancer and the possibility of dying, finds a new perspective through the strength and optimism of a new friend.

Rachel's Daughters: Searching for the Causes of Breast Cancer (documentary), 1997, USA.

Seven women who currently have or have survived breast cancer travel across the country asking researchers and experts about the possible causes of breast cancer.

A Woman's Tale (motion picture) 1991, AFFC.

An older woman diagnosed with cancer is determined to live her last days with the dignity she displayed her entire life. In this courageous performance, the actress portraying the main character herself had cancer while making the film.

The list below represents a few of the best-selling educational movies listed by type of cancer as indicated by sales from popular retail stores and websites.

BREAST CANCER

Between Us: A First Aid Kit for your Heart and Soul, 1999, USA.

Focus on Healing through Movement & Dance for the Breast Cancer Survivor, 1999, USA, Tapeworm.

Initial Discovery and Diagnosis of Breast Cancer, 2000, USA.

Man's Guide to Women's Breast Cancer: Partners in Hope, 2001, USA.

No Hair Day: Laughing (and Crying) Our Way Through Cancer, 2001, USA, WGBH Boston.

Options in the Treatment of Breast Cancer, USA, Pathway Video, LLC.

Three Days Out: A Breast Cancer Odyssey, 2000, USA, PBS.

Women's Health: Breast Cancer—Replacing Fear with Facts, 1999, USA, Parade.

PROSTATE CANCER

Not Alone—Couples Share Candidly About Prostate Cancer, 1998.

Prostate Cancer: A Journey of Hope, 1999, USA, PBS.
COLON AND RECTAL CANCER
Detecting Colon Cancer: Knowledge is Power, 2000, USA, Health Talks at The Cleveland Clinic.
Today—Confronting Colon Cancer 2001, USA, A&E Home video.
SKIN CANCER
A Doctor in Your House: Vol 3—*Skin Cancer: Our Dangerous Day in the Sun*, 1999, USA, United American Video.
Melanoma And Other Skin Cancer, 2000, USA, HealthInfo.
CHILDHOOD CANCER
My Hair's Falling Out . . . Am I Still Pretty? A Childhood Cancer Education Video, 1992, USA, PBS.
CANCER—NONSPECIFIC
Cancer: Increasing Your Odds of Survival, 1999, USA, PBS.
Cancer: A Turning Point—An Interview with Dr. Lawrence LeShan, 2000, USA, Tapeworm.
Health: Great Minds of Medicine: Cancer, 1997, USA, Unapix Inc.
Living & Laughing With Cancer, 1998, USA, Tapeworm.
Living with Cancer: A Message of Hope, 1998, USA, Wellspring Media.
When Cancer Touches Your Life: Meeting the Needs of Patients and Families, 2000, Health Talks at The Cleveland Clinic.

CHAPTER 29

Living Wills and Health Care Proxies

LAURA M. PRAGER, M.D.
FRED H. MILLHAM, M.D., M.B.A.

OUTLINE

WHAT ARE LIVING WILLS AND
HEALTH CARE PROXIES?

COMPONENTS OF AN ADVANCE
DIRECTIVE

WHY SHOULD I CREATE AN
ADVANCE DIRECTIVE?

HOW SHOULD I DECIDE WHO WILL
BE MY HEALTH CARE PROXY?

WHEN SHOULD I CREATE AN
ADVANCE DIRECTIVE AND
DESIGNATE A HEALTH CARE
PROXY?

HOW DO I CREATE AN ADVANCE
DIRECTIVE?

WHAT DECISIONS WILL A HEALTH
CARE PROXY NOT COVER?

WHAT ARE LIVING WILLS AND HEALTH CARE PROXIES?

A living will is a document that delineates what types of medical care and treatment you will want to have in the future should you become incapacitated or incompetent and unable to communicate your wishes. Living wills can be simple or complex, limited or far-reaching. You do not need a lawyer to write one. Most living wills state, in simple language, under what circumstances life-sustaining medical treatments should be continued, limited, or withheld; such a document serves as a guide for your physicians and family members.

However, because a living will is a document written at one point in time and clinical situations may change rapidly and unpredictably, it is important to choose a person who can serve as your advocate and help your doctors interpret your living will. Such a person is said to hold your *health care power of attorney* or to be your *health care proxy*. The term *health care proxy*, in addition to referring to such a person, also refers to a legal document that designates a person you know and trust to make health care decisions for you if, for any reason, you are unable to make decisions for yourself. The combination of a living will and a health care proxy is called an advance directive. As it is impossible to anticipate all of the specific clinical issues that may arise, having a health care proxy is of more practical importance than having a living will. Having your general wishes spelled out in a living will, though, makes the job of the health care proxy easier during potentially difficult times.

Under federal law (the Patient Self-Determination Act of 1990), all patients entering a hospital must be offered the opportunity to create an advance directive. Each state has laws governing advance directives; some provide specific forms while others set only general guidelines. Some advance directives are simple and specify only the identity of your health care proxy; others are made up of many sections and offer more guidance to the person granted power of attorney (Table 29-1).

COMPONENTS OF AN ADVANCE DIRECTIVE

1. *Instructional section:* This section allows you to make explicit statements about what you would or would not want to be done for you under specific circumstances.
2. *Durable power of attorney section (health care proxy):* This section allows you to designate a specific person to make medical decisions for you in the event that

TABLE 29-1 Components of an Advance Directive

Instructional section
Durable power of attorney section (health care proxy)
Values statement section
Organ donation section
Illness scenarios section

you should become mentally and/or physically incapacitated. The authority of the power of attorney is limited to medical decisions. Most people choose a family member, trusted colleague, or close friend. The person who is given power of attorney will be the one to authorize or refuse any procedures or therapies for you in the event that you are unable to express your desires. As long as you are competent to make your own decisions, the power of attorney remains inactive. The person to whom you give power of attorney should have a thorough understanding of your wishes and desires, as it will be that person's responsibility to see that your wishes govern the decisions of your caregivers.

3. *Values statement section:* This section allows you to state specific values and expectations you have regarding your treatment. For example, if you wish to have life-sustaining treatments continued under all circumstances, such a statement can be made in this section. Or you may prefer to limit some life-sustaining measures but to ensure continued pain control and other forms of comfort care.

4. *Organ donation section:* The organ donation sections allow you to indicate whether you want any of your organs to be used for purposes of transplantation after your death. While this statement is not binding on the next of kin, it is useful to have your preference stated in writing.

5. *Illness scenarios section:* Many advance directives have a section in which specific scenarios are described; you may indicate what you would like to have done if such a situation arises.

WHY SHOULD I CREATE AN ADVANCE DIRECTIVE?

An advance directive will help those caring for you to follow your wishes. Reviewing your advance directive with your caregivers and loved ones can facilitate discussion of your fears and expectations as you confront serious illness. Many people find that discussing end-of-life issues openly, well in advance of trouble, lessens their worry about the future. Undoubtedly, your family members or other loved ones will be anxious about how best to help you through the course of your illness.

Making medical decisions for a loved one can be an intimidating and frightening task. Family members often feel comforted when you give them clear instructions regarding your medical care. If you have made your wishes clear ahead of time, your family and friends will be better able to manage both your care and their feelings if and when the time arrives for them to do so.

If you do not create an advance directive, your next of kin will be placed in the position of making decisions about your care when you are unable to do so. In some cases, family members with equal claim as your next of kin may differ in their thoughts about what you do or do not want (including what treatments you should or should not have). Disagreements among family members can result in conflict with caregivers around medical decision making and worsen an already extremely difficult and tense situation.

HOW SHOULD I DECIDE WHO WILL BE MY HEALTH CARE PROXY?

While most people appoint a spouse, significant other, or family member to be their health care proxy, anyone who is not an employee or representative of the health care facility in which a person is treated can be a proxy. The person you appoint should be someone you trust, who understands your needs and wishes, and who will be able to advocate for you during a time in which you cannot advocate for yourself. Sometimes, a discussion with family and friends about advance directives is a good way to help you decide who would be the best person to represent you and to hold your health care power of attorney.

Although it is important for you to discuss your needs and wishes with your physicians, you should not appoint one of your doctors as your health care proxy. Your doctor's job is to help your health care proxy understand the medical issues and to inform him or her of the decisions that must be made. Because your physician will be in the position of carrying out the decisions of your health care proxy, it is inappropriate for him or her to be in the position of making those decisions.

WHEN SHOULD I CREATE AN ADVANCE DIRECTIVE AND DESIGNATE A HEALTH CARE PROXY?

As life-threatening illnesses can occur unexpectedly, it is a good idea to work on an advance directive as soon as you feel ready to think about these issues. Should your wishes change regarding your living will or your health care proxy, you can simply amend the existing document or create a new advance directive. Remember, the advance directive does not take effect (i.e., it is not active) as long as you are well enough to make your own decisions.

You should not assume that once you have prepared an advance directive, your physician or other caregivers would know about it. You should discuss it with your physician and leave a copy of it with him or her. If you are admitted to the hospital, be sure that another copy is placed in your medical record. Also, make sure your close friends and family members either have a copy of your advance directive or know where one is located.

HOW DO I CREATE AN ADVANCE DIRECTIVE?

You can obtain the general form accepted by your state from the admitting department of any local hospital or from agencies such as the American Association of Retired Persons (AARP), the American Bar Association (ABA) on Legal Problems of the Elderly, or the American Medical Association (AMA). You may also wish to look at forms used by other states in order to learn more about potential directives. An example of an advance directive is given in Fig. 29-1.

FIGURE 29-1 Sample advance directive form

I, _____, write this document as
a directive regarding my medical care.

Initial those sections you wish to be included in your Advance Directive. You may cross out or change any words or sentences you wish.

PART 1. My Durable Power of Attorney for Health Care

_____ **I appoint the person named below to make decisions about my medical care if I cannot make those decisions myself. I want the person I have appointed, my doctors, my family and others to be guided by information I have included below.**

Name: _____

Home telephone: _____

Work telephone: _____

Address: _____

_____ **I have not appointed anyone to make health care decisions for me in this or any other document.**

PART 2. My Living Will

These are my wishes for my future medical care if there ever comes a time when I cannot make these decisions for myself.

A. These are my wishes if I have a terminal condition.

Life-sustaining treatments

_____ I want the life-sustaining treatments that my doctors think are best for me.

_____ I do not want life-sustaining treatment (including CPR) started. If life-sustaining treatments are started, I want them stopped.

_____ Other wishes: _____

Artificial nutrition and hydration

_____ I do not want artificial nutrition and hydration started if they would be the main treatments keeping me alive. If artificial nutrition and hydration are started, I want them stopped.

_____ I want artificial nutrition and hydration even if they are the main treatments keeping me alive.

_____ Other wishes: _____

Comfort care

_____ I want to be kept as comfortable and free of pain as possible, even if such care prolongs my dying or shortens my life.

_____ Other wishes: _____

(continued)

FIGURE 29-1 (*continued*)

B. These are my wishes if I am ever in a persistent vegetative state.

Life-sustaining treatments

_____   I want the life-sustaining treatments that my doctors think are best for me.

_____   I do not want life-sustaining treatment (including CPR) started. If life-sustaining treatments are started, I want them stopped.

_____   Other wishes:

_____

Artificial nutrition and hydration

_____   I do not want artificial nutrition and hydration started if they would be the main treatments keeping me alive. If artificial nutrition and hydration are started, I want them stopped.

_____   I want artificial nutrition and hydration even if they are the main treatments keeping me alive.

_____   Other wishes:

_____

Comfort care

_____   I want to be kept as comfortable and free of pain as possible, even if such care prolongs my dying or shortens my life.

_____   Other wishes:

_____

C. Other directions

You have the right to be involved in all decisions about your medical care, even those not dealing with terminal conditions or persistent vegetative states. If you have wishes not covered in other parts of this document, please indicate them below.

PART 3. Other Wishes

A. Organ donation

_____   I do not wish to donate any of my organs or tissues.

_____   I want to donate any or all of my organs and tissues which are appropriate for transplantation.

_____   I only want to donate these organs and tissues:

_____

_____   Other wishes:

_____

B. Autopsy

_____   I do not want an autopsy.

_____   I agree to an autopsy if my doctors and family wish it.

_____   Other wishes:

_____

(*continued*)

FIGURE 29-1 (*continued*)

C. Other statements about your medical care

Additional statements regarding my health care advance directive can be found on the attached sheets which number: _____ pages.

PART 4. Signatures

This document must be signed by at least two witnesses.

A. Your signature

By signing, I demonstrate that I understand the purpose and the effect of this document.

Signature: _____   Date: _____

Address: _____

B. Witnesses' signatures

I believe the person who has signed this advance directive to be of sound mind, that he/she signed or acknowledged this advance directive in my presence. The above does not appear to be acting under pressure, duress, fraud, or undue influence. I am not related to the person making this advance directive by blood, marriage, or adoption nor, to the best of my knowledge, am I named in his/her will. I am not the person appointed in this advance directive. I am not a health care provider or an employee of a health care provider who is now, or has been in the past, responsible for the care of the person making this advance directive.

Witness #1

Signature: _____   Date: _____

Printed

name: _____

Address: _____

Witness #2

Signature: _____   Date: _____

Printed

name: _____

Address: _____

Adapted with permission from the District of Columbia Hospital Association, 1250 Eye, NW, Suite 700, Washington, DC 20005; telephone: 202-682-1581; fax: 202-371-8151.

It is in your best interest to discuss your diagnosis and prognosis with your physician; such a discussion will help you decide which end-of-life treatments and life-sustaining measures you would be willing to agree to. Although this may be a challenging task, it is advisable to make a list of your wishes.

Choose the person you would like to designate as your health care proxy and make sure that that person understands what you are asking; make sure that he or she is willing to assume the responsibility inherent in the job.

Discuss specific circumstances with your health care proxy and determine how each circumstance should be handled. Examples of possible scenarios are listed below:

1. Would you want to be placed on a ventilator (a breathing machine) to extend your life if there is little hope of survival or a meaningful recovery?
2. Would you want to have all means possible (including chest compressions and electrical or chemical cardioversion) used to reverse a cardiac arrest, or would you prefer not to undergo such procedures?
3. Would you be willing to be dependent on dialysis if your kidneys failed?
4. If you were on a ventilator and there was little hope of recovery, would you want the doctors to remove you from it?
5. If you were no longer able to eat or to drink, would you want intravenous hydration and nutritional support?

Complete the advance directive. Most states require two witnesses and some states place a limit on who can act as a witness. Give one copy to your physician, one to your health care proxy, and others to family members.

WHAT DECISIONS WILL A HEALTH CARE PROXY NOT COVER?

Your health care power of attorney becomes inactive upon your death. Therefore, although you might have indicated that you wanted your organs used for transplantation, that decision will be made by your next of kin, not by your health care proxy (unless they are one and the same). However, your written document (which includes your preferences) should be used to guide the choices of your next of kin.

Your health care power of attorney does not extend to financial or other legal matters. Moreover, your health care proxy has no control over your estate.

CHAPTER 30

Treatment Decisions at the End of Life

Terry Rabinowitz, M.D., D.D.S.

WHAT ARE END-OF-LIFE DECISIONS?

As we face the end of our lives, many of us will assess what we have accomplished and what remains to be done. We may be satisfied with our achievements and at peace with approaching death, or we may feel disappointed or sad that we have not done more. Most of us will have mixed feelings: we may feel quite content with some of our successes, but probably there will be places where we wish we could have done more.

Knowing that death is approaching may cause some of us to feel pressured to accelerate the pace of our lives, so that each minute is consumed "doing" something. This urgency may lead to anxiety and stress that actually makes it more difficult to do anything. Taking the time to make important decisions about how we will be cared for when there is little time left is something that every one of us should do when there *is* sufficient time *and* when our mental functioning is as good as it can be. Thus, the ideal time to make end-of-life decisions is before we are faced with imminent death.

End-of-life decisions include those choices that each of us (or an appropriate designee) will need to make to help guide or direct the type of care we receive when we are dying. Some of these decisions might be made many years before we are faced with death. For example, a woman whose husband was on a ventilator (a respirator or breathing machine) for a long time before his death might decide that she would never wish such treatment, and she might make such a choice while still in the prime of her life. She then should appropriately document this decision so that, when her own death is imminent, no such treatment is administered. Others who are dying may not have had the opportunity or desire to make decisions about their terminal care so far in advance. Still, they should take the opportunity as soon as possible to make as many decisions about their care as they can or care to do. This chapter introduces some important end-of-life decisions that should be considered and presents information to help guide you in making choices.

WHO MAKES THE DECISIONS REGARDING MY CARE AT THE END OF LIFE?

Although many patients and those providing their care believe that others can make decisions about this care, this is not always the case; in fact, it is unlawful and unethical except in specific circumstances. For every adult, "decisional capacity" is assumed to be present unless sufficient evidence is available to support the notion that decisional capacity is impaired or absent.

Decisional capacity can be defined as the ability to understand relevant information concerning one's medical condition; the risks, benefits, and alternatives regarding a specific treatment; and the ability to communicate a choice (Table 30-1).

TABLE 30-1 Decisional Capacity

Decisional capacity is defined as
The ability to understand relevant information concerning one's medical condition
The ability to understand the risks, benefits, and alternatives regarding a specific
  treatment
The ability to communicate a choice

The capacity to make informed decisions is an essential criterion that must be ascertained early in a person's medical care so that his or her wishes are respected.

The terms *decisional capacity* and *competence* are often used interchangeably. In general, this poses no problem if one keeps in mind that *competence* is a legal term while *decisional capacity* has a less strict definition. When someone is found to be incompetent, this decision has been made by a judge after appropriate information has been brought before him or her by one or more persons who believe that the person in question lacks decisional capacity. Those who care for or about the person do not have the legal authority to judge that person as incompetent, although they may have formed an opinion about that person's competence.

Competence is a performance-specific term. That is, it defines the ability to perform or function in a particular situation or with respect to a certain task. Thus, a person may be incompetent to manage his or her finances but competent to refuse a surgical procedure or intubation (that is, placement of a breathing tube down the windpipe). It should be the standard of care for every patient that decisional capacity be assumed present or restored for as many situations as possible.

Capacity may change during the course of an illness. For instance, someone who is dying may develop an infection that causes temporary confusion. That person may have been clear-headed with full decisional capacity only a few hours earlier; now he or she is disoriented, cannot say why he or she is in the hospital, and cannot appreciate the severity of his or her medical condition. During this period of confusion, decisional capacity may be lacking, but may be restored once the infection is controlled and cognitive function—clear thinking—returns to normal.

Decisional capacity in someone who is dying can be affected by a concurrent mental disturbance. Profound depression, dementia, or anxiety, to name a few such conditions, may be severe enough to impair a person's ability to make a decision. Appropriate treatment of the accompanying symptoms may lead to restoration of decisional capacity.

The presence of one or more mental disorders, even chronic ones such as schizophrenia, bipolar disorder, or personality disorder, do not by their presence alone automatically lead to impaired decisional capacity. Most people with mental disorders who also have physical illnesses retain their ability to make a decision during most or all of their illness. In this patient population as in others, intact decisional capacity should be assumed until proven otherwise.

Decisional capacity should be assessed appropriately in every person for whom there is worry that such capacity is affected. Information from those close to the patient regarding functioning prior to illness onset, as well as expressed wishes regarding care, will be essential for this assessment. Additional studies of cognitive function (e.g., the Mini-Mental State Examination and clock drawing tests) and laboratory and diagnostic studies [such as blood tests and an electroencephalogram (EEG)] may be necessary. These tests can determine the nature and degree of cognitive disturbance and whether there is a treatable or reversible cause.

You can designate others to make health care decisions for you. That is, you may feel more comfortable having someone else make medical decisions for you although there is no question of your decisional capacity. Refer to Chap. 29 for information on how such decisions can be made and how you can increase the likelihood that those decisions will be respected.

CAN MY ABILITY TO MAKE DECISIONS REGARDING MY CARE BECOME IMPAIRED?

As stated earlier in this chapter, certain conditions might affect your ability to make decisions regarding your care. Some of these conditions might occur as a consequence of your cancer and others might result from preexisting conditions unrelated to cancer (Table 30-2). First, we will consider some conditions that can be caused by cancer that might lead to impaired decisional capacity.

Cancer has the potential to produce disturbances in any organ system in your body, either by affecting a particular organ directly or via indirect side effects. For example, cancer that has spread to the brain can compress it directly, which may result in mental status changes. On the other hand, a reduction in the red blood cell count (anemia), a side effect of some cancers, can lead to diminished delivery of oxygen to all cells of the body including those of the brain, which may also result in mental status changes.

Acute, or sudden-onset confusion is also called *delirium;* it typically evolves over a period of hours to days and represents a change from a previous, better level of mental functioning. In the setting of advanced cancer, delirium ranks among the most common causes of impaired decisional capacity.

Although the term *acute confusion* suggests that a person with such a condition would appear agitated and perhaps combative or threatening, this form of delirium is present in only about one-third of cases. The remaining two-thirds comprise depressed or mixed (i.e., agitated-depressed) forms. This makes the diagno-

TABLE 30-2 Conditions That Can Impair Decisional Capacity

Direct effects of cancer on an organ (e.g., cancer invading the brain)
Indirect effects of cancer on an organ (e.g., lymphoma that releases chemicals that cause flu-like symptoms)
Pre-existing psychiatric conditions (e.g., depression)

sis and treatment of the condition more difficult as some persons with the "quiet" form of delirium are not recognized as being delirious because they may not get someone's attention. Delirium does not always affect decisional capacity; however, when delirium is present, decisional capacity should be assessed carefully. If it is determined that the person with delirium has lost the ability to make decisions, appropriate decisions that are reflective of what that person would have wanted can be made on his or her behalf if necessary.

A preexisting mental condition also may impair the ability to make informed decisions. For example, depression in a person with cancer may be so serious that cognitive function is compromised. This is not specific to cancer, but instead may be a symptom of profound depression. The cognitive impairment may range from minimal to severe, and in some cases it may affect decisional capacity. In another person, symptoms of mania with psychotic features (involving a loss of the ability to distinguish between reality and fantasy) may be so extreme that the person no longer believes that cancer is present and begins to make decisions based upon that fallacy. This places his or her health in jeopardy.

Decisional capacity can be affected by cancer through the production of chemicals (e.g., cytokines) that may have psychotropic (mind-altering) properties or by the direct effects of cancer on any organ system of the body. Preexisting mental conditions may also affect decisional capacity in the person with cancer. When decisional capacity is in question, it is essential that all possible causes of diminished capacity be considered and ruled out or treated.

SHOULD I HAVE A "DO NOT RESUSCITATE" (DNR) ORDER WRITTEN ON MY BEHALF?

This is one of the hardest decisions that a dying person has to make. Some of the difficulty in making this decision arises from misunderstandings of what "resuscitation" involves. Miscommunications (between the person with cancer and those treating him or her, or between that person and family and friends) also contribute to difficulties in making a decision regarding resuscitation.

Many people who are unfamiliar with certain medical procedures or have only watched these procedures on television or at the movies imagine that resuscitation is a relatively simple process that is successful in a large number of patients. Unfortunately, this is not the case. Moreover, the term *resuscitation* is often taken to denote a specific process that comprises administration of medications and oxygen, intubation (placement of a breathing tube), and chest compressions. Resuscitation aims to restore an adequate airway, breathing pattern, and circulation (the "ABCs" of resuscitation) to a person.

In reality, resuscitation may require nothing more than administration of some sugar-containing liquid (in the case of a diabetic who took too much insulin) or placing someone who feels as if he or she might faint on an incline. At the other extreme, attempts at resuscitation may comprise a complex set of invasive treatments that may require considerable time and effort and which may produce significant discomfort and side effects [e.g., rib fractures or blood clots to the lungs or brain (embolism)]. Resuscitation may involve a large spectrum of treatments, some of which may be desired and some of which are refused. For decision making at the end of life, the term *resuscitation* usually refers to more complex treatments given to someone whose heart has stopped ("cardiac arrest"), whose breathing is compromised ("respiratory arrest"), or who may be experiencing symptoms that, if not treated, will lead to death.

Deciding whether you wish to be resuscitated first requires that you understand the nature and prognosis of your illness. This decision may be radically different for a person who has a potentially curable or slowly progressive cancer than for a person who has a life expectancy of only a few weeks.

Imagine that you have been admitted to a hospital for treatment of an acute (sudden-onset) problem (e.g., pneumonia, dehydration, or anemia), one that may or may not be related to your cancer. Your expectation is that once the acute problem has resolved, you will be discharged and continue your life as you had before. In such a case, you might not elect, request, or accept DNR status (because you have decided that if you are resuscitated, you might live a satisfactory life and you do not want to forgo such treatment at this time because your life might be shortened).

As a contrasting example, consider that you are facing a shorter life expectancy, say 2 months, and that you have been suffering because of your illness. You might develop pneumonia or an intestinal obstruction and be admitted to the hospital for treatment. Given that you have been suffering, you might decide that you do not wish resuscitation in the event of cardiac or respiratory arrest; *but* this may be an ideal opportunity to request better symptom control of, for example, pain or shortness of breath.

Deciding whether or not you will request or accept resuscitation requires more than the knowledge about your medical condition and its prognosis. It also requires that you understand fully what resuscitation comprises in the hospital or in your community so that you can decide among the various options presented.

For instance, many hospitals will present you with a relatively detailed list of options of what can be done for you as part of a resuscitation protocol; you may be given the opportunity to choose some and to decline others. Other hospitals may provide fewer details and may simply ask whether or not you wish to have a DNR status ordered.

For any situation in which you are asked to declare your "code status," you should make sure you know what each procedure comprising resuscitation involves *and* what consequences you might reasonably expect. For instance, resuscitation may lead to intubation (placement of a breathing tube) and to prolonged time on a ventilator (mechanical breathing machine), a treatment that you might not want but that is not expressly stated in the list of options presented to you.

There may be terms that are unfamiliar to you regarding DNR status. Unfortunately, many people unfamiliar with medical treatment may believe erroneously that they understand what these terms mean. Make sure you are completely satisfied that you understand everything you read; if you do not, ask your physician or nurse to define terms for you so that you can make the decision most appropriate for you.

Remember, in a best-case scenario, you will have made these decisions prior to ever coming to a hospital, in the comfort of your own home and with the support of your friends and family. Once you have made a decision regarding DNR status, make a copy of the form you have signed and keep it in a safe place, making sure your family is aware of its location if necessary.

SHOULD I ALLOW MYSELF TO BE PLACED ON A MECHANICAL VENTILATOR?

A mechanical ventilator is a machine that will assist your breathing or that will completely take over your breathing for you. This machine is flexible in that it can be set to "breathe" for you at a certain rate, providing a certain volume of oxygen and allowing you to breathe on your own if you are able. With this device, room air or oxygen is directed to the lungs by a tube placed in the trachea (the windpipe). For some patients, being on a ventilator is an acceptable treatment for short- or long-term management of breathing problems; for others, it is quite uncomfortable and unacceptable, even when used for short periods. Mechanical ventilation/intubation may increase the risk of developing a lung infection because it provides a more direct route for disease-causing bacteria (pathogens) to enter the lungs. Infection also may be facilitated because the normal gag and cough reflexes (two ways by which the lungs naturally protect us from foreign bodies) are bypassed.

Most of us who have had a surgical procedure have been placed on a ventilator briefly with few complications; because we were unconscious during the surgery, we remember nothing of the treatment. Problems with mechanical ventilation usually arise when someone is conscious during the treatment and experiences discomfort, either physical or psychological.

Receiving mechanical ventilation usually requires that someone remain in a hospital or a rehabilitation facility where the function of the ventilator (and the person receiving the treatment) can be monitored frequently and where necessary adjustments can be made. Speech is significantly compromised because air is diverted from the vocal cords. Many but not all people on ventilators require medications for sedation, discomfort, anxiety, or fear.

For some, it may be necessary to administer drugs that relax or paralyze the muscles to avoid interference with the ability of the ventilator to function. Conscious paralysis can be distressing; it requires use of more frequent or higher doses of antianxiety medications, which usually leads to increased sedation and decreased interaction with loved ones and care providers.

For more chronic breathing problems (generally, for people requiring a ventilator for more than 30 days), intubation may not be an acceptable or appropriate way to supply air or oxygen to the lungs, and a tracheostomy (a temporary or permanent opening in the neck to which a breathing tube is connected) may be required. A tracheostomy is a surgical procedure performed in an operating room under general anesthesia. Although this is a more complicated procedure than intubation alone, it may present the opportunity for better communication with friends and loved ones in that for some, the tracheostomy site may be temporarily blocked, allowing expired air to pass over the vocal cords, and resulting in relatively normal speech.

In considering intubation or mechanical ventilation, the following variables (stated in the form of questions for your physician) should be considered and weighed so that an informed decision about this treatment can be made:

What is my condition and prognosis?

Will my condition or prognosis be affected by intubation/mechanical ventilation/tracheostomy?

Will it be affected for better or worse?

How long is this treatment expected to continue?

Is it expected that I will die while on the ventilator?

Where will I have to be for this treatment?

For how long?

Are there other places where I can get the same treatment that are closer to home or to loved ones?

Can I have this treatment at home?

If I can go home, who needs to be there?

How often?

Is tracheostomy anticipated?

Will I require sedation, muscle relaxation, or paralysis?

Is it expected that I will have the same quality of interaction with loved ones as I do now?

If not, what changes are expected?

Can I have a consultation with the speech and language specialist?

What do you recommend?

Why?

SHOULD I ALLOW A FEEDING TUBE TO BE PLACED?

For one or more reasons, it may not be possible for you to receive adequate nutrition by eating. Possible causes of inadequate nutrition that might be due to cancer include:

Inability to swallow or painful swallowing

Loss of appetite or motivation to eat

Nausea or vomiting

Impaired absorption of nutrients

Weakness or fatigue

Your doctor may recommend that you have a feeding tube placed to help you receive adequate nutrition. Such a tube may be placed at different levels along your digestive tract. Starting at the highest point, a small-caliber, flexible tube might be inserted into your nose and passed into your esophagus (the natural tube in your body that connects your mouth to your stomach) and from there into your stomach. Sometimes this tube is advanced past your stomach into the first portion (duodenum) or second portion (jejunum) of your small intestine. The tube is taped to your nose and an x-ray usually confirms its position. It is inspected periodically for patency (making sure the opening is not clogged) by nurses or others. Usually, it is easily removed and reinserted. Some people do not like its presence and always feel as if something were caught in their throats, and for some, this feeling (or one of gagging) is intolerable.

Another type of feeding tube bypasses the mouth and esophagus and is inserted directly into the stomach via a small cut made in the abdomen. This type of feeding tube is needed for longer-term feeding needs or for situations in which it is impossible to use the type of tube described above (e.g., there may be a tumor that blocks the esophagus). This tube is placed while a person requiring such a tube is sedated or receives general anesthesia. There is usually mild to moderate discomfort which dissipates in a few days following placement of the tube.

As with any treatment, there are pros and cons to feeding tube placement. Table 30-3 lists some of these for you to consider.

To help you decide whether you want a feeding tube, it is important to consider the consequences of such treatment and to place them in the perspective of your cancer and its prognosis. Important variables that you should consider (again, stated as questions for your physician) before making your decision follow:

What is my condition and prognosis?

Will it be affected by feeding tube placement?

Will it be affected for better or worse?

How long is this treatment expected to continue?

Where will I have to be for this treatment?

For how long?

Can I have this treatment at home?

If I can go home, who needs to be there?

How often?

What do you recommend?

Why?

TABLE 30-3 Feeding Tube Placement: Some Pros and Cons

Variable	Pro	Con	Comments
Nutrition	In some people, nutrition may improve.		Improves access to important nutrients because certain impediments (e.g., mechanical obstruction) are bypassed.
Prognosis	May improve if poor nutrition is affecting health.		If there is a poor prognosis independent of nutritional status, better nutrition will produce only a modest positive effect if at all.
Comfort		May not improve with respect to the comfort derived from eating; food cannot be tasted; no mechanical "feedback" from the mouth	No social satisfaction associated with eating; hunger is usually transient and thirst may be treated with ice chips.

DO I WANT TO DIE AT HOME OR IN THE HOSPITAL?

For many people who are dying, where they will die is one of the few final decisions that will be under their control. It is possible to die at home even if your time at home will be short, and your choice to do so should be respected and supported. However, not everyone wants to die at home. For some, home evokes certain associations that they would rather leave "untouched" during dying; for these individuals, death in the hospital is preferred, and this choice should be respected.

You may feel that if you decide to die at home, you run the risk of receiving less care than you would in the hospital. For example, you may worry that you will experience more pain or anxiety. There is no way to guarantee that a home death will be better or worse than one in the hospital.

Much of what is important for many receiving terminal care—adequate pain control, closeness of loved ones, familiar surroundings, and "low-tech" treatment—may be obtained more easily at home. Also, with the generally increased availability of visiting nurses, patient-controlled analgesia (PCA) machines, and potent pain and anxiety medications, to name a few important variables, the person who decides to die at home need not worry that his or her care will suffer. In fact, it may turn out that patient preferences are respected and adhered to with greater frequency at home than they are at the hospital, as the potential for miscommunication is decreased.

HOW SHOULD I PREPARE MY FAMILY FOR MY DEATH?

Preparing your family for your death should not be your task alone. A dying person may not have the physical or emotional strength to ready loved ones for his or her impending death and may therefore need the help of others whom he or she can trust. The type, extent, and quality of the preparation will vary from family to family and will be influenced by their relationships with one another. There may be significant strengths and weaknesses in each relationship you have with someone close to you that may become more obvious when you are dying.

In preparing your family for your death, you should first make an honest appraisal of your relationship with each of the members with whom you have important "business." This appraisal might best be done in private or with the help of someone with whom you do *not* have a significant emotional attachment or long history—for example, a nurse at the hospital, a trusted member of the clergy, or a psychotherapist.

The appraisal does not have to be complex. Consider the important parts of your relationship with that other person and how you expect your death will affect him or her. Try to identify one or a small number of people who you believe will be able and willing to act as a liaison between you and all of those important to you if you choose not to, or cannot, be in contact with them. That person may be someone who will be terribly saddened by your passing but with whom you have a trusting and honest relationship.

WHICH ISSUE SURROUNDING MY DEATH SHOULD I ADDRESS FIRST?

It is impossible to say with certainty how much time any of us has left. If you expect to die shortly, try to prioritize your plans so that you have the best chance of getting the work you have identified as most important done before you die; keep in mind, though, that you may not be able to accomplish everything. Just about everyone has a personal set of priorities, and it is important that you consider all areas that you wish to address. A list of possible "domains" that you might consider follows:

Do I want a funeral?

What do I want done at the funeral?

Who should give the eulogy? Should there be music?

What do I want done with my remains?

Should I be buried or cremated?

Where?

Who will be in charge?

Do I have a will?

Is it in proper order?

What will I leave (e.g., money, possessions, property) and to whom?

Whom do I want to see before I die?

Whom do I *not* want to see before I die?

Most of us will have unfinished business with important family members or friends at the time of our deaths. As death approaches, it is not humanly possible to resolve all issues with everyone we know or care about, so it makes sense to

Work on the relationships or areas that have a chance of improving

Accept that some relationships will not improve before you die, accept your feelings about this "loss," and move on

Accept that those with whom you may not have made complete peace before you die will survive.

Many people who are dying and their families have the unfortunate fantasy that the dying process will mend seriously impaired relationships and that somehow all wounds will heal before death arrives. Commonly, such hopes or beliefs actually get in the way of some of the important work that a dying person might want to do before he or she dies.

WHAT IF MY PREFERENCES DIFFER FROM THOSE OF MY FAMILY?

There may be situations in which your end-of-life preferences are at odds with those of your family. Such differences might arise for several reasons. These include previously agreed upon (between you and your family) preferences that are no longer those that you wish to have, preferences of yours that were never acceptable to other family members, and a lack of awareness on the part of your family about your preferences (and distress after learning what they are).

Disagreements among loved ones are often uncomfortable; in the context of dying, these unpleasant conditions can deteriorate considerably, making the distress of dying even worse and causing increased friction among loved ones. Although your best interests may be paramount in the mind of a loved one, his or her feelings about what might be best for you may be different from what you want.

Others may place substantial pressure on you to change your preferences, using guilt or other feelings that may be painful and that may cause you to doubt your decision. You may decide that you will change your decision to "keep the peace" or you may try to reach a compromise with those who care about you so that all of you can live comfortably with the decision. On the other hand, you may decide to not make any changes and to live with whatever feelings your family may have. In any case, you should not feel that you have to do this alone; those caring for you should be available to help, even if they themselves do not agree with some or all of your decisions.

Remember that it is the responsibility/duty of your physician and of the other members of your health care team to respect *your* wishes and to make sure that they are carried out in every appropriate way. You also have a right to expect that your privacy will be respected and that no information will be shared with others without your consent.

CHAPTER 31

Palliative Care and Hospice

Amy E. Gagliardi, M.D.

OUTLINE

WHAT IS PALLIATIVE CARE?

Palliative care is a type of medical treatment intended to support people living with life-threatening illness. Although palliative care can be used alongside therapies aimed at curing the illness, it is most often used when the disease is progressive and cure is no longer possible. The focus of palliative care is on careful control of physical symptoms and both psychological and social (or psychosocial) issues to maximize quality of life. Optimal pain control, attention to psychological and spiritual issues, work to support the family, and coordination of medical services can have a tremendously positive impact on the experience of people living with cancer.

It is equally important to clarify what palliative care is *not*. Sometimes people believe that palliative care means that their doctor will "give up" on them or take a passive approach to their care. Palliative care is, in fact, an active process, in which physical symptoms are managed aggressively with a doctor's ongoing care. It is different from other forms of cancer treatment, however, in that the focus of care shifts from eliminating the disease to supporting people living with cancer as comfortably and as long as possible.

WHAT IS THE DIFFERENCE BETWEEN PALLIATIVE CARE AND HOSPICE CARE?

Although the terms are often used interchangeably, hospice care is really the final chapter of palliative medicine. As mentioned above, palliative care can be initiated at any point in a person's illness and becomes most important when the emphasis shifts from curing the disease to living with it comfortably. Palliative care is often initiated in the hospital and is usually coordinated by inpatient medical teams. Hospice care becomes important in the final stages of illness, when life expectancy is thought to be 6 months or less. Although it shares many goals with palliative care (e.g., pain control and management of physical symptoms), it usually is provided at home or in free-standing programs and focuses on managing treatment at the end of life.

WHAT IS THE HISTORY OF PALLIATIVE CARE?

In 1967, Dame Cicely Saunders opened St. Christopher's House in London, England, in response to what she saw as a deficit in the care of the terminally ill. Through the movement that followed, the importance of symptom management—as well as the psychological, social, and spiritual concerns of patients—was increasingly brought to the attention of health care providers. The development of continuous pain medication dosing schedules and other symptom-relief measures at St. Christopher's set an example for physicians of how to care more effectively for people living with terminal illness.

WHAT ARE THE ADVANTAGES OF PALLIATIVE CARE?

Despite many advances in medical technology, there is concern that people with terminal illnesses may not receive the quality of care they deserve. Many studies suggest that those who are dying and their families experience a wide range of unmet needs. One large U.S. study, the SUPPORT trial, highlights many of these problems. The study enrolled patients with a median survival of 6 months who were admitted to an academic hospital with advanced medical conditions. Many patients died without effective control of their pain and other symptoms, and doctors proved no better than chance in knowing whether their patients wanted life-sustaining procedures [e.g., cardiopulmonary resuscitation (CPR)]. This and other studies have highlighted the need for better management of physical symptoms and improved communication of a person's wishes.

Palliative care emphasizes good communication among a person with an illness, his or her family, and the medical team concerning control of pain and other symptoms. It incorporates an interdisciplinary approach that addresses the patient as a whole person and takes into account his or her individual needs and wishes. It allows the individual to tailor his or her care to address the physical, psychological, spiritual, and family issues that are most important to that person. And finally, it emphasizes advanced care planning that helps preserve an individual's autonomy and choice around the time of death (Table 31-1).

WHEN WILL I BECOME A CANDIDATE FOR PALLIATIVE CARE?

Palliative care becomes increasingly important as the focus of treatment shifts from curing the illness to palliation of symptoms. However, palliative care can be introduced into the medical treatment plan at any time. Some people choose to use palliative efforts earlier, in combination with curative efforts, to provide a greater

TABLE 31-1 **The Focus of Palliative Care**

Careful control of physical symptoms
Attention to psychosocial issues to maximize the quality of one's life
Optimal pain control
Attention to spiritual issues
Support of the family
Coordination of medical services and good communication
Advanced planning of care so as to preserve autonomy

focus on symptom management. The mix of curative and palliative efforts depends on the goals of care, which evolve as the disease progresses.

Another reason to consider palliative care earlier rather than later is that care at the end of life is improved if certain issues are addressed as early as possible. For example, it is much more effective to treat pain prophylactically, that is, before it starts, than to respond to the pain once it is present. The same is true for confusional states and malnutrition. In addition, emotional and psychosocial issues are easier to manage if they are addressed before one is mired in the late stages of the illness.

WHAT DO I NEED TO CONSIDER IN ORGANIZING MY PALLIATIVE CARE?

The focus of a particular palliative treatment evolves to meet a person's needs as the disease progresses. However, the treatment as a whole should be guided by specific goals of care that are determined by the person with an illness, his or her family, and the health care team (Table 31-2). The goals of care can be empowering because they provide a path to follow in times of uncertainty. They will also evolve as the disease progresses, but they can provide clarity when treatment choices become overwhelming. In developing treatment goals for palliative care, several areas should be considered.

Consider the Illness

What are my expectations about how my cancer will develop over time, and what is my expected prognosis? What are the different options for treatment, and what is the recommended treatment? Although the specific prognosis may not be clear (and it may depend on a number of factors that cannot be predicted), doctors can often provide some concept of prognosis on which to base treatment decisions.

TABLE 31-2 **Areas to Consider in Developing Treatment Goals of Palliative Care**

Consider the illness
   Prognosis
   Symptoms most likely to develop
Consider your personal values
   What is most important to you in planning for the time you have left?
   What aspects of your life do you most want to preserve?
   What are the particular circumstances of your life now and what would you
     like to see happen?
   What is possible, given the nature of your illness?

Prognosis can have significant implications for treatment planning. For example, if life expectancy is short, the goals of care will focus on the most immediate issues (e.g., comfort level, allowing for maximal time with one's family and for psychological preparation for death). It also is important to know what types of symptoms are likely to become most prominent if the cancer should progress. For example, cancer that spreads to the brain may cause confusion and loss of speech, while cancer that spreads to the digestive tract may cause other symptoms (e.g., abdominal pain, difficulty eating, or constipation), but it will not affect cognition. The development of specific treatment goals (e.g., to maximize the clarity of thinking and one's ability to communicate) should incorporate what is known about how a specific cancer spreads.

Consider Your Personal Values

What is most important to you in planning for the time you have left? What aspects of your life do you most want to preserve? What are the particular circumstances of your life now and what would you like to see happen? What is possible, given the nature of your illness? For example, someone who most values being at home with his or her family will have different treatment priorities than someone who most cares about being physically active. Target those symptoms that will interfere with the activities most important to you and develop a list of treatment priorities that protect what you care about most. Once the goals of care have been formulated, they can guide treatment decisions at any point in the course of the illness.

WHICH SYMPTOMS CAN BE TREATED BY PALLIATIVE CARE?

Several symptoms (e.g., pain, difficulty breathing, anorexia/weight loss, constipation, nausea/vomiting, neurologic changes, and psychological distress) require medical intervention near the end of life (Table 31-3). Medications can be used to control such symptoms and to enhance the quality of life at every stage of illness. In general, the goal should be to relieve symptoms while maintaining alertness as much as possible.

Pain

Although many people fear pain at the end of life above all else, almost all pain experienced by those with a terminal illness can be relieved by simple regimens that can be taken by mouth. Medication for pain should be taken at whatever dose relieves distress. When the pain is continuous, the medications can be used around-the-clock. This can be supplemented by a "breakthrough" dose that is given as

TABLE 31-3 Symptoms
That Can Be
Controlled with
Palliative Care

Pain
Shortness of breath
Digestive tract ailments
Confusional states
Depression

needed to control pain that occurs between the usual times that the medication is given.

The World Health Organization has implemented an "analgesic ladder" used in many palliative care programs to control cancer pain. In this approach, people with cancer pain are treated first with nonopioid (nonnarcotic) medications. If this is not sufficient, opioid medications are used. Finally, adjuvant (or supplementary) medications can be added to augment the effect of the opioids.

The nonopioid medications [nonsteroidal anti-inflammatory drugs (NSAIDS), and acetaminophen] often are effective for mild levels of pain. If the pain is more severe, opioid analgesics (e.g., morphine, codeine, oxycodone, hydromorphone, fentanyl, and methadone) can be used, possibly in conjunction with nonopioids. Many of the opioids cause sedation and constipation as side effects, so additional medications may be needed to counter these effects. Opioids come in a variety of forms, including long-acting (i.e., they last more than 4 hours), transdermal (administered through a skin patch), intravenous (i.e., given by vein), local anesthetic, and nerve block.

Opioid analgesics may not control pain completely in all patients; occasionally they need to be augmented with an additional "adjuvant" medication. These medications include tricyclic antidepressants (TCAs), anticonvulsants, and steroids, which may be added depending on the type of pain. Bisphosphonates also can be used to treat pain that is caused by cancer affecting the bones. Ultimately, a variety of medications can be used alone or in combination to control cancer pain and reduce suffering at the end of life. It is important to keep in mind that a person with cancer pain will not become a "drug addict" from using appropriate doses of opioid medications to relieve that pain.

Shortness of Breath

Also called dyspnea, shortness of breath can be caused by a variety of mechanisms and can be frightening to people with cancer and to their families. It can be treated in a variety of ways depending on the cause. The mainstays of treatment are supplemental oxygen and opioid medications. When the sensation of being short of breath causes anxiety, benzodiazepines can be added to reduce feelings of fear.

Symptoms Related to the Digestive Tract

Many cancers affect the digestive tract at some point in the course of illness; as a result, a variety of symptoms can develop. These may include mouth pain (from oral lesions), constipation, diarrhea, nausea, and vomiting. Ascites is caused by the accumulation of fluid in the abdomen; it can cause bloating and discomfort. Anorexia, or decreased appetite with weight loss, can result from a number of factors and is common in people with advanced cancer. There are a variety of palliative measures, including some new and some not-so-new medications for the management of mouth pain, constipation or diarrhea, nausea, and vomiting; there are also procedures to remove the fluid that builds up in ascites as well as steroids and other medications to alleviate poor appetite and weight loss. Palliation should target the specific symptoms causing the distress.

Confusional States

"Delirium" is a state of confusion that can occur in people with advanced cancer; it can be caused by a variety of factors related to either the cancer itself or to treatment of the cancer or its symptoms. Often the confusion is subtle; even when it is not, it can be treated. Psychiatric medications called *neuroleptics* (e.g., haloperidol) can be used to clear up thinking and to reduce feelings of agitation. Other palliative strategies—such as decreasing the dose of sedating medications, increasing hydration, and managing infectious or metabolic abnormalities—may help treat the underlying cause of the delirium.

Depression

Many people assume that depression is a normal or expected reaction in people with advanced cancer. They may not realize, however, that depression is a treatable illness that is different from sadness. Depression is often difficult to diagnose because many of the usual symptoms of depression (e.g., low energy, poor concentration, decreased sleep, reduced interests, and appetite) can also be caused by medical illnesses. When symptoms such as hopelessness, feelings of worthlessness, and suicidal thinking are present, however, a biological depression may be implicated. Palliative treatment should be initiated with antidepressants and possibly with stimulants [e.g., methylphenidate (Ritalin)] that can help improve mood, energy, and appetite. See Chap. 25 for further details on this topic.

CAN I INITIATE OTHER TREATMENTS WHILE RECEIVING PALLIATIVE CARE?

Yes. Often, people believe that palliative care means the cessation of treatment. In fact, it refers to the active and aggressive management of symptoms. Specific treatments and procedures may be used to address the symptoms that are causing distress. Artificial feeding, transfusion, hydration, antibiotics, chemotherapy, radiation therapy, and surgery are all interventions that can enhance the quality of life for some people. These interventions are used not to cure the underlying disease but to control or eradicate specific symptoms. For example, radiation may be used to shrink a tumor that is compressing a nerve and causing pain. Antibiotics may be used to treat an infection that is causing fever and confusion. Consideration should be given to the burden of these interventions versus the expected benefit to the person with cancer, keeping in mind the goals of care most important to the individual.

WHAT IF I WANT TO STOP A PARTICULAR TREATMENT?

Often, interventions (such as intravenous fluid administration and the monitoring of vital signs) seen as common in the hospital setting become burdensome to the person with advanced disease. Decisions regarding stopping or not initiating a treatment, however, should not be made in haste; they require careful consideration of the goals of the palliative treatment and the wishes of the person with cancer. Common issues that people often struggle with are possible use of CPR, support on a ventilator, kidney dialysis, and use of hospital admissions or emergency room visits. The competent person has the right to refuse treatment, but these decisions should be made in consultation with the medical team and with some deliberation.

Because many people with terminal cancer at some point become unable to make decisions, it can be helpful to designate a "health care proxy" (an individual, often a family member, who is legally charged with making medical decisions for you). This person can continue to advocate for your health care wishes if you become unable to do so. See Chap. 29 for more details on this topic.

WHERE SHOULD I RECEIVE PALLIATIVE CARE?

You can receive palliative care in a number of places. You can remain in an acute care hospital, return home with or without home-care services, enter a long-term-care facility with or without hospice services, or enter inpatient hospice care (Fig. 31-1). Once again, this is an extremely personal decision and is best made by considering the factors specific to your situation. Factors that may be considered include your need for symptom control, the availability of caregivers, and the level of caregiver support you require (e.g., 24-hour care, nighttime care only, or the need for help with heavy lifting). Other factors include the level of support technology required (e.g., medications taken by mouth versus intravenous infusions), the emotional supports available to you and to your caregiver, and financial considerations. The important decision of where to receive palliative care should be

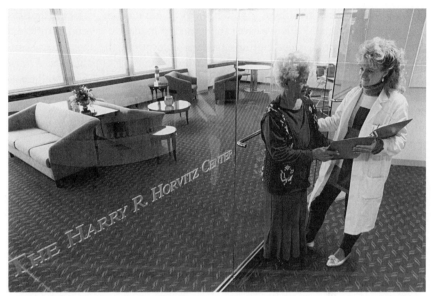

FIGURE 31-1 You can receive palliative care in a number of places, including an acute care hospital.

made with your priorities in mind and with combined input from you, your family, the medical staff, and the discharge planner or social worker.

HOW CAN I FIND OUT MORE ABOUT PALLIATIVE CARE IN MY COMMUNITY?

Many medical centers have a division of palliative medicine or a palliative care doctor on staff who can be consulted for treatment decisions. Most oncologists will be knowledgeable about palliative care and hospice services in their community as well. Resources available on the Internet include websites that can direct you to palliative care services in your area. The National Hospice and Palliative Care Organization (*www.nhpco.org*) offers information and resources for individuals looking to learn more about palliative care.

SUMMARY

Palliative care is a type of medical treatment designed to manage symptoms and to enhance quality of life. It can be implemented at any point in the course of cancer treatment, but is most often used when cure is no longer possible. The focus of treatment then shifts toward living with cancer as long and as comfortably as possible. The goals of treatment should be tailored to reflect the values and priorities of the individual. Palliative care can be used to manage a myriad of different physical and psychological symptoms and may incorporate the use of many procedures and interventions that can help to achieve the goals of palliation. A variety of options exist regarding how to incorporate palliation into the overall treatment plan, how to target symptoms, and where to receive palliative care. Most importantly, palliative care offers people the opportunity to shape their terminal care in a way that can maximize the quality of their lives.

CHAPTER 32

Rational Suicide and Euthanasia

TERRY RABINOWITZ, M.D., D.D.S.

WHAT IS "RATIONAL SUICIDE"?

Dying may be accompanied by intense, unremitting suffering that can affect your ability or desire to go on with life. You may feel that, given your terminal illness, the suffering you are experiencing cannot be justified, and you may wish to die sooner than might be expected from your illness, either by your own hand or with the assistance of someone else. This chapter covers the difficult and controversial topic of suicide or physician-assisted suicide.

Suicide is the act of intentionally killing oneself. For the purposes of this chapter, *euthanasia* is defined as physician-assisted suicide. Many, if not most, of those who study such behavior believe that suicide is the end product of irrational thinking in someone who was psychologically impaired at the time of his or her death. However, in the past one to two decades, an increasing number of experts in the field as well as many lay persons have been promulgating the notion of "rational suicide." If we believe that suicide is an irrational act, how can we place this belief in the context of the concept of rational suicide? If we believe that suicide may potentially be a rational act, can we identify criteria that, if met, would help us to decide if the act were or were not rational?

Rational suicide is a suicide that occurs with a realistic understanding of one's condition in the absence of a treatable psychiatric illness; moreover, the majority of uninvolved observers from the individual's community would find the decision acceptable.

Some physicians have proposed that the following elements be present in defining a rational suicide/physician-assisted suicide:

1. The request to die must be freely, clearly, and repeatedly made.
2. The person's judgment must not be impaired.
3. The person's condition must be incurable and associated with severe, unrelenting, intolerable suffering.
4. The suffering and the request must not result from inadequate hospice care.

Moreover, if physician-assisted suicide is planned, it should be carried out only in the context of a meaningful doctor–patient relationship, after consultation with another experienced physician. Clear documentation should offer proof that the above conditions were met.

Element 1 requires that your decision be made freely, without undue pressure, either internal or external. In deciding whether this requirement is met, you should consider what may be driving your decision. Have you ever felt suicidal when you have not been ill? If yes, what stopped or prevented you from acting on your feelings? Is that deterrent no longer present? If not, why not?

Element 2 specifies that judgment be intact. In brief, adequate judgment in the context of terminal illness and contemplation of suicide can be defined as the ability to understand the seriousness and potential for recovery from the disease in question; the risks, benefits, and types of treatment available; and the ability to identify and make a choice—in this case, not only for a particular treatment but specifically for suicide or physician-assisted suicide.

Judgment can be impaired by one or more conditions associated with your illness; every effort should be made to correct any reversible cause of impaired judgment. It is very important to remember that judgment may be compromised when depression is present. Depression is a state of chronic sadness or despondency that may be so severe that it impairs your ability to think rationally (see Chaps. 17 and 25 for more details).

Depression can be problematic in terminal illness because it may not be recognized by you or by those caring for you; as a result, you may not know that your judgment is adversely affected. Thus, you may mistakenly assume that your thinking and decision-making capacity are normal, and you may make decisions that you would not have made had you not been depressed.

Elements 3 and 4 can be addressed together. It is assumed that the suffering you are experiencing cannot be relieved; otherwise, you would, according to element 4, be receiving adequate hospice care. This is an area that you may want to explore more deeply before you finally decide that you want to take your own life.

Suffering is a domain that is inadequately addressed or treated in the large majority of those who ultimately decide they wish to hasten death. It makes sense to some that, given a terminal prognosis and intractable suffering, suicide or physician-assisted suicide is justifiable or even preferable. Before accepting that this element is present, however, you might wonder whether the suicide would be justifiable if the suffering could be managed.

A rational process (that includes discussion with your physician and a consulting physician) should be maintained to prevent decisions from being made in the heat of battle or distress. With a better understanding and better treatment of your condition, it is hoped that you will decide not to pursue suicide.

CAN THE AVOIDANCE OF SUFFERING BE GUARANTEED AS DEATH APPROACHES?

When people with cancer describe physical suffering, they usually refer to an emotional response to pain. Physical suffering can also include, for example, extreme fatigue or shortness of breath. This agony, although due to some physical cause, may also (and usually does) manifest itself as mental distress. While some who are dying have an enormous capacity to deal with both physical and emotional forms of suffering, others do not. The relative amount of suffering a person can endure is not an indicator of that person's emotional or physical hardiness but is, unfortunately, often taken to indicate how "tough" one can be when faced with adversity. By some, the admission of suffering is viewed as childish or as an indication of weakness; unfortunately, this belief leads to humiliation, a feeling that some find far worse than pain. For these people, death is preferable to shame.

Before you can discuss whether it is possible to avoid suffering as death approaches, you must first acknowledge to yourself and to others that you *are* suffering. Then, you must hope that the people listening to you will appreciate that your suffering must be addressed; it should not merely be brushed off as a "natural" response to dying that everyone eventually experiences. Admitting that you are suffering may actually take more strength than "tucking it in"!

Several powerful classes of drugs can be used to help treat physical and emotional pain in someone who is dying. Treatment is complicated in many situations, however, when these drugs are not used appropriately and/or they are used too late. In addition, some of the drugs, when administered at doses sufficient to provide effective symptom control, may cause sedation as a side effect. This brings up the concept of trade-offs in terminal care.

WHAT ARE SOME OF THE TRADE-OFFS IN MY CARE THAT I SHOULD BE AWARE OF, AND HOW MIGHT THESE AFFECT MY DECISION ABOUT SUICIDE?

The concept of trade-offs, for our purposes, is based upon the assumption that all suffering associated with dying can either be eradicated or reduced to tolerable levels. However, there will, in some instances, be a "cost" associated with the treatment—this is the trade-off. Costs may include increased somnolence, diminished mental alertness, or even an inability to control normal bodily functions.

Some people do not want their interactions with loved ones or their mental clarity to be affected adversely during their last days. They opt for increased lucidity at the expense of suboptimal pain control. While this choice should be supported, it is possible that some of these people suffer needlessly. In many cases, it is possible to treat suffering with drugs that have a long duration of action, making it possible to be comfortable, though sedated, for most of the day. When the effects of these drugs wear off and mental alertness improves, pain and suffering may become worse but tolerable. During this time of improved mental alertness, interactions with those important to you can take place, and the medication can be given again once you are alone.

Some experience humiliation when symptom control is optimized because mental clarity, appropriate behavior, continence, and other parameters may be affected. This change is remembered by the person with cancer or reported to him or her by others at a later time. This embarrassment is difficult to abide and may lead to a decision to forgo beneficial treatment, perhaps to the point where suicide looks like the only viable option.

Another decision that involves trade-offs is the question of where you will die and who will care for you. You may believe that you might not receive the same competent care at home that you would in a hospital; you may therefore decide that you want to die in the hospital (so that you won't suffer). Similarly, you may feel that dying at home will be too burdensome for others because they will have to care for you and may, in the process, suffer themselves. On the other hand, others believe that dying in the hospital is too costly and could become financially burdensome. Thus, the only "reasonable" solution seems to be to choose an early death so that others will be spared some emotional or financial expense. This logic may seem sound, but it is important to consider how your early death might affect others.

People with cancer should have frank discussions with their physicians and families regarding the trade-offs outlined above, as well as their needs and desires in their final days. These discussions should occur early in their care if possible. In this way, one's preferences can be explored and misconceptions about symptom control and other domains can be addressed and corrected during a period when urgent treatment is not required. When these matters are discussed early in the course of illness, there is time to consider alternative options and to make informed decisions.

The wish for suicide may be driven by suffering; exacerbated by depression, anxiety, or some other mental problem; and decided upon hastily or mistakenly because of impaired judgment. In the vast majority of cases, the wish for suicide is the product of the failure to recognize or to treat suffering appropriately and/or of a person's inability or unwillingness to relinquish control to others. You should confront this problem head-on so that you, your family, and your caregivers will be empowered and can work together to optimize your treatment.

WHAT IS EUTHANASIA?

Euthanasia is the intentional putting to death of a person with an incurable or painful disease; it is intended as an act of mercy. This is differentiated by some from physician-assisted suicide where a patient may actively participate in causing his or her own death, aided by a physician; in euthanasia, a patient's participation may not be necessary.

IS EUTHANASIA OR PHYSICIAN-ASSISTED SUICIDE LEGAL?

Euthanasia has been practiced for many centuries; it has been supported and embraced by some cultures and reviled by others. For many, euthanasia, suicide, or physician-assisted suicide is unacceptable because of religious or ethical convictions. In 1997, the U.S. Supreme Court ruled that there is no constitutional right to physician-assisted suicide; however, the Supreme Court did affirm a constitutional right to appropriate palliative care. Also in 1997, the people of the state of Oregon voted by a substantial majority to legalize physician-assisted suicide under certain conditions. Other states have been considering similar legislation.

In the year 2000, Oregon physicians wrote 39 prescriptions for lethal doses of medications, compared with 24 in 1998 and 33 in 1999. Of the 39 patients who received the prescriptions, 26 died after ingesting the medication, 8 died from their underlying disease, and 5 were still alive as of December 31, 2000. The 27 patients who died in the year 2000 represent a rate of 9 deaths from lethal medication per 10,000 deaths in Oregon that year. No other state has made physician-assisted suicide/euthanasia legal. In the past 5 years, ten states have passed bills making euthanasia or physician-assisted suicide illegal.

In the Netherlands, where euthanasia and, to a lesser extent, physician-assisted suicide have been socially accepted and openly practiced, euthanasia was recently legalized. An estimated 3600 cases of voluntary euthanasia are carried out each year in the Netherlands.

A survey of 3102 physicians about physician-assisted suicide and euthanasia showed that, of 1902 (61 percent) completing the survey, 11 percent reported that, in view of the current legal climate, there were circumstances under which they would consider hastening a person's death by prescribing medication; 7 percent said they would provide a lethal injection. On the other hand, 36 and 24 percent, respectively, said they would do so if it were legal. A request for physician-assisted suicide had been received by 18.3 percent and a request for a lethal injection by 11.3 percent. Some 6 percent of the responding physicians reported that they had complied with such requests at least once.

WHAT DRIVES A PERSON TO CONTEMPLATE SUICIDE?

In the year 2000, a survey of terminally ill patients and their caregivers about their desires and attitudes concerning physician-assisted suicide and euthanasia was conducted. It showed that, of the 998 terminally ill patients queried, 60.2 percent supported euthanasia or physician-assisted suicide in a hypothetical situation, but only 10.6 percent reported that they would seriously consider these options for themselves. Factors associated with being *less* likely to consider euthanasia included feeling appreciated, being 65 years of age or older, and being African American. Factors associated with being *more* likely to consider physician-assisted suicide or euthanasia included the presence of depressive symptoms, having substantial care needs, and being in pain (Table 32-1). One can infer from this study that the likelihood of requesting physician-assisted suicide or euthanasia will diminish if certain symptoms are better controlled.

The study cited above and others that deal with suicide, physician-assisted suicide, and euthanasia show that there is a cluster of symptoms, attitudes, and beliefs that predict a desire to commit suicide or to request physician-assisted suicide. Some of these important determinants are as follows:

Experiencing pain or suffering

Feeling depressed or despondent

TABLE 32-1 Factors Associated with the Consideration of Euthanasia

---

Factors making people *less* likely to consider physician-assisted euthanasia
Feeling appreciated
Being 65 years of age or older
Being African American

Factors making people *more* likely to consider physician-assisted suicide or euthanasia
Presence of depressive symptoms
Having substantial care needs
Being in pain

Being short of breath

Feeling alone or abandoned

Feeling worthless

Feeling hopeless

Many or all of these symptoms, attitudes, and beliefs have the potential to respond to appropriate treatment. When they are corrected, the wish to hasten death may fade. For instance, depressive symptoms may respond quickly (after one or two doses) to psychostimulant medications (such as dextroamphetamine or methylphenidate). When depression improves, pain and suffering may also improve, and the wish for euthanasia or physician-assisted suicide may disappear (see Chaps. 17, 22, and 25 for more information on this subject).

WHAT IS THE "RULE OF DOUBLE EFFECT" AND HOW COULD IT APPLY TO ME?

Although many patients and physicians are opposed to physician-assisted suicide or euthanasia, most believe that suffering must be treated aggressively. This may cause emotional conflict for both patients and doctors, who might worry that by treating pain aggressively with medications that may depress the drive to breathe, death will be hastened. For patients opposed to suicide, physician-assisted suicide, or euthanasia, and for those physicians who don't wish to cause a patient's death or to contribute to it (for ethical and/or legal reasons), it may be difficult to accept (patient) or to prescribe (physician) appropriate doses of medications. The result may be that suffering continues, although it could have been alleviated.

According to the rule of double effect, however, this line of thinking is misguided. The rule of double effect states that, if there was no intent to kill but only to relieve suffering, no ethical principle was violated. For example, administering high doses of opioids (e.g., morphine) to treat a terminally ill patient's pain is morally justifiable even if it contributes to or causes the patient's death. Another example would be a physician who attempts to treat a dying patient's depression aggressively with an antidepressant or psychostimulant and, as a result, produces a fatal cardiac arrhythmia. In determining whether a given action was acceptable, the rule relies on the *intent* of the treatment, not the result.

The rule of double effect, developed by Roman Catholic theologians, has its origins in the Middle Ages. For this reason, some feel that it is too religion-based to be a useful guide for treatment of patients in the United States, comprising people who have such varied ethnic, religious, and social backgrounds. However, the principle of intent can be applied in any circumstance in which suffering and potentially fatal treatment is being considered. It is a good opportunity for a person with cancer and his or her physician to discuss treatment options frankly and for physicians to let their patients know, "I won't kill you or contribute to your killing yourself, but I will do *everything* necessary to stop your suffering."

CHAPTER 33

Grief and Bereavement

Paul Hammerness, M.D.
Ned H. Cassem, M.D., S.J.

OUTLINE

WHAT IS GRIEF?

Grief is a natural reaction to loss; it does not in itself suggest the presence of an illness. It is the beginning step of the process of mourning, which follows such losses as death, personal injury, illness, isolation, or deprivation. Grief may be influenced by religion, culture, and personality, as well as by the nature and significance of the loss experienced.

WHAT DO MOST PEOPLE EXPERIENCE WHEN THEY SAY THEY ARE GRIEVING?

Signs and symptoms of grief may include crying, wailing, pleading, and making statements of hopelessness, as well as experiencing feelings of loneliness, helplessness, and despair. Poor appetite, difficulty sleeping, and anhedonia (a lack of pleasure or a decreased interest in one's usual activities) may follow. Emotional numbing or a lack of feeling may occur (Table 33-1). While the person or function that has been lost may be thought of or presented to others in an idealized way, mixed feelings typically exist. However, emotions such as anger may be more difficult to admit or to share openly. If so, guilt may then follow, as a consequence of conflicted, unexpressed feelings.

WHAT IS THE DIFFERENCE BETWEEN GRIEF, BEREAVEMENT, AND MOURNING?

While not consistently or universally applied, grief has been defined as the feelings and behaviors associated with loss, bereavement as the fact of loss, and mourning as the social expressions of loss, as observed in funerals or cultural rituals. Symptoms of grief can be similar to those of major depressive disorder (MDD); these include poor sleep, decreased appetite, and feelings of sorrow.

TABLE 33-1 Signs and Symptoms of Grief

Crying
Wailing
Pleading
Making statements of hopelessness
Experiencing feelings of loneliness, helplessness, and despair
Poor appetite
Difficulty sleeping
Anhedonia (a lack of pleasure or a decreased interest in one's usual activities)
Emotional numbing or a lack of feeling

WHAT ARE THE PHASES OF GRIEF AND RECOVERY?

Not every person mourns in the same manner. However, phases of grief frequently proceed as follows: shock, disbelief, denial, gradual realization, and eventual return to function (Fig. 33-1). There may be moments or periods of return to prior phases along this path of recovery. Before one can adjust to the reality of a loss (e.g., the loss of a loved one or a diagnosis of cancer, which represents the loss of health), with a return to full function, the loss must be accepted, both intellectually and emotionally.

Using the example of the loss of a loved one, in the first step, one must develop an intellectual account or understanding of how the loss occurred. The next step brings emotional acceptance of the loss, with a gradual reduction of the intensity of feelings of loss and/or pain. This emotional acceptance is accomplished slowly over time, with repeated exposure to memories of the lost one and reminders of him or her, accompanied by a renewal of acute grief. The pangs of recalled conflict with anger or harsh words intensify and prolong grief. Eventually, as balance between love and anger is achieved, pain in recollection is replaced by feelings of fondness and comfort. This gradual transformation may be

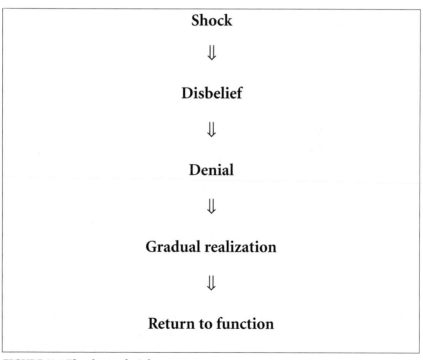

FIGURE 33-1 *The phases of grief.*

accompanied by such moments, as when one imagines that the lost person is still present.

Finally, function returns, with less distancing and denial despite reminders of the loss. This process has also been described as moving from disorganization to reorganization. Patterns of thinking, acting, and living are reorganized into a new existence. Yet, in the best sense, one carries the lost person forever as a positive force for self-esteem and facing obstacles.

WHAT IS MEANT BY "DENIAL"?

Denial is a defense used to protect one's immediate consciousness against difficult or unbearable realities. At times, some degree of denial is healthy; it may allow you to function without the chaos fueled by anxiety, anger, or despair. Denial typically evolves over time. However, on occasion, denial can be unyielding and problematic and can jeopardize one's safety (e.g., preventing one from seeking timely medical care or leading one to take unnecessary risks).

HOW LONG DOES BEREAVEMENT TYPICALLY LAST?

Symptoms of bereavement vary and can last for several months. When bereavement has proceeded well, you may achieve a new equilibrium and function by the end of the first year. However, despite the resumption of normal duties or employment within a few months, it may take 2 or 3 years for you to develop comfort with your new reality or identity.

WHAT ELSE COULD IT BE IF IT IS NOT GRIEF? (COULD IT BE DEPRESSION?)

A person who is grief-stricken may also be suffering from an ongoing medical or psychiatric illness or a substance abuse or dependence problem. A loss also may exacerbate a prior problem or an illness that was in remission. Of special importance is determining whether what appears to be grief is in fact major depression. An episode of major depressive disorder (MDD) may signify a recurrence of major depression, or it may represent the first episode in reaction to a significant stressor: in this case, a loss. This topic is covered in greater detail in Chap. 25.

Major depression is defined as a change of functioning marked by either depressed mood (though it can be an irritable mood in children or adolescents) or diminished interest or pleasure in activities most of the day, nearly every day, over a 2-week period. It is also characterized by four or more of the following symptoms: disturbed sleep, worthlessness or guilt (about things other than actions taken or not taken by the survivor at the time of death), diminished ability to concentrate, disturbed appetite or weight change, thoughts of death (other than the survivor feeling that he or she would be better off dead or should have died with the deceased person) or suicide, marked psychomotor retardation (slowed mentation and physical movements) or agitation (restlessness), and fatigue or loss of energy. Hallucinatory experiences may occur in the context of an episode of MDD, beyond thinking that one hears the voice of the deceased person or transiently sees his or her image, as may occur with grief.

Major depression is not an appropriate reaction to a loss or stressor. It is a serious illness (despite seeming so "understandable"), and it requires treatment. Left untreated, it may lead to other medical conditions, to impaired function, or to death by suicide. In the setting of major depression, medical and/or psychiatric attention is well advised. The diagnosis of major depression after a loss is not given unless the signs and symptoms meet the standard criteria as listed above and last for more than 2 months from the moment of loss. Exceptions to this general rule include reactions to the loss of a partner or spouse or to the loss of a child.

WHAT IS CONJUGAL BEREAVEMENT?

Conjugal bereavement is bereavement due to loss of a spouse or partner. Researchers of older populations have studied this specific loss. Conjugal bereavement is commonly associated (in up to 15 percent) with symptoms of major depression up to 13 months after loss and has been associated with an increased rate of suicide. Despite the clear impact of bereavement on the mental health of older adults, therapy for conjugal bereavement fails to meet rigorous evidence-based standards.

However, clinicians do know that treatment regularly works. In one recent study involving 80 persons over the age of 50 years with bereavement (following death of a spouse), the combination of nortriptyline (a tricyclic antidepressant) and interpersonal therapy was more effective than placebo (a sugar pill) or either treatment alone. In other words, a clinician should offer a depressed, grieving patient standard treatment for major depression as soon as the person meets the diagnostic criteria outlined in the preceding section.

WHAT HAPPENS WHEN A CHILD DIES?

When a child dies, the parent may feel that his or her future has died as well. Parents may mourn unmet expectations for the child, feel a sense of failure as a protector, or feel that the world seems unfair, uncertain, and out of control. As with other forms of grief, the loss of a child is best understood within a family's social and cultural context. In parents of fatally ill children, early phases of numbing and disbelief occur, as the parents face the impending loss. Anger may be voiced at the physicians or others bearing the news, or it may be turned inward, in self-reproach.

While each parent may experience loss in a different way, a healthy mourning process will follow for those couples able to somehow unite in grief. Sadly, divorce is common following the death of a child. In addition, the health of the surviving children may depend on the ability of the parents (alone or apart) to mourn together.

HOW DO CHILDREN COPE WITH LOSS?

The study of grief in children can be traced back to the 1960s, when John Bowlby presented attachment and loss as pivotal to the study of human development. Bowlby wrote a series of three volumes on attachment, separation, grief, and mourning, in which he described children's responses to loss under favorable and unfavorable conditions. Favorable conditions include the presence of a secure relationship prior to loss, the provision of prompt and accurate information, the chance to ask questions and to participate in family grief, and the knowledge of a surviving parent or substitute (Table 33-2). A clear difference between an adult and a child's grief is the child's dependence on others to assist with this process.

Despite the complex influences of present cultures, religions, and family systems on childhood grief, emotional and/or behavioral symptoms of distress following loss typically include nonspecific symptoms, such as a depressed or anxious mood and somatic symptoms (e.g., physical complaints; feeling ill). Temper outbursts, acting-out behaviors, and difficulties with peer or sibling relationships may occur. Despite (and because of) the significant impact of loss, children may quickly return to play or to school as a means of coping.

Those persons who sustain a loss in childhood may have an increased risk of developing a psychiatric condition later in life. A recent in-depth review of the outcome in children suffering a loss found dysphoria (unhappiness) commonly reported (in up to 70 percent), but the prevalence of a clinical diagnosis of depression varied (8 to 26 percent). Other symptoms included anxiety (of separation, and manifested as fears about the safety of the surviving parent), somatic complaints (e.g., headache and abdominal pain), and symptoms consistent with posttraumatic stress disorder, when the loss was associated with trauma (e.g., a parent

TABLE 33-2 Children's Responses to Loss

Favorable responses depend on the following:
The presence of a secure relationship prior to loss
The provision of prompt and accurate information
The chance to ask questions and to participate in family grief
The knowledge of a surviving parent or substitute

who dies in a car accident). The gender of the child may also influence the expression of grief; higher rates of acting out and psychiatric difficulties were observed in boys, while girls tended to internalize their feelings. The presence of dysfunctional mental health symptoms in the surviving parent appeared to influence outcome for the child. No clear influence on outcome was found in association with the type of death (as in murder or suicide), sudden loss compared to expected death, the death of a mother versus that of a father, the age of the child, the attendance of the child at the parent's funeral, or general levels of family function.

The American Academy of Child and Adolescent Psychiatry (AACAP) has published several public service "Facts for Families" booklets; these include *Children and Grief, When a Pet Dies,* and *Helping Children After a Disaster.* These guides discuss common developmental reactions to loss and include warning signs of problems with the grieving process or responses to other stressors. Practical advice can also be found in guidebooks, published by the National Center for Grieving Children and Families, such as *35 Ways to Help a Grieving Child.*

HOW DO CHILDREN COPE WITH THE LOSS OF A PARENT?

Bereavement may be particularly long and complicated following the uniquely difficult loss of a parent, and it may be reexperienced throughout a child's life. An understanding of the developmental principles of how children at different ages grieve as well as the commonalities among all children will help guide caregivers in this process (Table 33-3). In addition, the loss of a parent may leave a child with a heightened sense of vulnerability (and perhaps with symptoms of posttraumatic stress).

TABLE 33-3 Helping Children Cope with the Loss of a Parent

Infants	Meet immediate needs with consistency, as the infant will be most affected by the sorrow and functioning of the survivors. Create memorabilia, such as letters, tapes, or photographs of the dead or dying parent to provide a bridge to recollections in later years.
Preschoolers	Explore likely misconceptions about feelings of responsibility for the death of a parent and a surviving parent's withdrawal and sadness.
School-age children	Communicate to provide an understanding of the circumstances, without overwhelming the child with detail. Allow children at this age to visit a dying parent in the hospital or to attend a funeral, but don't force them to do so.
Adolescents	Support teens in turning to each other for support, and in finding an adult with whom to share feelings of loss. Adolescents will be interested in the meaning of life and death.

Overall, it is important for all children to continue age-appropriate activities. It is critical for the surviving adult(s) to assess the children for depression. While physical activities, art work, and play may provide outlets for a child's energy and emotion, perhaps the most valuable gift to a child suffering a loss is to listen to his or her story.

For infants, meeting immediate needs with consistency is the primary task of caregivers, as the infant will be most affected by the sorrow and functioning of the survivors. Creating memorabilia—such as letters, tapes, or photographs of the dead or dying parent—may provide a bridge to recollection in later years.

Because a preschooler may feel responsible for the death of a parent and may misunderstand a surviving parent's withdrawal and sadness, exploration about likely misconceptions will help to reduce guilt in this age group. Communication with school-age children should provide an understanding of the circumstances without overwhelming the child with detail. Children at this age may wish to visit a dying parent in the hospital or to attend the parent's funeral. A familiar adult, with proper explanation of the emotional and physical setting, should guide the child through these events. The child should not be forced to touch the parent, whether living or dead, or to attend the funeral.

While teens often turn to each other for support, it is important for the adolescent to find an adult with whom to share feelings of loss; this may include a teacher, clergy, friend, or mental health professional. Teenagers are more interested in the meaning of life and death than are younger children. Yet, with their egocentric view of the world, teens may be more focused on their own personal grief.

HOW DO DIFFERENT CULTURES GRIEVE?

While there may be certain universal patterns or themes in grief and bereavement, individuals understand death and dying within their own cultures and therefore manifest grief in unique ways. It is important to allow people to express or conduct mourning practices or rituals; in so doing, they honor the loss according to these cultural norms.

Death may be understood as a social affair, affecting to varying degrees the community as well as the individual. However, direct involvement by family or by the community in the process of death varies widely. In western societies, there often is a process of distancing oneself from direct contact with the deceased. In other cultures, young children are directly exposed to death, with death occurring at home more often than in a hospital setting. Distancing from the reality of death, as well as trends toward secularization, are influential factors in shaping grief in western societies. Bereavement counselors, mental health specialists, or educators in schools may play increasingly important roles in the process of loss and mourning.

Discussions on culture and grief have included articles on Latino cultures, on rural Mexican families, on Asian and Tibetan expressions of bereavement, on traditional healers and bereavement in Cambodia refugee populations, and on Ethiopian immigrants. A comprehensive textbook on this topic by Parkes and associates (1997) presents bereavement and mourning practices across several major world systems, including Hindu, Tibetan Buddhist, Jewish, Christian, and Islamic cultures.

HOW CAN I BEST HELP SOMEONE ELSE WHO IS GRIEVING?

Despite the strong pressure from others to end the grieving process prematurely (with overt or subtle cues to "move on"), the goals of intervention and support are not to force an end to this process. Interventions for those who are grieving should focus on being present and supportive in words and deeds. Listening should allow an open expression of grief. Some people may not wish to speak soon after a loss; instead, finding a quiet place in which to commune in silence may serve as an adequate initial intervention.

In addition, one should assess the level of social supports, including those immediately available; this may include an intervention as practical as offering a ride home from the hospital if that is where the loss occurred. It also is useful to remember that the deceased may have been a caregiver for a child, a spouse, an elderly parent, or another individual who is now in need of medical or other functional assistance.

Grief-stricken individuals should be encouraged to attend to their usual activities of daily living and to partake in basic self-care. The continued presence and support of helpful others, and not just early support in accomplishing basic tasks, is of utmost importance. Grief may alter individual relationships and family systems dramatically and leave those who are afflicted even more isolated.

Help with grief is most effective when it is tailored to the individual's experience of loss. For example, those suffering from sudden loss may benefit from open disclosure and the sharing of feelings, thereby making the loss real. Loss following a conflicted relationship may be helped best through the promotion of early grieving, sharing self-reproach and guilty feelings, and helping the family reorganize and support each other. Increasing the survivor's self-esteem and efficacy may help after a loss of a highly dependent relationship. Finally, understanding the cultural context may be the most valuable first step in assisting an individual with his or her grief.

WHAT FEATURES OF GRIEF SUGGEST THE NEED FOR TREATMENT? WHAT IS PATHOLOGIC OR COMPLICATED GRIEF?

Most grief resolves without medical or psychiatric intervention. However, grief may stray from its normal, healthy course and be considered "pathologic" (pathology is the study of disease processes, and the term *pathologic* relates to a disease state). Presence of the following symptoms for more than a year after a loss may indicate a complicated grief disorder: pangs of intense emotion, feelings of being excessively alone or empty, social withdrawal, severe intrusive thoughts, unusual sleep disturbance, distressed yearnings, maladaptive loss of interest, and avoidance of tasks reminiscent of the deceased.

Grief syndromes that may benefit from professional interventions include unexpected or sudden loss with an inability to accept the loss, grief associated with a conflicted relationship before the loss (manifest by little early grief, then later by worsening of symptoms and painful yearnings), and dependent grief from faulty attachments, which results in subsequent chronic grief. A recent study of mid- to late-life bereaved spouses found traumatic grief to be predictive of not only psychiatric symptoms but also of physical illness.

WHAT CAUSES COMPLICATED, PATHOLOGIC, OR CHRONIC GRIEF?

Grief is an expression of attachment. Therefore, observed patterns of grief can be traced to the relationship lost and perhaps to earlier childhood patterns of attachment. In addition, social influences may play a role through inhibition of the expression of grief or its resolution (e.g., "carrying the torch" forever).

For example, in a study of approximately 70 Boston widows and widowers under the age of 45, predictors of a failure to recover from conjugal bereavement included yearning (often associated with dependency), sudden loss, and anger or self-reproach, which seemed to be associated with an ambivalently held or conflicted relationship.

Difficulty and fears of living independently following a loss may be associated with true dependency, not just simply with missing one's companion. People in such relationships may also complain of the struggle to accept the reality of the loss, of poor concentration, of fears of mental collapse, of desires for someone to "take over," of feelings that the deceased person is watching over them, and of increased feelings of loneliness. These characteristics may have childhood antecedents in fears of separation or in seeing the world as a dangerous place. Isolation may prolong the grief reaction, as can an imagined continued relation with the deceased, lack of self-confidence, and a lack of solace and continued support from others.

Sudden loss may result in another form of chronic or complicated grief, particularly if accompanied by an inability to accept reality or by anger and guilty feelings. At 2 to 4 years of follow-up, this subset of Boston widows/widowers often made statements such as "It's not real," "I wouldn't care if I died," and "I feel that I could have done something to prevent the death." This sense of randomness and unpredictability in the world may breed fear and isolation.

Loss of an ambivalent or conflicted relationship may result in a complicated and chronic bereavement as well. Delayed expressions of grief, with guilt and remorse, may occur, as anger may interfere with the expression of early grief. This form of grief may be experienced by individuals with generalized insecurity or difficulties with attachment.

HOW CAN DOCTORS BEST HELP SOMEONE WHO IS EXPERIENCING GRIEF?

As doctors struggle with an inherent desire to fix or to cure, they may neglect the areas of death and suffering. The more a physician understands and evaluates his or her own reactions to loss and suffering, the more he or she will be available to a patient.

The physician can play a special role in this difficult process. In confronting the person who has sustained a loss or in breaking bad news about a death or other loss, it is crucial to keep certain fundamentals in mind. One must be able to speak freely and openly with the person/family in an appropriate setting, at eye level, and in a place where the words may be heard. One must anticipate projected anger and be able to accept this as part of the grieving process. Acknowledging and allowing for a person's spirituality may suggest individual understanding and provide great comfort.

Little has been published regarding how physicians actually conduct grief work. A recent poll of 400 primary care physicians in Ohio provided some insights into this area. Doctors reported that addressing grief is both important and satisfying, and that patients are interested in talking with them about their reactions. Doctors typically identified grieving patients following a known loss, when the patient appeared depressed, or when physical symptoms did not "add up." The physicians decided how to respond primarily based on the relationship that the patient had to the deceased or to the loss, on the nature of the available supports, on whether death was a sudden one or a suicide, and on whether the doctor knew the patient well.

Treatment involved expressing condolences, encouraging the grief-stricken person to talk about his or her loss with family and friends, providing anticipatory guidance, touching the patient (the most common gesture—83 percent), and arranging for more frequent appointments. When the patient raised the topic, 60 percent of the physicians discussed spiritual concerns; roughly half would ask about spirituality.

Regarding treatment, 71 percent of this sample of primary care physicians would prescribe medications for insomnia, 68 percent would prescribe medications if the person were "clinically depressed," and 55 percent would prescribe treatment to newly bereaved patients for a short period. Medications used included antidepressants (63 percent), benzodiazepines (for sedation or anxiety; 43 percent), antihistamines (25 percent), and low-dose antidepressants for sedation (20 percent). A barrier to treatment voiced by a majority of primary care physicians was inadequate time (87 percent).

Most of the physicians sampled had learned how to perform grief work through clinical or personal experience, whereas only one-third reported contact with mental health professionals about this topic. Responsiveness of the doctor was more likely if he or she perceived that the patient wanted to talk and if the physician felt it was helpful, rewarding, and important to do so. In addition, increased physician comfort with crying patients, more comfort with expressions of personal loss, involvement in spiritual pursuits, and continuity of care were factors that improved the doctor's responsiveness.

WHAT MEDICATIONS ARE USEFUL IN TREATING GRIEF OR BEREAVEMENT?

When medications are used for the state of grief, they should be taken with specific goals in mind and for a limited time. In general, medications are not the primary treatment for grief. Low doses of medications (such as lorazepam 0.5 mg) may be used to promote sleep. Even low-dose benzodiazepines (such as lorazepam), however, may leave a person feeling groggy in the morning and unable to participate in activities or to think or process information clearly. Antidepressants may be prescribed when the diagnosis of major depression is made or for related underlying psychiatric and/or medical conditions.

HOW CAN I BEST PREPARE OTHERS FOR IMPENDING LOSS?

In assisting people with an impending loss, through cancer or another illness, communication is paramount. The single most important topic is conflict resolution, both for the dying person and for loved ones. This should be empathically and aggressively addressed, long before the patient is too ill or disabled to forgive, to thank, and to tell family members that he or she loves them.

In first communicating difficult news (of any sort), information should be delivered clearly and must be received and understood. It should be given in familiar terms, in a language that fits with the person's understanding of the illness. Such communications should be rehearsed; they should be brief and designed to give reassurance regarding continued care and attention as well as to encourage further open dialogue.

Open communication with the person who is dying is preferable; yet one must acknowledge the pace at which he or she wants this information. The goal of enhanced communication is an improved quality of life with maintained hope, not forced acceptance. A dying person can support close family and friends who are grieving as well, with supportive statements that might convey that they are forgiven, will survive, can function independently, and can form new identities and relationships.

Finally, one should be given a chance to process ongoing relationships. Family and friends should be given the opportunity to care fully for the person who is facing an impending death. People should be allowed to hold a vigil or to care for the dying based upon their upbringing, religion, or culture.

Glossary

ABCD rule: an acronym standing for **a**symmetry, **b**order irregularity, **c**olor variegation, and **d**iameter; each of these signs makes a skin lesion more likely to be a melanoma.

Abulia: lack of will or motivation.

Accuracy: a statistical term that describes the proportion of a test's results that correctly identifies the tested individual as either having or not having the relevant cancer.

Acupressure: a Japanese practice, also known as Shiatsu massage, that uses finger pressure instead of needles to stimulate specific points along the body in order to restore the body's life energy and bring it back into balance.

Acupuncture: a Chinese practice that uses fine needles inserted into specific areas along the body; when these areas are stimulated, they help rebalance natural energy flow within the body.

Acute pain: a new-onset pain that typically is accompanied by physical signs of pain, such as sweating, an increase in blood pressure and heart rate, and facial grimacing.

Adenocarcinoma: a type of cancer that originates in glands; it is a common cancer of the breast, colon, stomach, prostate, and pancreas.

Adjuvants: medications that enhance the effects of analgesics.

Adrenaline: a chemical produced by the adrenal glands; it stimulates the heart to beat faster and the lungs to breathe harder.

Advanced directive: a combination of a living will and a health care proxy; it guides caregivers to make the health care decisions you would make for yourself if you become incapacitated.

Agnosia: lack of ability to recognize familiar objects despite intact sensory function.

Akathisia: restlessness; the inability to sit still.

Alkylating agent: a type of cancer chemotherapy that either causes DNA to become too sticky, so it cannot be copied, or causes breaks in the DNA, which prevents it from being copied.

ALL: acute lymphoid (or lymphoblastic) leukemia.

Allogeneic bone marrow transplantation (BMT): the bone marrow transplantation procedure in which the person with cancer receives normal bone marrow from a healthy donor.

Alopecia: loss of hair.

Alternative medicine: sometimes called integrative or nontraditional therapy; it comprises a large number of health-related therapies, behaviors, and practices that are considered outside the realm of traditional western medicine.

Amenorrhea: a lack of menstruation.

AML: acute myeloid (or myelogenous) leukemia.

Amniocentesis: a technique that samples the amniotic fluid surrounding a fetus for the purpose of analyzing cells, in order to determine the gender of the fetus and to look for the presence of several genetic conditions.

Analgesic ladder: a graduated approach to the selection and administration of analgesics for pain control.

Analgesics: medications that treat pain.

Anemia: the state of having a low red blood cell count.

Angiogenesis: the formation of new blood vessels.

Angiogenesis inhibitors: a class of cancer-fighting drugs that prevent growth of new blood vessels into a tumor, thereby preventing the tumor's growth.

Anhedonia: a lack of pleasure or a decreased interest in one's usual activities.

Anorexia: a decrease in or absence of appetite.

Antibodies: proteins made by white blood cells, which protect the body from infections.

Anticonvulsant: an antiseizure medication with mood-stabilizing and adjunctive analgesic effects.

Antiemetic: an antinausea medication.

Apathy: absence of emotion; indifference.

Aphasia: a difficulty with the transmission of language (e.g., speaking, reading, writing, or repeating).

Apoptosis: the process of programmed cell death.

Aprosodia: lack of pitch, rhythm, and modulation of speech.

Aromatherapy: the use of highly concentrated plant extracts to balance and restore the body, mind, and spirit.

Ascites: the accumulation of fluid in the abdomen.

Auditory cortex: that portion of the brain that receives auditory information (sounds) and then sends that information to the temporal lobe for processing.

Autologous bone marrow transplantation (BMT): the bone marrow transplantation procedure in which the person with cancer is both the donor and the recipient of the bone marrow.

Autopsy: an examination of a body by a pathologist to determine the cause of death.

Autosomal dominant inheritance: a type of transmission of genetic cancer risk that gives each child a 50 percent chance of developing cancer.

Autosomal recessive inheritance: a type of transmission of genetic cancer risk in which both parents must pass on to the child a cancer-causing gene for the child to develop cancer; each child has a 25 percent chance of developing the cancer.

Azoospermia: the prolonged absence of sperm in the semen.

Barrett's esophagus: precancerous changes in the lining of the esophagus that may result in adenocarcinoma of the esophagus, a type of cancer.

Basal ganglia: a structure within the brain that helps to regulate coordinated movements.

Baseline tests: tests (e.g., radiographic or chemical) that measure tumor size or the level of function of normal organs (e.g., of a tumor marker, or liver or kidney function) before a medication or treatment is begun.

Basophils: white blood cells that help regulate allergic responses.

B cells: white blood cells that make a particular type of antibody.

Benign: noncancerous or not harmful.

Benzodiazepine: a class of medication that relieves anxiety.

Biofeedback: a technique that helps shape behavioral and physiologic responses by informing the person about his or her state of arousal and muscle tension.

Biopsy: a surgical procedure (often minor) in which tissue is obtained from an organ thought to be involved with cancer.

Bladder: an organ in the pelvis that stores urine; it is shaped like a triangular balloon.

Blood-brain barrier: a filter that purifies the blood that reaches the brain; this barrier prevents many chemicals that might be toxic to the brain from reaching it, as well as many medications.

Bone marrow: a large liquid organ responsible for production of blood components; it is found inside most long and flat bones of the body.

Bone marrow biopsy: a procedure in which a needle is placed into the bone marrow to remove cells for analysis by a pathologist, often performed on the hip.

Bone marrow collection: the bone marrow from a donor that is administered to a recipient.

Bone marrow recipient: the person who receives the harvested bone marrow.

Bone marrow suppression: inhibition of bone marrow function that leads to diminished production of red blood cells, white blood cells, and platelets.

Bone marrow transplantation (BMT): a treatment that uses high doses of chemotherapy and often radiation to eliminate most of the bone marrow stem cells; this is followed by the infusion of new stem cells from another person of from the person with cancer.

Brachytherapy: high-energy radiation from a radiation source, such as radiation seeds, placed within the body and delivered into a small area; the radiation source is placed as close as possible to the cancer cells, e.g., in the prostate.

***BRCA1* and 2:** cancer genes that predispose a woman to developing breast or ovarian cancer.

Bronchoscopy: a procedure in which a tube with a fiberoptic camera is inserted through the mouth and down the throat into the lungs; it allows examination of the trachea and bronchi and can be used to biopsy lung tissue.

Burnout: a term used to describe a syndrome of fatigue, temper outbursts, substance use, bodily complaints, and other manifestations of stress.

Cancer: an abnormal growth of cells; often referred to as a mass, growth, tumor, nodule, spot, lump, lesion, or malignancy.

Cancer in the bones: a nonspecific phrase referring to cancer that has spread to the bones or has originated in the bones.

Cancer screening: performing tests for cancer on people who have no symptoms of cancer and have not already been diagnosed with the cancer for which they are being tested.

Cancer susceptibility gene: a gene that causes a person to be more prone to developing cancer.

Carcinogen: a cancer-causing agent, e.g., cigarette smoke or radiation.

Cardiac arrest: the state when the heart has stopped beating.

Case manager: a member of the health care team who deals with insurance issues and coordinates home services if needed; such a person may serve as a link between a person with cancer and his or her health care team.

CEA: Carcinoembryonic antigen, a type of tumor marker used most commonly to follow colon or lung cancer.

Central line: an intravenous (IV) catheter placed in the chest wall or neck; it tunnels into large veins at the base of the neck or under the collarbone.

Cerebral cortex: the outermost section of the brain, associated with higher-level thinking.

Chemotherapy: the use of chemicals (drugs) in the treatment or control of cancer.

Chi Kung: a Chinese mind-body technique that uses different positions to facilitate using the body effortlessly; in doing so it aims to unite the body and mind.

Child-life specialist: a mental health professional who specializes in the care of children.

Cholangiocarcinoma: cancer of the gallbladder.

Chromosome: the carrier of genetic information in the form of genes and DNA and thus the "blueprints" for a cell's function; chromosomes are located within the cell's nucleus.

Chronic pain: unlike acute pain, this type of pain typically occurs in the absence of physical signs; it is pain that has lasted for more than 6 months.

Clinical trial: a research study in which participants help doctors improve health by agreeing to possibly receive an experimental medicine, procedure, or screening test.

CLL: chronic lymphoid (or lymphocytic) leukemia.

CML: chronic myeloid (or myelogenous) leukemia.

Code status: the decision about whether a person would wish to be resuscitated in the event of a cardiac or respiratory arrest.

Cognitive-behavioral therapy (CBT): a technique that reviews a person's way of thinking and develops new skills that will better prepare the individual for managing particular concerns.

Cohort: a patient group.

Colon: a muscular tube approximately 10 ft long that connects the small intestine to the anus.

Colonoscopy: a screening test in which a tube carrying a fiberoptic camera is used to inspect the interior aspects of the colon in order to search for the presence of colon cancer.

Competence: a synonym for decisional capacity—i.e., the ability to understand relevant information (including the risks, benefits, and alternatives to a treatment) concerning one's medical condition and the ability to communicate a choice.

Complementary medicine: sometimes called integrative or nontraditional therapy, it refers to a large number of health-related therapies, behaviors, and practices that are considered outside the realm of traditional western medicine; complementary medicine is practiced alongside western medicine.

Complete remission: the total disappearance of cancer from all parts of a person's body, as detected by radiologic tests, blood tests, or other special tests.

Computed tomography (CT): a high-tech type of x-ray in which images are taken of "slices" of the body to view internal structures.

Confabulation: the making up of tales and a readiness to give a fluent answer with no regard to the facts.

Congenital mole: a precancerous skin lesion.

Cryotherapy: a type of therapy that uses a cold probe to kill tumors.

Cure rate: the percentage of people in a given population who are permanently rid of their cancer.

Cystectomy: surgery to remove the bladder.

Cystoscopy: a test that uses a fiberoptic catheter inserted into the urethra and from there into the bladder to look for cancer of the bladder.

Cytokines: chemicals released by cancers; they may cause fevers, chills, sweats, fatigue, loss of appetite, nausea, or vomiting.

Cytopenia: a low blood cell count.

Cytoplasm: the substance within a cell that surrounds the nucleus; it contains a cell's machinery and carries out its functions.

Decisional capacity: the ability to understand relevant information (including the risks, benefits, and alternatives regarding a treatment) concerning one's medical condition and the ability to communicate a choice.

Delirium: a syndrome involving a disturbance of attention, cognition, and affect, with a fluctuating course that develops over hours to days; it often is associated with perceptual disturbances and difficulty with sleep.

Delusion: a fixed, false belief.

Denial: a psychological defense used to protect one's consciousness against difficult or unbearable realities.

Depression: a mood, affect, or diagnosis associated with disturbance of sleep, appetite, concentration ability, and energy, as well as with feelings of worthlessness, hopelessness, guilt, and thoughts of suicide.

Diagnostic radiology: the science of interpreting radiology images of internal structures.

Disease-free survival: the proportion of people whose cancer has never returned at a specific time after diagnosis.

DNR: an acronym for "**do n**ot **r**esuscitate." That is, in the event of a catastrophic event (e.g., a cardiac arrest), the person who is declared DNR will not undergo heroic or lifesaving efforts to prolong life (usually because the person's chances of regaining a meaningful existence after a catastrophic medical event would be exceedingly low).

Donor lymphocyte infusion (DLI): the procedure in which a subset of white blood cells (called lymphocytes) is collected from the bone marrow donor and given to the recipient in the form of a blood transfusion.

Dose-response effect: the effect that relates a higher drug dose with a greater effect; e.g., a smoker with a greater number of cigarette pack-years is more likely to develop cancer; similarly, cancer cells exposed to higher levels of chemotherapy are more likely to die.

Durable power of attorney: a legal document that allows you to specify a specific person to make decisions (including medical decisions) for you if you are mentally or physically incapacitated to make decisions for yourself.

Dysarthria: disturbance of articulation due to paralysis, incoordination, or spasticity of the muscles of speech.

Dyscalculia: difficulty in computing or calculating.

Dysgraphia: difficulty in writing.

Dyslexia: difficulty in reading.

Dysplastic nevi: precancerous skin lesions.

Dyspnea: the experience of shortness of breath.

Echopraxia: involuntary imitation of movements made by another person.

ECT: electroconvulsive therapy, also known as shock therapy.

Egocentricity: a perspective of being at the center of everything; common in children.

Electroencephalogram (EEG): a noninvasive test that measures electrical activity of the brain.

Eligibility criteria: guidelines under which subjects can participate in a clinical trial.

Embolism: a blood clot (which usually travels to the lungs or brain).

Embryo cryopreservation: a technique that involves freezing eggs for up to several years for later use.

EMLA cream: a local anesthetic, applied to the skin to ease discomfort; topical procaine (Novocain).

Engraftment: the process that results when newly transplanted bone marrow or stem cells take residence within the bone marrow and begin producing new blood cells.

Environmental carcinogen: a cancer-causing chemical found in the environment (i.e., not genetic).

Enzymes: proteins necessary to make DNA or its building blocks or to metabolize (break down) medications.

Eosinophils: white blood cells that protect against parasites and are associated with allergic responses.

Esophagus: a long muscular tube that carries chewed food from the mouth to the stomach.

Euthanasia: often considered to be synonymous with physician-assisted suicide.

Ewing's sarcoma: a type of tumor of the bone or soft tissue.

Executive function: the function of the frontal lobes of the brain, which, like an executive, must make decisions based on the information at their disposal; they compare, contrast, and plan courses of action.

Experimental procedures: nonstandard tests or treatments administered during a clinical trial.

External beam radiation: high-energy rays originating from outside the body that are applied to a cancer and to a small margin of normal tissue surrounding it.

False negative: a test result that fails to discover an abnormality when that abnormality (e.g., cancer) is in fact present.

False positive: a result of a screening test that appears to find a cancer when in fact none exists.

Feeding tube: a tube placed into a person at different levels of the digestive tract (either through the nose, mouth, or abdomen) to ensure adequate nutrition.

Field cancerization: a process by which a large area of the body can develop invisible genetic changes that make it easier for cancer to occur in that area, analogous to a primer that makes it easier for paint to stick to a surface such as metal.

Frontal lobe: the part of the brain closest to the forehead; it plays a crucial role in the maintenance of attention to ongoing experiences and in the formulation of a response.

Gene therapy: a treatment that involves modification of a gene's function with the hope of treating a disease.

Genes: the structures within a cell's nucleus into which deoxyribonucleic acid (DNA) is packed; many genes form a chromosome and encode the "blueprints" for a cell's function.

Genetic discrimination: the use of genetic information (such as the results of a cancer susceptibility gene test) by insurers or employers in a negative way (including increasing premiums or changing coverage to eliminate care for cancer).

Graft-versus-host disease: a condition that results when newly transplanted bone marrow recognizes protein labels on tissues in the recipient (including the skin or gut) as being foreign and therefore attacks them.

Graft: the marrow that is collected from a bone marrow donor.

Graft-versus-tumor effect: the condition that results when tumor cells are recognized as foreign by the newly transplanted bone marrow and are attacked; it occurs only in the setting of an allogenic BMT.

Granulocytes: white blood cells that capture bacteria and destroy them.

Grief: a natural reaction to loss; it is the beginning of mourning.

Group psychotherapy: the process of having several people meet with a mental health professional to work on one or more psychological issues.

Guided imagery: a technique that involves imagining certain situations and responses to prepare for what lies ahead and to alter the body's response to stress; it is a process of relaxed yet deliberate concentration to refocus attention away from a stressful situation.

Hallucination: a subjective perception in any of the five sensory modalities of something that does not exist objectively.

Harvest: a collection of bone marrow from a donor that is administered to a recipient.

Health care proxy: a legal document that designates a person you know and trust to make health care decisions for you if for any reason you should be unable to make such decisions for yourself.

Historical control group: a group of patients who have been treated previously with a standard therapy and are used as a comparison group for patients treated with a new therapy or a new combination of therapies.

HLA (human leukocyte antigen): a collection of genes found on the sixth chromosome that provides the code for the unique self-label found on all cells.

Holistic therapy: a multidisciplinary or supplemental approach to care that includes the psychological, emotional, and spiritual life of a person as well as his or her physical well-being

Homeopathy: a practice that uses a combination of small quantities of herbal and/or mineral-based medications specifically tailored to a person's symptoms.

Hormonal therapy: a group of cancer treatments that either add a hormone or block a hormone's production or function; this type of therapy suppresses the stimulus for certain types of tumor growth.

Hospice care: often synonymous with palliative care; the final chapter of palliative care, with an emphasis on comfort.

Host: the person who receives a harvested bone marrow.

H. pylori: short for *Helicobacter pylori;* a type of bacteria that commonly causes gastritis or peptic ulcer disease; it may also be a risk factor for gastric cancer.

Human research subject protection: a system designed to protect the rights of voluntary subjects (people) in a clinical study.

Hyperalgesia: an increased response to painful stimuli.

Hyperesthesia: an exaggerated pain response.

Hyperpathia: a persistent pain that occurs beyond the location of the stimulus.

Hypnosis: a technique that focuses attention to induce relaxation or to modify selected behaviors or thought patterns.

Idiosyncratic: unpredictable.

Illusion: a sensory misperception.

Immunosuppression: a state in which a person's immune system is depressed or functions poorly, making that person susceptible to simple infections.

Immunotherapy: a type of therapy that tries to activate the body's immune system to fight off cancer.

Impotence: inability to get and to maintain an erection.

Incontinence: inability to keep urine or stool from leaking.

Incurable cancer: a cancer that cannot reasonably be expected to disappear, even with the best therapy available; incurability does not imply that rapid death or rapid growth of a cancer will occur.

Individual psychotherapy: the process of one-on-one meetings with a mental health professional to work through psychological issues.

Informed consent: a process ensuring that patients are made aware of and understand the potential risks and benefits of a given study.

In situ carcinoma: an early stage of cancer that is visible only microscopically; e.g., a tumor sitting on top of the bladder lining that has not penetrated into the bladder wall.

Intercessory prayer: prayer on behalf of others.

Interferon: a class of medication that modulates immune function; it is used in the treatment of melanoma, leukemia, and lymphoma.

Internal beam radiation: high-energy rays originating from within the body that are delivered into a small area; the radiation source is placed as close as possible to the cancer cells.

Interstitial brachytherapy: the use of radioactive implants in the form of needles, wires, or seeds placed directly within a tumor.

Intracavitary radiation: radiation from a radioactive energy source that is placed within a body cavity or orifice.

Intracytoplasmic sperm injection (ICSI): a technique in which, under the microscope, a single sperm is injected directly into an egg. Later, the fertilized egg is implanted in the uterus.

Intrathecal pump: a device that can deliver medications to a specific area around the spinal cord.

Intrauterine insemination: a technique whereby sperm are inserted into the uterus after hormone-induced ovulation.

Intravenous (IV): by vein.

Intubation: placement of a breathing tube down the windpipe.

In vitro fertilization (IVF): a technique that brings egg and sperm together in a test tube; once the egg has been fertilized, it is later implanted in the uterus.

IRB: an acronym for institutional review board; a committee that reviews a plan for a study prior to its initiation and ensures that the study plan is logical, scientifically sound, and safe for the patients enrolled in the study.

Jaundice: the condition that occurs when bile in the blood causes a person's skin to turn yellow.

Kidneys: a pair of organs located in the back of the abdomen near the bottom of the rib cage; they help to control the amount of water in the body and either retain or excrete water, as well as remove some toxins and medications from the circulation.

Lead-time bias: a statistical term describing the time between the point at which a cancer becomes detectable by screening and the point at which it becomes symptomatic.

Length-time bias: a statistical term describing the tendency of screening tests to detect slow-growing tumors.

Lentigo maligna: a precancerous skin lesion.

Leukemia: a cancer of the cells in the bone marrow and bloodstream; also, a liquid tumor.

Leukopenia: the state of having a low white blood cell count.

Libido: sex drive.

Liver: an organ with an enormous sponge-like network of small blood vessels called sinusoids; the cells that line these sinusoids break down the toxins and drugs in the bloodstream.

Living will: a document that delineates what types of medical care and treatment you will want to have in the future should you become incapacitated or incompetent and unable to communicate your wishes.

Logorrhea: garrulousness.

Lumbar puncture (LP): a procedure that involves placing a needle in the lower back to obtain some of the fluid surrounding the spinal cord and brain; commonly called a "spinal" or "spinal tap."

Lymph: the fluid, comprising water and some chemicals, that leaks out of blood vessels after coursing through organs and tissues; it is returned to the bloodstream through the lymph ducts.

Lymph nodes: the "way stations" of the immune system where foreign objects (including bacteria) are "presented" to immune cells to determine whether these objects should be attacked; lymph nodes are scattered throughout the body.

Lymphoma: a cancer of the lymph nodes; also, a type of liquid tumor.

Magical thinking: a type of thinking characterized by a mixture of reality and fantasy; common in children.

Magnetic resonance imaging (MRI): a high-tech type of x-ray in which images are taken of "slices" of the body to view the internal structures; unlike a computed tomography or regular x-ray, MRI uses magnets and does not emit radiation.

Malignant melanoma: the most dangerous type of skin cancer; it arises from sun-damaged melanocytes.

MALT: an acronym for mucosa-associated lymphoid tissue; a type of lymphoma caused when immune cells in the stomach wall overreact to the presence of a bacterium in the stomach.

Mammography: a special x-ray of the breasts used to detect cancer.

Massage therapy: the use of touch and techniques of stroking and kneading the body's muscles to improve body structure and function.

Match: a suitable candidate for a bone marrow transplantation.

Maximally tolerated dose: the highest dose of a medication that can be tolerated; this dose is usually limited by side effects.

Mechanism of action: the way something works.

Median survival: similar to the average time for survival with an illness; an equal number of people live a shorter time than the median survival time as live longer.

Medical oncologist: an internist who specializes in the treatment of cancer.

Meditation: a technique involving relaxed breathing and focused attention or mindfulness intended to induce calm.

Mental status change: a change in a person's mental functioning (involving disturbances in affect, mood, behavior, perception, and cognition).

Mental status examination: a system of evaluation of a person's mental abilities (involving assessment of cognition, memory, affect, mood, judgment, and perceptions).

Metastasis: a cluster of tumor cells that have spread to another organ or lymph node distant from their site of origin.

Minitransplantation: also termed nonmyeloablative transplantation; a type of bone marrow transplantation that uses reduced-dose conditioning regimens that are not designed to kill all remaining tumor cells in the body.

Mixed chimerism: the coexistence of two bone marrows (the newly transplanted bone marrow and the recipient's marrow).

Motor cortex: a territory of the brain that regulates movement; the right half (hemisphere) of the brain controls the left side of the body, while the left side of the brain controls the right side of the body.

Mourning: the social expression of loss, as observed in funerals or cultural rituals.

Mourning prayer: in the Jewish faith, Kaddish is recited by a rabbi or by family members to pray for the deceased.

Mucositis: an irritation of the lining of the gastrointestinal tract; also, sores of the mucous membranes that line the mouth and throat.

Multidisciplinary care: care provided by different members of a health care team, often comprising surgical oncologists, medical oncologists, radiation therapists, rehabilitation specialists, plastic surgeons, nutritionists, social workers, psychiatrists, and others.

Multiple myeloma: a cancer of cells (called plasma cells) in the bone marrow; also, a type of liquid tumor.

Mutation: a change or mistake in the DNA pattern in any gene, which may cause the gene to malfunction.

Negative predictive value: a statistical term describing the probability that a negative test result will correctly identify the absence of cancer in the person tested.

Negative test result: a test result that discovers no abnormality.

Neuroblastoma: a type of tumor of the nervous system; a type of brain cancer.

Neuroleptic: a class of medication that treats agitation, perceptual disturbances, and psychosis.

Neuropathic pain: often difficult to describe, these pains are derived from nerves that carry pain signals; symptoms often are characterized as burning, shooting, stabbing, or tingling.

Neuropsychiatric testing: a compilation of tests to assess in great detail how a person thinks, remembers, and perceives the world.

Neutropenia: the state of having a reduced level of one type of white blood cell, the neutrophil; often defined as having a neutrophil "count" of less than 500 cells per cubic milliliter of blood.

Nociception: the perception of pain.

Nonopioid medication: nonnarcotic medications (e.g., acetaminophen and nonsteroidal anti-inflammatory drugs) taken for pain relief.

NSAIDs: nonsteroidal anti-inflammatory drugs; a class of medications that diminish inflammation, thereby minimizing swelling and pain.

Nuclear medicine scans: a class of tests that use safe radioactive chemicals to image parts of the body; these include positron emission tomography (PET) scans and gallium scans.

Nucleus: the central structure of a cell that houses the chromosomes, the "blueprints" for cell function.

Nutritionist: a health care professional who focuses on nutrition and on adequate caloric intake.

Occipital lobe: the back part of the brain, which houses the visual cortex.

Oncologist: a cancer specialist.

Opioid analgesic: a narcotic (e.g., morphine, codeine, oxycodone, hydromorphone, fentanyl, methadone, and meperidine) taken for pain relief.

Organ donation: the process by which one can authorize the removal of an organ for use by another person.

Osteosarcoma: a type of tumor of the bone.

Ovarian failure: a permanent absence of ovulation.

Ovaries: a pair of organs that make up part of the female reproductive system; they produce eggs once a month, as well as some female hormones.

Overall survival: the proportion of patients who are alive after a given number of months or years following a cancer diagnosis; in other words, simply a head count of the number of living cancer patients without regard to whether the cancer has disappeared or still exists.

Ovum banking: the storage of eggs for later use.

Pack-year: the terminology used to incorporate the duration of exposure to smoking and the dose of smoking; a person who smokes two packs of cigarettes per day for 20 years has a 40-pack-year (2 packs × 20 years) smoking history.

Pain specialist: a physician who specializes in the diagnosis and treatment of pain.

Palliative care: a type of medical treatment intended to support a person living with a life-threatening illness; it is most often used when an illness is progressive, cure is no longer possible, and the focus of care shifts to minimizing symptoms.

Pancreas: an organ in the abdomen, adjacent to the stomach; it produces enzymes that help to digest food and produces insulin, which allows the body to store sugar.

Paraneoplastic syndrome: a condition in which a cancer produces a chemical unrelated to the usual function of the organ in which the cancer arises; the chemical causes side effects and unusual symptoms. For example, a lung cancer cell may produce a chemical causing a person to experience profound muscle weakness.

Parenchyma: tissue within the lung that gives lungs their substance.

Partial remission: significant, though incomplete, shrinkage of a tumor.

Patient-controlled analgesia (PCA): analgesia (e.g., morphine, dilaudid) administered by a machine that the patient controls, to provide pain relief as needed.

Peer review: a process of critical review carried out by the editors of a medical journal before a study is accepted for publication.

Penetrance: the degree to which people with altered cancer susceptibility genes actually develop cancer.

Performance status: a measure of how functional a person is while living with cancer.

Peripheral blood stem cells: bone marrow cells found in the bloodstream.

Perseveration: the repetition of a word, phrase, or action.

Petechiae: tiny bleeds under the skin that resemble pinpricks; they are due to low platelet counts.

Petitionary prayer: prayer in which one "petitions" for a particular intervention.

Pharmacist: a health care professional who dispenses medications and acts as a source of information on medications.

Phase I trial: the first study in humans used to evaluate a drug; it asks basic questions regarding drug delivery, including dosing and toxicity (side effects).

Phase II trial: a study of a drug's safety and its spectrum of efficacy; e.g., how well the drug works in shrinking a tumor or in improving a person's outcome.

Phase III trial: a study of a drug's efficacy; this study also compares new treatments or new combinations of existing treatments to the current standard of treatment in a specific cancer.

Phase IV trial: a postmarketing surveillance study.

Photon energy: a measure of the intensity of an x-ray beam, described as the number of "packets" of energy released into cells.

Physical dependence: a syndrome of physical changes that occurs after chronic use of some medications, e.g., opiates and benzodiazepines.

Physical therapist: a health care specialist who helps a person regain strength so that he or she can return to normal levels of activity.

Physician-assisted suicide: a suicide facilitated by a physician, often through a prescription of lethal medicines.

Placebo: a dummy pill that contains no active ingredient; it is designed to look, taste, and even smell like the active drug to which it is being compared.

Platelet: a cell in the bloodstream that facilitates blood clotting.

Polyps: small bunches of tissue that grow on the walls of the colon; they may develop into colon cancer.

Positive predictive value: a statistical term describing the probability that a positive test result will correctly identify the presence of cancer in the person tested.

Positive test result: a test result that discovers an abnormality.

Positron emission tomography (PET): a special type of imaging study that assesses the function of an organ, such as the brain.

Postmarketing surveillance study: also known as a phase IV trial; such a trial evaluates a drug's side effects and efficacy after it has been approved by the Food and Drug Administration (FDA) and while it is being used in the general population.

Predisposition gene: an inherited gene that can make a person more likely to develop cancer.

Premalignant conditions: abnormal growths that are thought to represent cells having a high likelihood of becoming cancerous over time.

Prevention trial: a trial to test a new approach to lowering the risk of a certain type of cancer in people who have never had cancer; to prevent cancer from coming back in a patient who has already had cancer; or to prevent the development of a new cancer in a patient who has already had cancer.

Priapism: a prolonged state of erection.

Principal investigator (PI): the person in charge of a study.

p.r.n.: short for the Latin term *pro re nata,* or as may be needed.

Progressive muscle relaxation: a technique involving muscle relaxation to induce a state of calm.

Prophylactic surgery: the removal of healthy (noncancerous) tissue before cancer can develop in that tissue.

Prosopagnosia: difficulty in recognizing faces.

Prostate: a gland about the size of a walnut located below the bladder and in front of the rectum, at the base of the penis; it surrounds part of the urethra. The prostate makes fluid that becomes part of semen.

Prostate-specific antigen (PSA): a chemical made by the prostate gland and secreted into the bloodstream; elevated levels of PSA may indicate the presence of prostate cancer.

Protocol: the plan for a study.

Psychiatrist: a mental health professional who also holds a medical degree.

Psychological dependence: a condition associated with a craving for a drug and its effects; it involves compulsive seeking and using of the drug.

Psychologist: a mental health professional.

Psychomotor agitation: a state of heightened tension, restlessness, and fidgeting.

Psychomotor retardation: a state of being slowed down, like a "couch potato."

Quality of life (QOL): how well a person functions and feels.

Quality-of-life (QOL) trial: a study that explores ways to improve the functional, social, and emotional well-being of a person with cancer.

Radiation: a type of energy that causes errors in a cell's ability to copy DNA accurately and subsequently to divide.

Radiation oncologist: a physician who treats cancer with radiation.

Radiation oncology: the discipline that uses radiation to treat cancer.

Radiation therapist: a health care professional with special training in radiation physics and the effects of radiation on bodily tissues; this person administers radiation therapy.

Radiation therapy: the science of eradicating tumor cells with radiation.

Radiofrequency ablation: a type of therapy that uses radio waves to kill tumorous cells.

Randomized controlled trial: a type of research study in which two groups are assigned different interventions or different therapies randomly (e.g., one group is screened by a test and the other is not screened by the test) and then are compared to determine which group fares better.

Rational suicide: suicide resulting from a rational thought process.

"Reasonable man" approach: similar to the legal concept: if a reasonable man or woman were to agree that the amount of improvement in a cancer for a specific length of time was meaningful, then it would be considered a remission.

Red blood cells: cells that carry oxygen from the lungs to the rest of the body.

Reduplicative paramnesia: a delusion that an impostor has replaced a known person.

Referred pain: this type of pain occurs at a site distant from the part of the body involved with cancer in the absence of spread of the cancer to that distant body part.

Regression: a return to an earlier psychological stage of development, often precipitated by stress.

Reiki: a Japanese technique that involves the laying on of hands to serve as a conduit for the life force or energy that flows through the body; it promotes relaxation, stress reduction, and improved immune system function.

Relapse rate: the percentage of people in a population in whom a cancer that has been in complete remission will come back.

Relaxation response: a technique, like meditation, used to induce or facilitate a state of calm.

Remission: the improvement (i.e., the shrinkage or disappearance) of a cancer.

Respiratory arrest: the state when breathing has stopped.

Resuscitation: a process that may include the administration of medications and oxygen, placement of a breathing tube down the windpipe, and chest compressions.

Retinoblastoma: a type of tumor of the eye.

Rhabdomyosarcoma: a type of tumor of the soft tissues.

Rule of double effect: a rule that relies on the intent of a treatment to determine if an action was acceptable (e.g., when high doses of narcotics are administered to treat a terminally ill person's pain and they result in a person's death from respiratory failure, the prescription is still considered appropriate).

Screening trial: a study that assesses the best way to find cancer in its early stages, when the cancer is still potentially curable.

Sensitivity: a statistical term that describes the proportion of people who actually have cancer in whom a given test would have correctly identified them as having the cancer.

Shiva: a period of mourning observed by members of the Jewish faith.

Side effects: reactions (other than intended effects) to medications or other treatments (e.g., radiation therapy).

Sigmoidoscopy: a test involving a direct visual inspection of the sigmoid colon through a tube inserted through the rectum; some colon cancers can be detected using this test.

Social worker: a health care professional who works with families and social systems.

Solid tumors: cancers affecting the tissue organs of the body, including the lung, breast, prostate, colon, rectum, or bladder; distinguished from liquid tumors.

Somatic pain: a pain that comes from the skin and from other tissues (excluding pain from internal organs).

Specificity: a statistical term that describes the proportion of people who do not have cancer who are correctly identified by a given test as not having the cancer.

Sperm banking: a technique whereby sperm are frozen and saved for future use.

Stable disease: a cancer that has not substantially increased or decreased in size.

Stage: a method of describing how far a tumor has spread, either within an organ, to nearby body structures, or distantly to other lymph nodes or body structures.

Statistical power: the ability to mathematically demonstrate effects of a treatment in an experimental group and in a control group.

Stem cell: a type of cell located in the bone marrow, from which other blood cells—including the red blood cells, white blood cells, and platelets—are created

Stem cell transplantation (SCT): a type of bone marrow transplantation in which the important component of a bone marrow transplantation, the stem (or grandfather) cell, which gives rise to the components of blood, is given to a person with cancer; stem cells can be collected from the bloodstream or from the bone marrow.

Stomach: a large muscular pouch at one end of the esophagus; the stomach produces acid and uses a grinding action to help digest food.

Stool guaiac: hemoccult testing; a screening test for microscopic amounts of blood in the stool.

Supportive care trial: a trial that explores ways to improve the comfort and quality of life of a person with cancer.

Surface molds: casts specially prepared to conform to the external surface of a specific cancer; used to administer radiation therapy.

Survivor guilt: the guilt experienced by some who have "escaped" cancer while others in a family or other group have not.

Tamoxifen: a widely used hormonal treatment that blocks the effects of estrogen.

T-cell depletion: a procedure whereby T cells, the cells involved in graft-versus-host disease following an allogeneic bone marrow transplant, are removed from the transplant using specialized machines and techniques.

Temporal lobe: a deep brain structure involved in the processing of auditory information and feelings.

TENS (transcutaneous electrical nerve stimulation): a technique that decreases the sensation of pain via stimulation by electrodes attached to the skin.

Teratogenic: able to cause birth defects.

Thalamus: a structure within the middle of the brain that serves as the central relay point for information; the gateway of the senses.

Therapeutic touch: a process of energy exchange in which the practitioner holds his or her hands a few inches from the body to correct the energy imbalance caused by disease.

Thrombocytopenia: the state of having a low platelet count.

TNM staging system: a system used for the evaluation and description of a cancer's size, spread to lymph nodes, location, and spread to other organs; **T** stands for tumor, **N** for lymph node involvement, and **M** for the presence of metastases.

Tolerance: a condition in which higher levels of medication are needed to achieve the same effect because of physiologic changes.

Total response rate: the proportion of people who have experienced either a partial or complete remission (or response) to a specific therapy.

Tracheostomy: a surgical procedure whereby a temporary or permanent opening in the neck is created to allow for placement of a breathing tube.

Transdermal: through the skin. For example, a medication may be administered transdermally.

Transfusion: the intravenous (by vein) replacement of a type of blood product or cell line (e.g., red blood cell or platelet transfusions).

Transitional cell carcinoma: cancer that arises from cells that line the bladder and ureters; the most common type of bladder cancer.

Treatment trial: a study that tests new therapies for cancer.

Tricyclic antidepressant (TCA): a class of antidepressant that has adjunctive analgesic (pain-relieving) effects.

Tumor marker: a type of protein that can be produced by a cancer and whose level can be measured in the bloodstream.

Tumor necrosis factor: a chemical released by a cancerous cell; it is associated with cachexia, anorexia, or wasting.

Tumor stage: the size, spread, and location of a tumor.

Tumor suppressor gene: a gene that keeps a cell healthy and prevents that cell from turning into a cancer.

Ultrasound-guided needle biopsy: a surgical procedure (often minor) in which tissue is obtained from an organ thought to be involved with cancer; placement of the biopsy needle is guided by ultrasound for more accuracy.

Ureter: a tube that carries urine from the kidney to the bladder.

Urethra: a tube that empties urine from the bladder.

Visceral pain: pain from internal organ injury.

Visual cortex: the portion of the brain involved in the recognition of lines and shapes; these stimuli are then sent to other brain regions for emotional processing.

Wilms' tumor: a type of tumor of the kidney that is more common in children.

Yoga: from India, this exercise technique helps balance and harmonize the body and mind to create a sense of well-being.

Selected Resources

INTERNET RESOURCES

Advance Directives

www.vh.org/Patients/IHB/Misc/AdvanceDirective.html/
www.ama-assn.org/public/booklets/livingwill.htm/

American Cancer Society

www.cancer.org/
http://www.cancer.org/eprise/main/docroot/PUB/PUB_1?sitearea=PUB

American Society for Cancer Research

http://www.aacr.org/

American Society of Clinical Oncology

http://www.asco.org/

Cancer Resource Room at the MGH

http://cancer.mgh.harvard.edu/resources.

Oncolink (University of Pennsylvania)

http://cancer.med.upenn.edu (click on "Psychosocial Support and Personal Experiences")

National Cancer Institute (NCI)

http://cancernet.nci.nih.gov

Association of Cancer Online Resources, Inc. (ACOR)

http://www.acor.org (This site offers extensive lists of e-mail discussion and support groups.)

Local chapter of the American Cancer Society

(check phone book)

USA TODAY
Associated Press (accessed 8/5/2001): Colon cancer screening worth the cost.
http://www.usatoday.com/life/health/cancer/colon/lhcco017.htm
Associated Press (accessed 8/5/2001): Experimental leukemia drug wins praise.
http://www.usatoday.com/news/healthscience/health/2001-07-25-leukemia-drug.htm
Associated Press (accessed 8/5/2001): Gene test offers better breast cancer treatment
http://www.usatoday.com/news/health/2001-02-21-breast-cancer.htm
Associated Press (accessed 8/5/2001): Green tea may not prevent stomach cancer after all.
http://www.usatoday.com/news/health/2001-02-28-green-tea.htm
Associated Press (accessed 8/5/2001): Lung cancer surgery: Practice makes perfect.
http://www.usatoday.com/news/healthscience/health/2001-07-18-lung-cancer.htm
Associated Press (accessed 8/5/2001): Women smokers may get more bladder cancer.
http://www.usatoday.com/news/health/2001-04-03-bladder-cancer-women.htm
Friend T (accessed 8/5/2001): Histamine doubles survival with melanoma.
http://www.usatoday.com/life/health/cancer/skin/lhcsk011.htm
Rubin R (accessed 8/5/2001): Viral test could aid detection of cervical cancer.
http://www.usatoday.com/news/health/2001-02-20-cervical.htm

THE NEW YORK TIMES
Altman LK: Chemotherapy before surgery aids bladder cancer. *New York Times* (electronic version) 5/15/2001.
Ames L: Milestones: A father's triumph over cancer. *New York Times* (electronic version) 10/15/2000.
Brody J: Personal health: Lung cancer cure? Try prevention instead. *New York Times* (electronic version) 11/24/2000.
Cancer drug shows promise, but is no panacea, tests find. *New York Times* (electronic version) 11/11/2000.
Christensen J: Scientist at work: John Reed—Running hot in pursuit of cancer treatment. *New York Times* (electronic version) 12/12/2000.
Grady D: New treatment offers promise against kidney cancer. *New York Times* (electronic version) 9/13/2000.

Kirby D: More options, and decisions, for men with prostate cancer. *New York Times* (electronic version) 10/3/2000.

Kolata G: Studies report no links to cancer in cell phones' use. *New York Times* (electronic version) 12/20/2000.

Wade N: Swift approval for a new kind of cancer drug. *New York Times* (electronic version) 5/11/2001.

THE WASHINGTON POST

Applied orally, missile defense technology may work: A new high-tech test can help target early mouth cancers. *Washington Post* (4/24/2001, p T6).

Help yourself: resources for alternative and complementary cancer treatment. *Washington Post* (9/4/2001, p HE06).

Too young to die: media images aside, breast cancer usually hits after 50. *Washington Post* (5/1/2001, p T7).

Who wants to know? A simple biopsy technique can detect more prostate cancers than are usually caught, but is this really useful? *Washington Post* (8/4/2001, p F4).

THE BOSTON GLOBE

Foreman J: When drugs are the only choice for a mother to be. *Boston Globe* (electronic version), 9/26/2000.

Mishra R: Drug found to be effective in 2 cancers. *Boston Globe* (electronic version), 4/5/2001.

Reucroft S, Swain J: Nicotine and cancer. *Boston Globe* (electronic version), 11/28/2000.

Rosenberg R: Vaccines to treat, not prevent, cancer: Products in test phase aim to help patients live longer. *Boston Globe* (electronic version), 10/15/2001.

Saltus R: A new look at cancer treatment. *Boston Globe* (electronic version), 11/14/2000.

Saltus R: Diet no help: A cancer study finds breast risk unchanged by healthy eating habit. *The Boston Globe* (electronic version), 2/14/2001.

NEWSWEEK

A cure for cancer? *Newsweek Magazine* (electronic version), May 28, 2001.

Begley S: Made-to-order medicine. *Newsweek Magazine* (electronic version), June 25, 2001.

Cowley G: Can we overcome cancer? *Newsweek Magazine* (electronic version), fall/winter 2001.

Greenberg SH, Springen K: Keeping hope alive. *Newsweek Magazine* (electronic version), fall/winter 2001.

Kalb C: A cancer "smart bomb." *Newsweek Magazine* (electronic version), December 18, 2000.

Laschever A: When the unthinkable happens. *Newsweek Magazine* (electronic version), August 13, 2001.

TIME MAGAZINE

Can food fend off tumors? *Time Magazine* (electronic version), July 19, 1999.

Cancer made to order. *Time Magazine* (electronic version), August 9, 1999.

Closing in on cancer. *Time Magazine* (electronic version), May, 21, 2001.

Curing cancer: The hope and the hype. *Time Magazine* (electronic version), May 18, 1998.

Everything you need to know about colon cancer and how to prevent it. *Time Magazine (electronic version), March 20, 2000.*

Cancer Research Foundation

The Cancer Research Foundation of America (CRFA) has the following educational materials and resources for the general public.
These brochures are concise yet informative. They list easy lifestyle changes and habits that can help decrease the risk of developing certain types of cancer. All can be found through the website *http://www.preventcancer.org/educcrfa.cfm* or ordered via phone (1-800-227-CRFA), or e-mail at info@crfa.org. The brochures and fact sheets can be downloaded free from the website.

> *Colorectal Cancer: Preventable, Treatable, Beatable!*
> *Healthy Kids: 7 Steps to Cancer Prevention for Parents*
> *Healthy Men: Self Help for Cancer Prevention*
> *Healthy Women: Self Help for Cancer Prevention*
> *Living Healthy: 7 Steps to Cancer Prevention*
> *The Cancer Research Foundation of America: Breaking the Codes*

Bladder Cancer

AMERICAN FOUNDATION FOR UROLOGIC DISEASE
http://www.afud.org/

Brain Tumors

AMERICAN BRAIN TUMOR ASSOCIATION (ABTA)
http://www.abta.org/

THE BRAIN TUMOR SOCIETY
http://www.tbts.org/

NATIONAL BRAIN TUMOR FOUNDATION
http://www.braintumor.org/

Breast Cancer

THE SUSAN G. KOMEN BREAST CANCER FOUNDATION
http://www.breastcancerinfo.com/

Y-ME NATIONAL BREAST CANCER ORGANIZATION
http://www.y-me.org/

Cervical Cancer

NATIONAL CERVICAL CANCER COALITION
http://www.nccc-online.org/

Childhood Cancer

www.squirreltales.com
http://cancernet.nci.nih.gov/occdocs/KidsHome.html
http://www.cancersourcekids.com/

Colon Cancer

COLORECTAL CANCER NETWORK
http://www.colorectal-cancer.net/

COLON CANCER ALLIANCE
http://www.ccalliance.org/

Death, Dying, and Grief

ASSOCIATION FOR DEATH EDUCATION AND COUNSELING
http://www.adec.org/

BEYOND INDIGO: GRIEF AND LOSS
http://www.beyondindigo.com/

CANCER RESOURCE ROOM AT MASSACHUSETTS GENERAL HOSPITAL
http://cancer.mgh.harvard.edu/resources

COMPASSIONATE FRIENDS: GRIEF FOLLOWING THE DEATH OF A CHILD
http://www.compassionatefriends.org/

DOUGY CENTER, THE NATIONAL CENTER FOR GRIEVING CHILDREN AND FAMILIES
http://www.dougy.org/

GRIEFNET: DEATH AND DYING RESOURCES
http://rivendell.org/

GROWTHHOUSE: GRIEF AND BEREAVEMENT, DEATH AND DYING
http://www.growthhouse.org/

GUIDELINE PUBLICATIONS, CHILDRENS' QUESTIONS ABOUT DEATH
http://www.guidelinepub.com/

INTERNATIONAL PSYCHO-ONCOLOGY SOCIETY: PSYCHOSOCIAL
DIMENSIONS OF CANCER
http://www.ipos-aspboa.org/

NATIONAL CANCER INSTITUTE INFORMATION ON CHILDREN AND GRIEF
http://www.graylab.ac.uk/cancernet/506750.html/

NATIONAL HOSPICE AND PALLIATIVE CARE ORGANIZATION
http://www.nhpco.org/

ONCOLINK, UNIVERSITY OF PENNSYLVANIA
http://cancer.med.upenn.edu/

General Information Regarding Cancer

www.acor.org
http://oncolink.upenn.edu/
http://cancer.med.upenn.edu/
http://cancer.mgh.harvard.edu/resources
http://www.acor.org/
http://www.pbs.org/wgbh/nova/cancer/
http://oncology.com/
http://www.preventcancer.org/educcrfa.cfm/

Genetic Testing

http://nhgri.nih.gov/Policy_and_public_affairs/Legislation/insure.htm
www.geneticalliance.org

Head and Neck Cancer

http://www.spohnc.org/

Hereditary Colon Cancer Association

www.hereditarycc.org

Kidney Cancer

KIDNEY CANCER ASSOCIATION
http://www.kidneycancerassociation.org/

AMERICAN FOUNDATION FOR UROLOGIC DISEASE
http://www.afud.org

Leukemias/Lymphomas

CURE FOR LYMPHOMA FOUNDATION
http://www.cfl.org/

LEUKEMIA AND LYMPHOMA SOCIETY
http://www.leukemia-lymphoma.org/

LEUKEMIA RESEARCH FOUNDATION
http://www.leukemia-research.org/

LYMPHOMA RESEARCH FOUNDATION OF AMERICA
http://www.lymphoma.org/

Lung Cancer

ALLIANCE FOR LUNG CANCER ADVOCACY, SUPPORT, AND EDUCATION
(ALCASE)
http://www.alcase.org/

Melanoma

THE SKIN CANCER FOUNDATION
http://www.skincancer.org/

Multiple Myeloma

INTERNATIONAL MYELOMA FOUNDATION
http://www.myeloma.org/

THE MULTIPLE MYELOMA RESEARCH FOUNDATION
http://www.multiplemyeloma.org/

National Alliance of Breast Cancer Organizations

www.nabco.org

National Cancer Institute

www.nci.nih.gov/
http://cancer.gov/ (main NCI web page)
http://cancernet.nci.nih.gov (CancerNet)
http://cancertrials.nci.nih.gov/ (clinical trials information)

National Comprehensive Cancer Network (NCCN): offers treatment guidelines

http://www.nccn.org

National Society of Genetic Counselors

www.nsgc.org

Ovarian Cancer

NATIONAL OVARIAN CANCER COALITION
http://www.ovarian.org/

OVARIAN CANCER NATIONAL ALLIANCE
http://www.ovariancancer.org/

Pain

http://www.oncologychannel.com.pain/

Pancreatic Cancer

PANCREATIC CANCER ACTION NETWORK (PANCAN)
http://www.pancan.org/

Prostate Cancer

CAP CURE
http://www.capcure.org/

AMERICAN FOUNDATION FOR UROLOGIC DISEASE
http://www.afud.org/

Risk Assessment for Cancer

www.nci.nih.gov
www.nsgc.org
www.cancer.mgh.harvard.edu/CancerCare/genetics.htm
www.facingourrisk.org
http://cissecure.nci.nih.gov/ncipubs/

Sarcomas

AMSCHWAND SARCOMA CANCER FOUNDATION
http://www.sarcomacancer.org/

Testicular Cancer

THE LANCE ARMSTRONG FOUNDATION
http://www.laf.org/

USA Today Online

http://www.usatoday.com/life/health/cancer/hainer/hainer.htm
The Associated Press (accessed 8/5/2001): Gene test offers better breast cancer treatment.
http://www.usatoday.com/news/health/2001-02-21-breast-cancer.htm
The Associated Press (accessed 8/5/2001): Women smokers may get more bladder cancer.
http://www.usatoday.com/news/health/2001-04-03-bladder-cancer-women.htm
Rubin R (accessed 8/5/2001): Viral test could aid detection of cervical cancer.
http://www.usatoday.com/news/health/2001-02-20-cervical.htm
The Associated Press (accessed 8/5/2001): Colon cancer screening worth the cost.
http://www.usatoday.com/life/health/cancer/colon/lhcco017.htm
The Associated Press (accessed 8/5/2001): Experimental leukemia drug wins praise.
http://www.usatoday.com/news/healthscience/health/2001-07-25-leukemia-drug.htm
The Associated Press (accessed 8/5/2001): Lung cancer surgery: Practice makes perfect.
http://www.usatoday.com/news/healthscience/health/2001-07-18-lung-cancer.htm
Friend T (accessed 8/5/2001): Histamine doubles survival with melanoma.
http://www.usatoday.com/life/health/cancer/skin/lhcsk011.htm
The Associated Press (accessed 8/5/2001): Green tea may not prevent stomach cancer after all.
http:www.usatoday.com/news/health/2001-02-28-green-tea.htm

BIBLIOGRAPHY

Alternative and Complementary Therapies

Cohen A: Treatment of antidepressant-induced sexual dysfunction: A new scientific study shows benefits of Ginkgo biloba. *Healthwatch* 5(1), 1996.

Davidson JR, Morrison RM, Shore J, et al: Homeopathic treatment of depression and anxiety. *Alternative Ther Health Med* 3:46–49, 1997.

LeBars PL, Katz MM, Berman N, et al: A placebo-controlled, double-blind, randomized trial of an extract of Ginkgo biloba for dementia. North American EGb Study Group. *JAMA* 278:1327–1332, 1997.

Sack RL, Hughes RJ, Edgar DM, Lewy AJ: Sleep-promoting effects of melatonin: at what dose, in whom, under what conditions, and by what mechanisms? Sleep 1997; 20:908-915.

Schulz V, Hänsel R, Tyler VE: *Rational Phytotherapy: A Physicians' Guide to Herbal Medicine,* 4th ed. Berlin: Springer-Verlag, 2001.

Stoll A, Severus WE, Freeman MP, et al: Omega 3 fatty acids in bipolar disorder. *Arch Gen Psychiatry* 56:407–412, 1999.

Boukoms A, et al: Chronic pain patients: Clues in the clinical interview. *Psychiatr Med* 4(1):, 1987.

Cherny NI, Portenoy, RK: The management of cancer pain. *Cancer J Clin* 45:63–64, 259–303, 1995.

Eckhardt K, Ammon S, Hofmann U, et al: Gabapentin enhances the analgesic effect of morphine in healthy volunteers. *Epilepsia* 40(Suppl 6):S66–S72; discussion S73–74, 1999.

Gatchel RJ: *Psychosocial Factors in Pain.* New York: Guilford Press, 1999.

Hyman SE, Cassem NH: Pain. *Scientific American Medicine, Current Topics in Medicine,* Subsec II. New York: Scientific American, 1989, pp 1–17.

Hackett TP: The pain patient: Evaluation and treatment. *MGH Handbook of General Hospital Psychiatry.*

Lefkokwitz M: *A Practical Approach to Pain Management.*

Massie MJ: *Pain: What Psychiatrists Need to Know.* American Psychiatric Press, 2000.

Miotto K, et al: Diagnosing addictive diseases in chronic pain patients. *Psychosomatics* 37:223–235, 1996.

Shvartzman P: Pharmacological treatment of cancer pain. *IMAJ* 2:536–539, 2000.

Oncologychannel.com. Website on the World Wide Web.
http://www.oncologychannel.com/pain/

Stieg RL, et al: Roadblocks to effective pain management. *Med Clin North Am* 83(3):810–821, 1999.

Scimeca MM, Savage SR, Portenoy RK, Lowinson J: Treatment of pain in the methadone-maintained patients. Pain Management. *Anesth Analg* 91(1):185–191, 2000.

USHHS: *Clinical Practice Guideline Number 9. Management of Cancer Pain. Washington, DC: US Department of Health and Human Services, March 1994.*

Books and Cancer

Books from the American Cancer Society book list:
All of these titles can be ordered online at *http://www.cancer.org/eprise/main/docroot/ PUB/PUB_1?sitearea=PUB* or by calling 1-888-227-5552.

Ackerman A, Ackerman A: *Our Mom Has Cancer.*

American Cancer Society: *A Breast Cancer Journey—Your Personal Guidebook.*

American Cancer Society: *American Cancer Society's Guide to Complementary and Alternative Cancer Methods.*

American Cancer Society: *Cancer in the Family: Helping Children Cope with a Parent's Illness.*

American Cancer Society: *Colorectal Cancer.*

American Cancer Society: *Consumers Guide to Cancer Drugs.*

American Cancer Society: *Informed Decisions: The Complete Book of Cancer Diagnosis, Treatment and Recovery.*

Bostwick DG, MadLennan GT, Larson TR: *Prostate Cancer: What Every Man—and His Family—Needs to Know.*

Houts PS, Buchner JA: *Caring-A Step-By-StepResource for Caring for the Person with Cancer at Home.*

Murphy GP, Morris SB, Lange D: *Informed Decisions: The Complete Book of Cancer Diagnosis, Treatment, and Recovery.*

Runowicz CD, Petrek JA, Gansler TS: *Women and Cancer: A Thorough and Compassionate Resource for Patients and Their Families*

For books on specific stages and experiences of cancer in general, below is a list of some of the top ranked books on these topics:

COPING

Fiore NA: *The Road Back to Health: Coping with the Emotional Aspects of Cancer.*, MI: Celestial Arts, 1990.

Holland JC, Lewis S: *The Human Side of Cancer: Living With Hope, Coping With Uncertainty,* New :York: Harper Collins, 2000.

Moore K, Schmais L: *Living Well With Cancer: A Nurse Tells You Everything You Need to Know About Managing the Side Effects of Your Treatment.*, NJ: Putman, 2001.

Todd AD: *Double Vision: An East-West Collaboration for Coping with Cancer.* Middletown, CT: Wesleyan University Press, 1995.

GENERAL INFORMATION AND GUIDES FOR PATIENTS AND FAMILIES

Anderson G, Simonton C: *Cancer: 50 Essential Things to Do.*, NJ: Plume, 1999.

Babcock EN: *When Life Becomes Precious.* New York: Bantam Books, 1997.

Canfield J (ed): *Chicken Soup for the Surviving Soul: 101 Inspirational Stories to Comfort Cancer Patients and Their Loved Ones.*, FL: Health Communications, 1996.

Girard V, Zadra D (eds): *There's No Place Like Hope: A Book of Hope, Help and Inspiration for Cancer Patients and Their Families.*: Compendium, 2001.

THERAPIES AND TREATMENTS

Cukier D, McCollough VE, Gingerelli F: *Coping with Radiation Therapy: A Ray of Hope.* New York: McGraw Hill, 2001.

Dollinger M et al: *Everyone's Guide to Cancer Therapy.*, MO: Andrews McMeel, 1998.

Frahm AE, Frahm DJ: *The Cancer Battle Plan: Six Strategies for Beating Cancer from a Recovered "Hopeless Case.",* NJ: Tarcher, 1998.

Zakarian B, Greenspan EM: *The Activist Cancer Patient: How to Take Charge of Your Treatment.* New York: Wiley, 1996.

DIAGNOSIS

Diamond WJ, Cowen WL, Goldberg B: *Cancer Diagnosis: What to Do Next.* Alternativemedicine.com

Harpham WS, Pilcher AB: *Diagnosis Cancer: Your Guide through the First Few Months.* New York: Norton, 1997.

Levine M: *Surviving Cancer: One Woman's Story and Her Inspiring Program for Anyone Facing Cancer.* : Broadway Books, 2001.

Breast Cancer

DIAGNOSIS

Austin S, Hitchcock C: *Breast Cancer: What You Should Know (But May Not Be Told) About Prevention, Diagnosis, and Treatment.* : PrimaCommunications, 1994.

Link J: *The Breast Cancer Survival Manual: A Step-by-Step Guide for the Woman Newly Diagnosed with Breast Cancer.* New York: Holt, 2000.

COPING AND LIVING WITH BREAST CANCER

Bruning N. *Coping with Chemotherapy.* New York: Ballantine Books, 1993.

Greenberg M. *Invisible Scars: A Guide to Coping with the Emotional Impact of Breast Cancer.* 1998.

Mayer M, Lamb Linda (eds): *Advanced Breast Cancer: A Guide to Living with* Metastatic Disease, 2d ed. Cambridge, MA: O'Reilly & Associates, 1998.

Muschal-Reinhardt R et al. *Rituals for Women Coping with Breast Cancer.* New York: Prism Collective, 2000.

Phillips RH, Goldstein P: *Coping with Breast Cancer: A Practical Guide to Understanding, Treating, and Living with Breast Cancer.* New York: Avery Penguin Putnam, 1998.

GENERAL INFORMATION AND GUIDES

Braddock S et al: *Straight Talk About Breast Cancer : From Diagnosis to Recovery: A Guide for the Entire Family.*, NB: Addicus Books, 1994.

Kneece JC, Brown T (ed): *Your Breast Cancer Treatment Handbook: Your Guide to Understanding the Disease, Treatments, Emotions and Recovery from Breast Cancer.*, SC: Edu Care, 2001.

Love SM, Lindsey K: *Dr. Susan Love's Breast Book.* Cambridge, MA: Perseus Publishing, 2000.

Stone B: *Cancer As Initiation : Surviving the Fire : A Guide for Living With Cancer for Patient, Provider, Spouse, Family, or Friend.*, IL: Open Court, 1994.

Chemotherapy

Karnofsky DA, Ableman WH, Craver LF, et al: The use of nitrogen mustards in the paliative treatment of carcinoma. *Cancer* 1:634–656, 1948.

Zubrod CG, Scheiderman ME, Frei E III, et al: Cancer—Appraisal of methods for the study of chemotherapy of cancer in man: thiophosphoramide. *J Chronic Dis* 11:7–33, 1960.

Lansky S, List M, et al: The measurement of performance in childhood cancer patients. *Cancer* 60:1651–1656, 1987.

Children and Cancer

COPING AND LIVING WITH CHILDHOOD CANCER

Adams DW: *Coping with Childhood Cancer: Where Do We Go from Here?*: Kinbridge Publishing, 1993.

Connolly H, Clancy T, Civi C: *Fighting Chance: Journeys through Childhood Cancer.*: Woodholm House Publishing, 1998.

Dorfman EV: *The C-Word: Teenagers and Their Families Living with Cancer.*, 1998.

Ekert H: *Childhood Cancer: Understanding and Coping.* New York: Gordon & Breach Science Publishing, 1989.

Fromer MJ: *Surviving Childhood Cancer.* Washington, DC: American Psychiatric Press, 1995.

Wolford CB, Wolford F, Moscow J: *My Story about Cancer.* Seven Locks Press, 1999.

GENERAL INFORMATION AND GUIDES FOR PATIENTS AND FAMILIES

Breen DL, Sion M, Mogul M (eds): *Cancer's Gift.*: Rock Wren Publishing, 2000.

Keene N, Lamb L (eds): *Childhood Leukemia: A Guide for Families, Friends & Caregivers (Patient-Centered Guides).* Cambridge, MA: O'Reilly & Associates, 1999.

Keene N, Ruccione K, Hobbie W: *Childhood Cancer Survivors: A Practical Guide to Your Future.* Cambridge, MA: O'Reilly & Associates, 2000.

Steen G, Mirro J Jr (eds): *Childhood Cancer: A Handbook from St. Jude Children's Research Hospital.*, Cambridge, MA: Perseus Press, 2000.

Colorectal Cancer

GENERAL INFORMATION AND GUIDES

Dunitz M, Rougier P, Wilke H (eds): *Management of Colorectal Cancer.* Malden, MA: Blackwell Science, 1998.

Johnston L: *Colon & Rectal Cancer: A Comprehensive Guide for Patients & Families.* Cambridge, MA: O'Reilly & Associates, 2000.

Marcet JE: *Colorectal Cancer : A Guide for Patients.*: Health Information Network, 1996.

Miskovitz PF, Betancourt M: *What to Do If You Get Colon Cancer : A Specialist Helps You Take Charge and Make Informed Choices.* New York: Wiley, 1997.

Pazdur R, Royce M: *Myths & Facts About Colorectal Cancer,* 2d ed.: Publisher Research & Representation, Inc. 2001.

Delivering the News

Buckman R: Living with cancer, in *What You Really Need to Know about Cancer: A Comprehensive Guide for Patients and Their Families.* Baltimore: Johns Hopkins University Press, 1997.

Kornblith AB: Psychosocial adaptation of cancer survivors, in Holland JC (ed): *Psychooncology.* New York: Oxford University Press, 1998.

Hamburg P: Breaking bad news, in Stern TA, Herman JB, Slavin PL (eds): *The MGH Guide to Psychiatry in Primary Care.* New York: McGraw-Hill, 1998.

Harpham WS: *Diagnosis Cancer: Your Guide Through the First Few Months.* New York: Norton, 1998.

Love SM: Fears, feelings, and ways to cope, in *Dr. Susan Love's Breast Book*. Cambridge, MA:Perseus Publishing, 2000.

Depression and Anxiety Associated with Cancer

American Psychiatric Association: *Diagnostic and Statistical Manual of Mental Disorders*, 4th ed. Washington, DC: APA, 1994.
Breitbart W, Krivo S: Suicide, in Holland JC (ed):*Psycho-oncology*. New York: Oxford University Press, 1998, pp 541–547.
Kaplan HI, Sadock BJ, Grebb JA: *Kaplan and Sadock's Synopsis of Psychiatry: Behavioral Sciences, Clinical Psychiatry*. Baltimore: Williams & Wilkins, 1994.
Massie MJ, Popkin MK: Depressive disorders, in Holland JC (ed): *Psycho-oncology*. New York: Oxford University Press, 1998, pp 518–540.
Noyes R, Holt CS, Massie MJ: Anxiety disorders, in Holland JC (ed): *Psycho-oncology*. New York: Oxford University Press, 1998, pp 548–563.
Pirl WF, Roth AJ: Diagnosis and treatment of depression in cancer patients. *Oncology* 13:1293–1301, 1999.
Weisman, AD: Coping with illness, in Cassem NH, Stern TA, Rosenbaum JF, Jellinek MS (eds): *Massachusetts General Hospital Handbook of General Hospital Psychiatry*, 4th ed. St. Louis: Mosby-Year Book, 1997, pp 25–34.

Fertility and Cancer

Schover LR, et al: having children after cancer. *Cancer* 86(4):696–709, 1999.

Grief and Bereavement

Association for Death Education and Counseling. *http://www.adec.org/*
Beyond Indigo: Grief and loss. *http://www.beyondindigo.com/*
Cancer Resource Room at Massachusetts General Hospital. *http://cancer.mgh.harvard.edu/resources*
Compassionate Friends: Grief following death of a child. *http://www.compassionate friends.org/*
Dougy Center, The National Center for Grieving Children and Families. *http://www.dougy.org/*
GriefNet: Death and dying resources. *http://rivendell.org/*
Growthhouse: Grief and bereavement, death and dying. *http://www.growthhouse.org/*
Guideline publications, Childrens' questions about death. *http://www.guidelinepub.com/*
International Psycho-Oncology Society: psychosocial dimensions of cancer. *http://www.ipos-aspboa.org*
National Cancer Institute information on children and grief. *http://www.graylab.ac.uk/cancernet/506750.html*
National Hospice and Palliative Care Organization. *http://www.nhpco.org/*
Oncolink, University of Pennsylvania. *http://cancer.med.upenn.edu/*
American Psychiatric Association: *Diagnostic and Statistical Manual of Mental Disorders*, Fourth edition. Washington, DC, American Psychiatric Association, 1994.

Bertrand D: [Mental health and cultural issues: the return of Khmers from France to Cambodia for healing purposes]. [French] *Sante* 7(5):330-334, 1997.

Birmaher B, et al. Childhood and adolescent depression: A review of the past 10 years. Part I. *J Am Acad Child Adolesc Psych* 35:1427-1439, 1996.

Bowlby J: *Loss: Sadness and depression.* New York, NY, Basic Books, 1980.

Braun KL, Nichols R: Death and dying in four Asian American cultures: a descriptive study. *Death Studies* 21(4):327-359, 1997.

Cassel EJ: The nature of suffering and the goals of medicine. *NEJM* 306:639-645, 1982.

Cassem NH: Care and management of the patient at the end of life, in Dale DC, Federman DD (eds): *Scientific American Medicine,* Sec 13, *Psychiatry,* Subsec IV. New York: Scientific American, 1998, pp 1–10.

Cassem EH: Care and management of the patient at the end of life, in Chochinov HM, Breitbart W (eds): *Handbook of Psychiatry in Palliative Medicine.* Oxford, UK: Oxford University Press, 2000, pp 13–23.

Dougy Center: *35 Ways to Help a Grieving Child.* Portland, OR: Western Lithograph, 1999.

Dowdney L: Annotation: Childhood bereavement following parental death. *J Child Psychol Psychiatry* 7:819–830, 2000.

Eisenbruch M: From post-traumatic stress disorder to cultural bereavement: diagnosis of Southeast Asian refugees. *Soc Sci Med* 33(6):673–680, 1991.

Eisenbruch M: Toward a culturally sensitive DSM: Cultural bereavement in Cambodian refugees and the traditional healer as taxonomist. *J Nerv Mental Dis* 180(1):8–10, 1992.

Fabrega H, Nutini H: Tlaxcalan constructions of acute grief. *Culture Med Psychiatry* 18(4):405–431, 1994.

Garber J, Hilsman R: Cognition, stress, and depression in children and adolescents. *Child Adolesc Psychiatr Clin North Am* 1:129–167, 1992.

Horowitz MJ, et al. Diagnostic criteria for complicated grief disorder. *Am J Psychiatry* 154(7):904–910, 1997.

Klass D: Tibetan Buddhism and the resolution of grief: The Bardo-thodol for the dying and the grieving. *Death Studies* 21(4):377–395, 1997.

Lemkau JP, et al: A questionnaire survey of family practice physicians' perceptions of bereavement care. *Arch Fam Med* 9:822–829, 2000.

Martinson IM: Funeral rituals in Taiwan and Korea. *Oncol Nursing Forum* 25(10):1756–1760, 1998.

Munet-Vilaro F: Grieving and death rituals of Latinos. *Oncol Nurs Forum* 25(10):1761–1763, 1998.

Parkes CM: Facing loss. *BMJ* 316:1521–1524, 1998.

Parkes CM, Weiss RA: *Recovery from Bereavement.* NJ: Jason Aronson, 1995.

Parkes CM, et al: *Death and Bereavement across Cultures.* London: Routledge, 1997.

Powell A: Adjustment disorders, grief and bereavement, in Stern TA, Herman JB (eds): *Psychiatry Update and Board Preparation.* New York: McGraw-Hill, 2000.

Prigerson HG, et al: Complicated grief and bereavement-related depression as distinct disorders: Preliminary empirical validation in elderly bereaved spouses. *Am J Psychiatry* 152:22–30, 1995.

Prigerson HG, et al: Traumatic grief as a risk factor for mental and physical morbidity. *Am J Psychiatry* 154:616–623, 1997.

Rauch PK: Death of a parent, in Finberg (ed): *Saunders Manual of Pediatrics.* Philadelphia: Saunders, 2001.

Reynolds, et al: Treatment of bereavement-related major depressive episodes in later life: A controlled study of acute and continuation treatment with nortriptyline and interpersonal psychotherapy. *Am J Psychiatry* 156:202–208, 1999.

Schreiber S: Migration, traumatic bereavement and transcultural aspects of psychological healing: Loss and grief of a refugee woman from Begameder county in Ethiopia. *Br J Med Psychol* 68:135–142, 1995.

Shapiro ER: Grief in family and cultural context: learning from Latino families. *Cult Div-Mental Health* 1(2):159–176, 1995.

Stoppelbein L, Greening LL: Posttraumatic stress symptoms in parentally bereaved children and adolescents. *J Am Acad Child Adolesc Psychiatry* 39:1112–1119, 2000.

Young B, Papadatou D: Childhood death and bereavement across cultures, in Parkes CM, et al (eds): *Death and Bereavement across Cultures.* London: Routledge, 1997.

Zisook S, Downs NS: Death, dying and bereavement, in Sadock BJ, Sadock VA (eds): *Kaplan & Sadock's Comprehensive Textbook of Psychiatry*, 7th ed. Philadelphia: Lippincott Williams & Wilkins, 2000.

Legal Issues and Cancer

Advanced Directives for Health Care: Deciding Today about Your Health Care in the Future. Iowa Health Book, *www.vh.org/Patients/IHB/Misc/AdvanceDirective.html*

Sabatino CP: *10 Legal Myths about Advance Medical Directives.* Commission on Legal Problems of the Elderly, American Bar Association, 740 Fifteenth Street, NW, Washington, DC 20005-1022 *abaelderly@abanet.org*

Shape Your Health Care Future with Health Care Advance Directives. American Medical Association, *www.ama-assn.org/public/booklets/livingwill.htm*

Massachusetts Health Care Proxy, Information, Instructions and Form, Massachusetts Health Decisions, P.O. Box, 417, Sharon, MA 02067.

Movies That Depict the Struggle with Cancer

Champions, 1984, USA, Embassy Pictures Corporation. The true story of Bob Champion (John Hurt), a British steeplechase jockey who, in the late 1970s, was diagnosed with cancer.

Closure, 2001, USA, Twenty One Productions. Based on a true story. A young married couple and their family struggle when the young woman is diagnosed with cancer.

Counting Days, 2000, USA, Emerald City Films. A young man struggles to bring his estranged family together and face the demons from his own past after his father is diagnosed with cancer.

Daibyonin (The Last Days), 1993, Japan. A Japanese movie director must come to terms with his terminal cancer. Despite many painful personal struggles and conflicts with those he loves, he realizes he does not want to die in the hospital and spends his last days peacefully at home.

Developing, 1995, USA. A short film about a single mother with breast cancer who must deal with her young daughter and help her understand what she is going through.

Dying Young, 1991, USA, Twentieth Century Fox Film Corp. A young woman looking for a new start in life takes a job tending to a man suffering from a blood cancer. They fall in love, knowing that it cannot last, for the man with cancer is destined to die.

Girls' Night, 1998, USA, Granada Film Productions. Two best friends fly to Las Vegas to fulfill the dream of one, who is dying of cancer.

God Said, "Ha!" 1998, Oh, Brother Productions Inc. Julia Sweeney talks about the period when her brother fought cancer and she also was diagnosed with a rare cancer.

My Life, USA 1993, Columbia Pictures. Diagnosed with cancer and with only a few months to live, a young man sets out to document his life and knowledge for his unborn son. The experience leads him on a voyage of self-discovery and reconciliation.

One True Thing, 1998, USA, Universal Pictures. A young, independent woman is forced to uproot her life to take care of a mother stricken with cancer. She makes discoveries about her parents and about her own life along the way.

The Politics of Cancer (documentary), 1995, USA, Healing Arts Documentary Productions. U.S. senators, scientists, doctors, pharmaceutical companies, CEOs, wives, and children confront a chaotic epidemic of cancer.

Princes in Exile, 1990, Canada, CBC. A young boy, angry at his diagnosis of brain cancer and the possibility of dying, finds a new perspective through the strength and optimism of a new friend.

Rachel's Daughters: Searching for the Causes of Breast Cancer (documentary), 1997, USA. Seven women who currently have or have survived breast cancer travel across the country asking researchers and experts about the possible causes of breast cancer.

A Woman's Tale (motion picture) 1991, AFFC. An older woman diagnosed with cancer is determined to live her last days with the dignity she displayed her entire life. In this courageous performance, the actress portraying the main character herself had cancer while making the film.

Purely educational movies are also available.

The list below represents a few of the best-selling titles listed by type of cancer as indicated by sales from popular retail stores and websites.

The list below represents a few of the best-selling educational movies listed by type of cancer as indicated by sales from popular retail stores and websites.

BREAST CANCER

Between Us: A First Aid Kit for Your Heart and Soul, 1999, USA.

Focus on Healing through Movement & Dance for the Breast Cancer Survivor, 1999, USA, Tapeworm.

Initial Discovery and Diagnosis of Breast Cancer, 2000, USA.

Man's Guide to Women's Breast Cancer: Partners in Hope, 2001, USA.

No Hair Day: Laughing (and Crying) Our Way Through Cancer, 2001, USA, WGBH Boston.

Options in the Treatment of Breast Cancer, USA, Pathway Video, LLC.

Three Days Out: A Breast Cancer Odyssey, 2000, USA, PBS.

Women's Health: Breast Cancer—Replacing Fear with Facts, 1999, USA, Parade.

CANCER—NONSPECIFIC

*Cancer: Increasing Your Odds of Survival,*1999, USA, PBS.

Cancer: A Turning Point—An Interview with Dr. Lawrence LeShan, 2000, USA, Tapeworm.

Health: Great Minds of Medicine: Cancer, 1997, USA, Unapix Inc.

Living & Laughing With Cancer, 1998, USA, Tapeworm.

Living with Cancer: A Message of Hope, 1998, USA, Wellspring Media.

When Cancer Touches Your Life: Meeting the Needs of Patients and Families, 2000, Health Talks at The Cleveland Clinic.

Prostate Cancer: A Journey of Hope, 1999, USA, PBS, Producer Julie D. Parker.

CHILDHOOD CANCER
My Hair's Falling Out . . . Am I Still Pretty? A Childhood Cancer Education Video, 1992, USA, PBS.

COLON AND RECTAL CANCER
Detecting Colon Cancer: Knowledge is Power, 2000, USA, Health Talks at The Cleveland Clinic.
Today—Confronting Colon Cancer

PROSTATE CANCER
Not Alone—Couples Share Candidly About Prostate Cancer, 1998.
Prostate Cancer: A Journey of Hope, 1999, USA, PBS.

SKIN CANCER
A Doctor in Your House: Vol 3—*Skin Cancer: Our Dangerous Day in the Sun*,1999, USA, United American Video.
Melanoma And Other Skin Cancer, 2000, USA, HealthInfo.

Palliative Care and Hospice

Abrahm J: Promoting symptom control in palliative care. *Semin Oncol Nurs* 14(2):95–109, 1998.
Billings JA: Recent advances: Palliative care. *BMJ* 321:555–558, 2000.
Bruere E,, et al: Management of specific symptom complexes in patients receiving palliative care. *CMAJ* 158 (13):1717–1726, 1998.
MacDonald N: Palliative care—An essential component of cancer control. *CMAJ* 158(13):1709–1716, 1998.
Weissman DE: Consultation in palliative medicine. *Arch Intern Med* 157:733–737, 1997.

Prostate Cancer

COPING AND LIVING WITH PROSTATE CANCER
Phillips RH: *Coping with Prostate Cancer: A Guide to Living with Prostate Cancer for You and Your Family.*, NJ: Avery Publishing Group, 1994.
Priest MW: *Diary of Courage Coping with Life-Threatening Illness.*: Strictly Books, 1990.

GENERAL INFORMATION AND GUIDES FOR PATIENT AND FAMILY
Berberich R: *Hit Below the Belt: Facing Up to Prostate Cancer.*, CA: Ten Speed Press, 2001.
Marks S, Moul J: *Prostate & Cancer: A Family Guide to Diagnosis, Treatment & Survival.* Cambridge, MA: Fisher Books, 2000.
Walsh PC, Worthington JF: *The Prostate: A Guide for Men and the Women Who Love Them.* New York: Warner Books, 1997.
Walsh PC, Worthington JF: *Walsh's Guide to Surviving Prostate Cancer.* New York: Warner Books, 2001.

Psychological Interventions and Support Groups

Fawzy FI, Fawzy NW, Arndt LA, Pasnau RO: Critical review of psychosocial interventions in cancer care. *Arch Gen Psychiatry* 52:100–113, 1995.

Fawzy FI, Fawzy NW, Hyun CS, et al: Malignant melanoma: Effects of an early structured psychiatric intervention, coping, and affective state on recurrence and survival 6 years later. *Arch Gen Psychiatry* 50:681–689, 1993.

Greer S: Psychological response to cancer and survival. *Psychol Med* 21: 43–49, 1991.

Holland JC, Lewis S: *The Human Side of Cancer.* New York: HarperCollins, 2000.

Ornish D, Brown SE, Scherwitz LW, et al: Can lifestyle changes reverse coronary artery disease? *Lancet* 336:129–133, 1992.

Spiegel D, Bloom JR, Kraemer HC, et al: Effects of psychosocial treatment on survival of patients with metastatic breast cancer. *Lancet* 2:888–891, 1989.

Spiegel D, Morrow GR, Classen C, et al: Group Psychotherapy for recently diagnosed breast cancer patients: A multicenter feasibility study. *Oncology* 8:428–493, 1999.

Skin Cancer

COPING AND LIVING WITH SKIN CANCER

Bishop B: *My Triumph over Cancer.* Chicago: Keats Publishing, 1986.

Long W: *Coping With Melanoma and Other Skin Cancers.:* Rosen Publishing Group, 1999.

Shuck C, Greenway HT: *Saving Face: My Victory Over Skin Cancer.:*
Pauls Eriksson, 2000.

GENERAL GUIDES AND INFORMATION

Kenet BJ et al: *Saving Your Skin: Prevention, Early Detection, and Treatment of Melanoma and Other Skin Cancers.* New York: Four Walls Eight Windows, 1998.

Poole CM, Guerry D: *Melanoma : Prevention, Detection, and Treatment.* New Haven, CT: Yale University Press, 1998.

Schofield JR, Robinson WS: *What You Really Need to Know About Moles and Melanoma (Johns Hopkins Press Health Book).* Baltimore:Johns Hopkins University Press, 2000.

Stress Reactions in Caregivers

Barraclough J: *Cancer and Emotion: A Practical Guide to Psycho-oncology,* 3rd ed. Chichester, UK: Wiley, 1999.

Houts PS, et al (eds): *Home Care Guide for Cancer: How to Care for Family and Friends at Home.:* American College of Physicians. 1994. (A user-friendly overview of strategies for success in caregiving, as well as potential pitfalls.)

McKhann CF: *The Facts about Cancer.* Engelwood Cliffs, NJ: Prentice-Hall, 1981.

O'Brien ME: *Spirituality in Nursing: Standing on Holy Ground.* Sudbury, MA: Jones and Bartlett, 1999.

Sekeres, MA, Gonzalez JJ, Stern TA: Recognition and management of staff stress in the intensive care unit, in Rippe et al (eds): *Intensive Care Medicine,* 5th ed. Philadelphia: Lippincott-Raven. In press.

The Impact of Cancer on the Family

Blanchard CG, Albrecht TL, Ruckdeschel JC: The crisis of cancer: Psychological impact on family caregivers. *Oncology* 11(2):189–194, 1997 (discussion, pp 196, 201–202).

Carter EA, McGoldrick M: *The Family Life Cycle: A Framework for Family Therapy.* New York: Gardner Press, 1980.

Covinsky KE, Goldman L, Cook EF, et al: The impact of serious illness on patients' families. *JAMA* 272:1839–1844, 1994.

Ell K, Michimoto R, Mantell J, Hamovitch M: Longitudinal analysis of psychosocial adaptation among family members of patients with cancer. *J Psychosom Res* 32:429–438, 1988.

Guidry JJ, Aday LA, Zhang D, Winn RJ: The role of informal and formal social support networks for patients with cancer. *Cancer Pract* 5(4):241–246, 1997.

Haggmark C, Theorell T, Ek B: Coping and social activity patterns among relatives of cancer patients. *Soc Sci Med* 25(9):1021–1025, 1987.

Kriesel HT: The psychosocial aspects of malignancy. *Primary Care* 42(2):271–280, 1987.

Kupst MJ: Family coping. Supportive and obstructive factors. *Cancer* 71(10 Suppl):3337–3341, 1993.

Lazarus RS, Folkman S: *Stress, Appraisal, and Coping.* New York: Springer-Verlag, 1984.

Lewis FM: Strengthening family supports: Cancer and the family. *Cancer* 65:752–759, 1990.

Manne S, Glassman M: Perceived control, coping efficacy, and avoidance coping as mediators between spouses' unsupportive behaviors and cancer patients' psychological distress. *Health Psychol* 19(2):155–164, 2000.

Meyers CA: The Blanchard/Albrecht/Ruekdeschel article reviewed. *Oncology* 11(2):201–202, 1997.

Mor V, Allen S, Malin M: The psychosocial impact of cancer in older versus younger patients and their family. *Cancer* 74(Suppl 7):2118–2127, 1997.

Morse SR, Fife B: Coping with a partner's cancer: Adjustment at four stages of the illness trajectory.*Oncol Nurs Forum* 25(4):751–760, 1998.

Northouse LL, Peters-Golden H: Cancer and the family: Strategies to assist spouses. *Semin Oncol Nurs* 9:74–82, 1993.

Tarraza HM, Ellerkmann RM: A view from the family: Years after a loved one has died of ovarian cancer. *Obstet Gynecol* 93(1):38–40, 1999.

Weitzner MA, Knutzen R: The impact of pituitary disease on the family caregiver and overall family functioning. *Psychother Psychosom* 67(3):181–188, 1998.

Zabora JR, Smith ED: Family dysfunction and the cancer patient: Early recognition and intervention. *Oncology* 5(12):31–35 (discussion 36, 38, 41), 1991.

The Role of Faith in the Lives of People with Cancer

O'Brien ME: *Spirituality in Nursing: Standing on Holy Ground.* Sudbury, MA: Jones and Bartlett, 1999.

Barraclough J: *Cancer and Emotion: A Practical Guide to Psycho-oncology*, 3d ed. Chichester, England: Wiley, 1999.

Carmody J: *Cancer and Faith: Reflections on Living with a Terminal Illness.* Mystic, CT: Twenty-Third Publications, 1994. (Personal reflections of a theologian on the role of faith following his diagnosis with multiple myeloma.)

Day SB: *Cancer, Stress, and Death.* New York: Plenum Press, 1986.

Kushner HS: *When Bad Things Happen to Good People.* 2d ed. New York: Avon Books, 1989.

Pearson K, Cassem NH: "Healthy-minded religion": The interface between psychiatry and religion. Lecture, 3/1999.

Cassem NH: Taking a spiritual history. Lecture, 1/1998.

Kuhn CC: A spiritual inventory of the medically ill patient. *Psychiatr Med* 6(2): 87–100, 1988.

Dossey L: *Special Report: The Role of Prayer and in Health and Healing.* New York: Boardroom Reports, 1994.

Sontag S: *Illness as Metaphor.* New York : Farrar, Straus and Giroux, 1978.

Dossey L: The return of prayer. *Alt Ther* 3(6), 1997.

The Use of Medications to Alter Mood and Behavior Associated with Cancer

American Psychiatric Association: *Diagnostic and Statistical Manual of Mental Disorders,* 4th ed., Washington, DC: APA, 1994.

Baede-van Dijk PA, van Galen E, Lekkerkerker JF: Drug interactions of *Hypericum perforatum* (St. John's wort) are potentially hazardous. *Ned Tijdschr Geneeskd* 144(17):811–812, 2000.

Baldessarini RJ, Tarazi FI: Drugs and the treatment of psychiatric disorders: Antipsychotic and antimanic agents, in Hardman JG, Limbird LE, Molinoff PB, et al (eds): *Goodman and Gilman's the Pharmacological Basis of Therapeutics,* 10th ed. New York: McGraw-Hill. In press.

Baldessarini RJ: Drugs and the treatment of psychiatric disorders: Antidepressant and antianxiety agents, in Hardman JG, Limbird LE, Molinoff PB, et al (eds): *Goodman and Gilman's the Pharmacological Basis of Therapeutics,* 10th ed. New York: McGraw-Hill. In press.

Fava M, Davidson KG: Definition and epidemiology of treatment-resistant depression. *Psychiatr Clin North Am* 19:179–200, 1996.

Fava M, Kaji K: Continuation and maintenance treatments of major depressive disorder. *Psychiatr Ann* 24:281–290, 1994.

George MS, Sackeim HA, Marangell LB, et al: Vagus nerve stimulation. A potential therapy for resistant depression? *Psychiatr Clin North Am* 23(4):757–783, 2000.

Holland JC, Breitbart W (eds). *Psycho-Oncology.* New York: Oxford University Press, 1998.

Hyman SE, Arana GW, Rosenbaum JF: *Handbook of Psychiatric Drug Therapy,* 3rd ed. Boston: Little, Brown, 1995.

Kaplan HI, Saddock BJ (eds): *Comprehensive Textbook of Psychiatry,* 6th ed. Baltimore: Williams & Wilkins, 1995.

Keck ME, Welt T, Post A, et al: Neuroendocrine and behavioral effects of repetitive transcranial magnetic stimulation in a psychopathological animal model are suggestive of antidepressant-like effects. *Neuropsychopharmacology* 24(4):337–349, 2001.

Lisanby SH, Datto CJ, Szuba MP: ECT and TMS: Past, present, and future. *Depress Anxiety* 12(3):115–117, 2000.

Mischoulon D, Rosenbaum JF: The use of natural medications in psychiatry: A commentary. *Harv Rev Psychiatry* 6:279–283, 1999.

Physicians' Desk Reference, 54[cf11]th ed. Montvale, NJ: Medical Economics Company, 2000.

Piscitelli SC, Burstein AH, Chaitt D, et al: Indinavir concentrations and St John's wort. *Lancet* 355:547–548, 2000.

Speer AM, Kimbrell TA, Wassermann EM, et al: Opposite effects of high and low frequency rTMS on regional brain activity in depressed patients. *Biol Psychiatry* 48(12):1133–1141, 2000.

Stahl SM: *Psychopharmacology of Antidepressants*. London: Martin Dunitz, 1997.

Treatment Issues at the End of Life

Bruera E, Neumann CM, Mazzocato C, et al: Attitudes and beliefs of palliative care physicians regarding communication with terminally ill cancer patients. *Pall Med* 14:287–298, 2000.

Buckman R: *How to Break Bad News. A Guide for Health Care Professionals*. Baltimore: Johns Hopkins University Press, 1992.

Jonsen AR, Siegler M, Winslade WJ: *Clinical Ethics: A Practical Approach to Ethical Decisions in Clinical Medicine*, 4th ed. New York: McGraw-Hill, 1998.

Haidet P, Hamel MB, Davis RB, et al: Outcomes, preferences for resuscitation, and physician-patient communication among patients with metastatic colorectal cancer. SUPPORT Investigators. Study to understand prognoses and preferences for outcomes and risks of treatment. *Am J Med* 105:222–229, 1998.

Gillick M: Rethinking the role of tube feeding in patients with advanced dementia. Sounding board. *N Engl J Med* 342:206–210, 2000.

Leff B, Kaffenbarger KP, Remsburg R: Prevalence, effectiveness, and predictors of planning the place of death among older persons followed in community-based long-term care. *J Am Geriatr Soc* 48:943–948, 2000.

Vollmann J, Burke WJ, Kupfer RY, et al: Rethinking the role of tube feeding in patients with advanced dementia. *N Engl J Med* 342:1755–1756, 2000.

Index